T0320693

# BIOTECHNOLOGY IN BLOOD TRANSFUSION

# DEVELOPMENTS IN HEMATOLOGY AND IMMUNOLOGY

Lijnen, H.R., Collen, D. and Verstraete, M., eds: Synthetic Substrates in Clinical Blood Coagulation Assays. 1980. ISBN 90-247-2409-0

Smit Sibinga, C.Th., Das, P.C. and Forfar, J.O., eds: Paediatrics and Blood Transfusion. 1982. ISBN 90-247-2619-0

Fabris, N., ed: Immunology and Ageing. 1982. ISBN 90-247-2640-9

Hornstra, G.: Dietary Fats, Prostanoids and Arterial Thrombosis. 1982. ISBN 90-247-2667-0

Smit Sibinga, C.Th., Das, P.C. and Loghem, van J.J., eds: Blood Transfusion and Problems of Bleeding. 1982. ISBN 90-247-3058-9

Dormandy, J., ed: Red Cell Deformability and Filterability. 1983. ISBN 0-89838-578-4

Smit Sibinga, C.Th., Das, P.C. and Taswell, H.F., eds: Quality Assurance in Blood Banking and Its Clinical Impact. 1984. ISBN 0-89838-618-7

Besselaar, A.M.H.P. van den, Gralnick, H.R. and Lewis, S.M., eds: Thromboplastin Calibration and Oral Anticoagulant Control. 1984. ISBN 0-89838-637-3

Fondu, P. and Thijs, O., eds: Haemostatic Failure in Liver Disease. 1984. ISBN 0-89838-640-3

Smit Sibinga, C.Th., Das, P.C. and Opelz, G., eds: Transplantation and Blood Transfusion. 1984. ISBN 0-89838-686-1

Schmid-Schönbein, H., Wurzinger, L.J. and Zimmerman, R.E., eds: Enzyme Activation in Blood-Perfused Artificial Organs. 1985. ISBN 0-89838-704-3

Dormandy, J., ed: Blood Filtration and Blood Cell Deformability. 1985. ISBN 0-89838-714-0

Smit Sibinga, C.Th., Das, P.C. and Seidl, S., eds: Plasma Fractionation and Blood Transfusion. 1985. ISBN 0-89838-761-2

Dawids, S. and Bantjes, A., eds: Blood Compatible Materials and their Testing. 1986. ISBN 0-89838-813-9

Smit Sibinga, C.Th., Das, P.C. and Greenwalt, T.J., eds: Future Developments in Blood Banking. 1986. ISBN 0-89838-824-4

Berlin, A., Dean, J., Draper, M.H., Smith, E.M.B. and Spreafico, F., eds: Immunotoxicology. 1987. ISBN 0-89838-843-0

Ottenhoff, T. and De Vries, R.: Recognition of *M. leprae* antigens. 1987. ISBN 0-89838-887-2

Touraine, J.-L., Gale, R.P. and Kochupillai, V., eds: Fetal Liver Transplantation. 1987. ISBN 0-89838-975-5

Smit Sibinga, C.Th., Das, P.C. and Engelfriet, C.P., eds: White cells and platelets in blood transfusion. 1987. ISBN 0-89838-976-3

Hendriksen, C.F.M.: Laboratory animals in vaccine production and control. 1988. ISBN 0-89838-398-6

Smit Sibinga, C.Th., Das, P.C. and Overby, L.R. eds: Biotechnology in blood transfusion. 1988. ISBN 0-89838-404-4

# Biotechnology in blood transfusion

Proceedings of the Twelfth Annual Symposium on Blood Transfusion,
Groningen 1987, organized by the Red Cross Blood Bank Groningen-Drenthe

*edited by*

**C.Th. SMIT SIBINGA and P.C. DAS**

*Red Cross Blood Bank Groningen-Drenthe, The Netherlands*

and

**L.R. OVERBY**

*Chiron Corporation, Emmeryville, California, U.S.A.*

KLUWER ACADEMIC PUBLISHERS

BOSTON / DORDRECHT / LONDON

ISBN 089838-404-4

Published by Kluwer Academic Publishers,
101 Philip Drive, Norwell, MA 02061, U.S.A.

Kluwer Academic Publishers incorporates
the publishing programmes of
D. Reidel, Martinus Nijhoff, Dr W. Junk and MTP Press.

In all other countries, sold and distributed
by Kluwer Academic Publishers Group,
P.O. Box 322, 3300 AH Dordrecht, The Netherlands.

Printed in The Netherlands

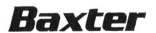

**Acknowledgement**

This publication has been made possible through the support of Baxter, which is gratefully acknowledged.

# CONTENTS

## III. Biotechnology and blood components

## IV. Clinical application and future directions

# MODERATORS AND SPEAKERS

## Moderators

| | |
|---|---|
| L.R. Overy (Chairman) | – Chiron Corporation, Emmeryville, CA, USA |
| P.C. Das | – Red Cross Blood Bank Groningen-Drenthe, Groningen, NL |
| B. Habibi | – C.N.T.S., Paris, F |
| G. Jacquin | – C.N.T.S., Paris, F |
| J. van der Meer | – Dept. of Internal Medicine, University of Groningen, Groningen, NL |
| C.Th. Smit Sibinga | – Red Cross Blood Bank Groningen-Drenthe, Groningen, NL |

## Speakers

| | |
|---|---|
| L.O. Andersson | – KabiVitrum, Stockholm, S |
| C.R. Bennett | – Merck Sharp and Dohme, West Point, PA, USA |
| E.J. Benz jr. | – Yale University, New Haven, CT, USA |
| E. Briët | – Dept. of Internal Medicine, University of Leiden, Leiden, NL |
| T.J. Hamblin | – Royal Victoria Hospital, Bournemouth, UK |
| P. Hervé | – C.R.T.S., Besançon, F |
| K.A. High | – The University of North Carolina at Chapel Hill, Chapel Hill, NC, USA |
| P.E. Highfield | – Wellcome Research Laboratories, Beckenham, UK |
| W.G. Ho | – University of California at Los Angeles, Los Angeles, CA, USA |
| S.L. Holbeck | – Fred Hutchinson Cancer Research Center, Seattle, WA, USA |
| D.J. Lutton | – New York Medical College, Valhalla, NY, USA |
| L. Messeter | – University Hospital Blood Bank, Lund, S |
| H.L. Ploegh | – Antoni van Leeuwenhoek Hospital, Amsterdam, NL |
| C.V. Prowse | – Edingburgh and South-East Scotland Regional Blood Transfusion Service, Edingburgh, UK |
| C. Rouzioux | – Necker Enfants Malades Hospital, Paris, F |
| A.B. Schreiber | – Rorer Central Research, Horsham, PA, USA |
| T.H. The | – Dept. of Internal Medicine, University of Groningen, Groningen, NL |
| D. Voak | – Regional Transfusion and Immuno-Haematology Centre, Cambridge, UK |

## Prepared Discussants

| | |
|---|---|
| G. Zettlmeißl | – Behringwerke AG, Marburg, FRG |

# FOREWORD

This symposium is devoted to Biotechnology in Blood Transfusion; there are 22 experts discussing the state of the art in the application of monoclonal antibodies, recombinant DNA technologies and heterologous expression systems to the improvement and sometimes replacement of blood products, characterization of blood constituents, and the effect of these developments on blood transfusion procedures.

Ten and maybe five years ago the title of a symposium such as this would have been *Biosciences in blood transfusion*, informing what basic developments in molecular biology, biochemistry and human physiology might pertain to blood transfusion in the distant future. That future is getting closer, and not only one is interested in basic developments in immunology, recognition and identification of viral and bacterial components and products, tissue and bloodgroup typing, but also in the potential application of these developments and their economic perspectives.

That is what biotechnology is all about: basic science tells us where and how we might look for new technologies, and the development of such technologies is only possible if there is a perspective for improvement in quality, safety, acceptance or performance to cost ratio. This means that working under the flag of biotechnology is both exciting and frustrating: exciting because there is much to be done over a very wide range, from very fundamental to applied studies, and even venturing into commercialization and new business development; frustrating because despite the seemingly endless possibilities, considerable energy and steadfastness are needed to realize the apparent economic potential. In the end economic feasibility is a harsher judge of reality than a granting committee.

Some of these prospects which are already being judged or will soon be judged, will be discussed during this symposium. They include such topics as:
1. large-scale production of monoclonal antibodies;
2. applications of monoclonal antibodies for quality control and the detailed characterization of blood and other tissues;
3. applications of monoclonal antibodies in the ultrapurification of blood proteins and other biologicals;
4. application of ultrapure blood proteins for therapeutic purposes, and
5. production of human blood proteins in large-scale mammalian cell bioreactors using heterologous recombinant DNA expression systems.

If we look a little further into the future, several other developments may well become important. For instance: the production of human blood proteins or appropriate substitutes not only in animals and in animal or microbial cell bioreactors, but also in suitable plants; the increased use of synthetic peptides and perhaps even proteins, as organic chemists improve their technologies inspired by the life sceinces and natural models; the application of protein engineering to alter blood proteins which are to be used therapeutically – I am thinking here of properties such as altered temperature or pH stability, smaller or larger size, antigenic epitopes tailored to specific patient groups and last but not the least, the development of ultrasensitive biosensing systems for the rapid and increasingly complete characterization of blood.

However, without the perspective of economic development biotechnology is nothing, and although this development can certainly occur spontaneously, it may be useful to create an atmosphere and an infrastructure which stimulate biotechnology based economic developments. Every industrial nation does this to some extent, using tax incentives, subsidies, specific programs or a combination thereof.

The Netherlands recognized this need in the late 70's and approached it in various formal and informal ways. University researchers came together and developed research and teaching programs in close co-ordination. This saved the government the unpleasant and difficult task of dividing limiting amounts of funds over large numbers of competing laboratories. Meanwhile, the Dutch Biotechnological Society was founded; its membership grew rapidly and is now well beyond 1000, which makes it one of the largest societies of the European Federation of Biotechnology. Contacts between universities, industries and government are intense, frequent and informal and the first phase of the government stimulated development can clearly be said to have been successfull.

The second phase is now upon us. Having established an excellent R&D infrastructure, the government has recently launched a program of support for industries which are interested in developing or expanding their R&D base in collaboration with university and institute laboratories. A similar approach is now being followed by the government in several other areas with economic potential, such as material sciences, information sciences, and of relevance to this symposium, biomedical technology.

In the university city of Groningen, a number of institutes and research centres has been developed and some of these are relevant to the topics discussed at this symposium. These include the Groningen Biotechnology Centre, the Biomolecular Science Centre, the BIOSON institute, the research laboratories of the Medical School, and of course, our host: the Red Cross Blood Bank Groningen-Drenthe.

Prof.Dr. Bernard Witholt
Dean Faculty of Biochemistry
President Science Park
University of Groningen

# I. Fundamentals of biotechnology

# OPPORTUNITIES FOR BIOTECHNOLOGY IN TRANSFUSION MEDICINE

L.R. Overby

Biotechnology is approaching its 15th anniversary. The importance of recombinant DNA technologies was recognized in 1974 when scientists recommended that ethical, environmental, technical and commercial issues surrounding genetic engineering should be assessed broadly before rapid exploitation of the impending breakthroughs. Most of these issues have been clarified and we have seen amazing progress in applying biotechnologies to problems in human health, to animal and plant life, and to areas of energy and the environment.

In this conference, we are highlighting existing and potential applications of biotechnology to blood transfusion and hemotherapy. If we look at progress in molecular biology over the past 15 years and its relation to blood transfusion issues, we can project that the future holds a bright promise for increased safety and efficacy for blood and blood products and for new discoveries that will increase the role of hemotherapy in human healt care.

In assessing the potential influences of biotechnology on blood transfusions, this review is organized into the following sections: (1) *Direct Products* that contribute to safety and efficacy of blood and blood products; (2) recombinant derived *Replacement Products* for materials purified from plasma; and (3) *Indirect Products and Knowledge* that may affect the supply and use of blood and blood products in hemotherapy. The review is not all-inclusive, but representative examples are discussed in each case that illustrate the positive role of biotechnology in transfusion medicine.

## Genetically engineered products that directly affect safety and efficacy

Transfusion-associated infections are major concerns of transfusion medicine. Most infections have been minimized over the last decade but have not been eliminated. Two major approaches have contributed to reduction in diseases transmitted by transfusion. In one case, blood is screened prior to use and interdicted from use if known infectious agents are probably present. Equally important is donor selection that minimizes donations from high-risk groups with the possibility of blood-borne infectious agents. In the case of infectious agent screening recombinant-derived antigen, antibodies and nucleic acids have led to improved diagnostic products that identify and diagnose blood donors with carrier states of hepatitis and AIDS viruses. In the case of high-risk donor groups recombinant-derived vaccines can serve to provide protective immunity and thereby ensure safety of blood from an immunized donor.

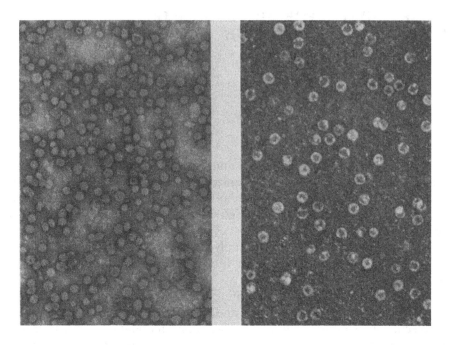

*Figure 1.* Electron microscope visualizations of HBsAg particles produced in yeast (left) and HBcAg particles produced in E. coli (right). Final magnification: 130,000×.

## HEPATITIS B SUBUNIT ANTIGENICITY

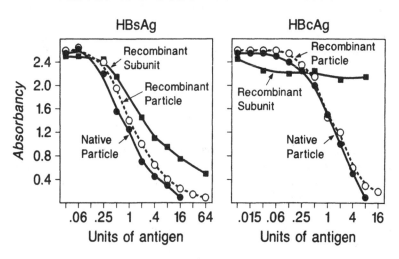

*Figure 2.* Comparison of native and recombinant HBsAg (left) and HBcAg (right) particles for reactivity with anti-HBs and anti-HBc, respectively, in human sera. Sera were tested for antibodies in an enzyme immuno assay using serum derived antigen. The sera were then retested after absorption with increasing quantities of native or recombinant antigens. A unit of antigen was arbitrarily defined as the quantity giving a 50% reduction in absorbancy.

# Hepatitis B and AIDS diagnostics and vaccines

*Hepatitis B.* The hepatitis B virus (HBV) was one of the first human pathogens to be cloned and sequenced and studied at the molecular level for producing viral antigens in heterologous organisms. Valenzuela et al., in 1982, cloned the subunit polypeptide gene for the surface antigen (HBsAg), and produced HBsAg particles in yeast, identical in all respects to native particles in plasma of infected individuals [1]. Earlier, Stahl et al. expressed the HBV core antigen (HBcAg) gene in E. coli and produced core antigen particles identical to the HBV nucleocapsid particles [2]. Electron microscopic visualizations of these two genetically engineered HBV antigens are shown in Figure 1. Biophysically the particles are identical to those found in human plasma during HBV infection.

The convenient sourcing of HBsAg and HBcAg by production in microorganisms has led to the use of the recombinant materials as diagnostic reagents. Immunologic identity of the native virus antigens and the corresponding recombinant antigens is illustrated in Figure 2. As shown in this comparison, native and recombinant HBsAg and HBcAg particles were equally competitive for anti-HBs and anti-HBc, respectively, in human antiserum. The dissociated HBsAg subunit protein was also reactive with anti-HBs. However, HBsAg subunit protein was not reactive with anti-HBc. Diagnostic accuracy and the quality of commercial products should be substantially increased through the use of genetically engineered antigen particles to test for anti-HBs and anti-HBc. Currently, all commercial tests for anti-HBc use E. coli produced HBcAg. This test is now being used in the United States as a surrogate screening marker for non-A non-B (NANB) hepatitis based on two prospective studies showing a correlation of HBcAg in donor blood and NANB hepatitis in recipients [3,4].

*Delta hepatitis.* The delta-hepatitis agent (HDV) does not appear to be a problem of safety in blood transfusions since the agent is found only during co-infection with HBV [5]. It is presumably a defective RNA virus that requires ongoing HBV replication for its own life cycle [6,7]. Superinfection of HBV with HDV almost always results in a more severe pathologic consequence. The agent appears to be a new class of human pathogen. The techniques of molecular biology have been key to understanding the nature of HDV. Wang et al. have cloned and sequenced the single stranded, circular RNA genome of HDV [8]. They also identified that the immunogenic 'delta antigen' was produced from the anti-genomic (positive) strand, and could be readily produced in bacteria. Figure 3 illustrates the possible open reading frames and candidate virus-coded proteins for HDV. Thus far, only the proteins derived from reading frame 5 in the anti-genomic strand have been found to react with antibodies present during HDV infection. Further work at the molecular level should lead to a more complete understanding of this new hepatotropic agent. Thus far, it appears that the agent represents a new class of mammalian viruses, with some properties suggestive of plant viroids and virusoids.

4

# POTENTIAL DELTA POLYPEPTIDE
# OPEN READING FRAMES

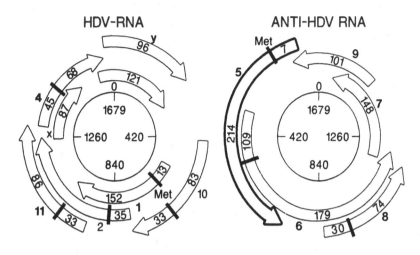

*Figure 3.* Map of the open frames of hepatitis delta virus genomic RNA (left) and the complementary RNA (right). Only the protein derived from reading frame in the complementary strand was found to react with human anti-delta sera.

# A.I.D.S. RETROVIRUS:
## Genomic Map

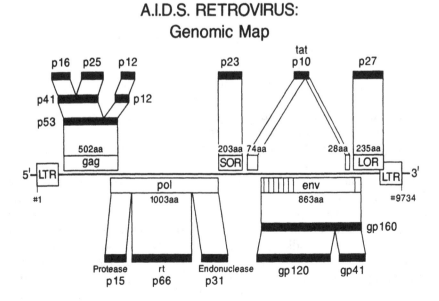

*Figure 4.* Genomic map of the typical human immunodeficiency virus showing the major virus proteins and their approximate molecular weight in kilodaltons.

*AIDS.* The Human Immunodeficiency Viruses (HIV) are currently one of the highest priority problems in public health. Transfusion associated AIDS is of special importance for blood transfusion services, and all blood collections in North America and Western Europe are routinely screened for antibodies to HIV. The initial commercial products for testing for anti-HIV have used partially purified viral lysates as antigen sources. Standardization of virus purity and control of false positive reactions have been difficult problems for these virus based tests. It is likely that recombinant derived proteins will be the method of choice for future generations of diagnostic tests for HIV antibodies and antigens.

Several HIV isolates were cloned and sequenced in 1985 [9]. The genomic map for HIV is illustrated in Figure 4, showing the major gene products of the virus. All of the virus protein studied thus far have been shown to induce antibodies in a large percentage of infected persons. These studies have been possible only as a result of producing each of the individual proteins through biotechnology processes and constructing immunoassays with the purified materials. Our laboratory estimated the percentage of sera from infected persons that reacted with each of nine HIV proteins [10]. As shown in Table 1, the reactive rates of sera varied from 37% to 99% for the individual antigens. We selected four recombinant proteins representing p-24 *gag*, p-31 *pol*, gp-41 *env* and gp-120 *env* as candidates for diagnostically relevant antigens. The four proteins were configured into a banded immunoblot format for detection of individual antibodies. Figure 5 shows the comparison of five sera tested with the recombinant immunoblot and a typical Western blot using purified HIV. The recombinant proteins showed equal immunoreactivity along with a simple and easily interpretable pattern. The procedure will be useful for rapid and sensitive confirmation of test results and for research on prognostic and diagnostic significance of antibody profiles. The availability of recombinant antigens will permit the procedures to be performed in many laboratories unable to routinely perform Western blots.

*Table 1.* Reactive rates of anti-HIV positive sera with individual virus proteins.

| Polypeptide designation | Gene source | Percentage of sera reactive |
|---|---|---|
| gp120 | env | 89 |
| gp41 | env | 98 |
| p53 | gag | 87 |
| p25 | gag | 76 |
| p16 | gag | 41 |
| p12 | gag | not tested |
| p31* | pol | 92 |
| p66** | pol | 80 |
| p15*** | pol | not tested |
| p27 | LOR | 37 |
| p20 | 3'ORF | 43 |
| p10 | tat | not tested |

* endonuclease; ** reverse transcriptase; *** protease

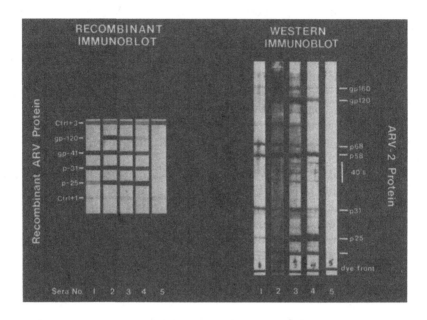

*Figure 5.* Comparisons of typical Western blot analyses using purified virus (right) and a recombinant immunoblot using four recombinant antigens (left) for antibodies in human immunodeficiency virus (HIV) sera. Sera 1-4 were from known infections. Serum 5 was a negative control.

*Table 2.* Comparison of anti-HIV reactive rates of 2013 normal blood donors in ELISA tests using recombinant antigens and purified virus.

|  | Recombinant antigen | Purified virus |
|---|---|---|
| No. of sera reactive | 5 | 14 |
| No. of sera confirmed positive | 1 | 1 |
| No. of sera non-reactive | 2007 | 1998 |

*Table 3.* Comparison of dilution sensitivity of ELISA tests for anti-HIV with recombinant antigens and purified virus.

| Serum dilution | Recombinant antigen | | Purified virus | |
|---|---|---|---|---|
|  | Absorbancy | +/− | Absorbancy | +/− |
| 0 | >3.000 | + | 2.320 | + |
| 1:2 | >3.000 | + | 2.163 | + |
| 1:4 | >3.000 | + | 1.542 | + |
| 1:8 | >3.000 | + | 0.990 | + |
| 1:16 | >3.000 | + | 0.520 | − |
| 1:32 | 2.025 | + | 0.361 | − |
| 1:64 | 1.323 | + | 0.230 | − |
| 1:128 | 0.570 | − | 0.157 | − |

A mixture of the same four HIV recombinant proteins was also used in a standard microtiter plate ELISA format for rapid screening for HIV antibodies. As shown in Table 2 we observed fewer false positive reactions in normal blood donor sera. The recombinant test was also more sensitive in detecting antibodies in several sequentially diluted sera (Table 3). These and other studies strongly imply that more reliable and accurate tests for screening blood for potential AIDS infectively will be possible by use of recombinant derived HIV proteins.

*Vaccines.* Transfusion transmitted infection can potentially be eliminated when donor blood from only immune individuals is transfused into immune recipients. Recombinant derived vaccines may in due time make this a possibility for hepatitis B. HBsAg produced in yeast is now commercially available as a vaccine and has a substantial history of safety and efficacy. Wide scale use of this vaccine in normal blood donor populations and in groups at high risk for transfusions and hemotherapy will inevitably reduce the incidence of transfusion-associated hepatitis B. Cost benefit analyses will be major issues. Jönsson has estimated that in a low risk general population the cost of preventing one case of hepatitis B by vaccination in over $20,000, and to avoid one death over $20 million [11]. The relative costs of HBsAg screening versus immunization of donors and recipients are challenges for biotechnology.

AIDS and non-A non-B (NANB) hepatitis represent more serious problems for all concerned with transfusion services and wide scale vaccinations may be the only recourse for controlling the diseases. The lack of success in discovering and characterizing the NANB hepatitis agent(s) despite an overwhelming effort during the past 10 years is difficult to explain in view of extensive knowledge about hepatitis A and hepatitis B. Conventional serologic and virologic techniques are probably unsuccessful because of knowledge gaps in the nature of the agent. We must now project that application of highly sensitive molecular biology techniques for cloning and discerning a rare nucleic acid in a universe of other host and foreign materials in a NANB infected liver or plasma will indeed be successful. Reconstruction experiments indicate that both HBV and HDV could have been discovered through 'blind' cloning without recourse to serology. In these cases serological methods led to identification of the viruses. Afterwards, the techniques of genetic engineering were applied to classify and clarify the replication mechanisms. For NANB the discovery will most likely come from a molecular approach, followed by clarification and control through serology. Because of the serious chronic sequelae of NANB hepatitis both a diagnostic to minimize transfusion transmission and a vaccine to give protective immunity for donors and recipients are urgently needed.

Immunization against HIV presents an ultimate challenge for molecular biologists and cellular immunologists, because the virus is a persistent and transforming retrovirus, and infects lymphocytic cells normally involved in events required for protective immunity. Studies are already underway evaluating immunogenic potential of recombinant produced HIV envelope proteins. Re-engineering the virus genome to circumvent pathogenicity and transforming potential with preservation of immunogenic potential is another approach that is well within the scope of current techniques. Biotechnology will play an important role in devising strategies for retrovirus immunizations.

### Recombinant derived replacement products

*Factor VIIIC.* Advances in broad use of stabilized blood components and purified plasma products have led to improvements in transfusion practices for controlling hemorrhage and coagulation disorders. Factor VIII and plasminogen activators, normal components of blood, are prime candidates for sourcing via genetic engineering. The genes for both Factor VIIIC and tissue plasminogen activator (TPA) have been identified, cloned, sequenced and expressed [12,13]. The active proteins have been produced in microorganisms and in mammalian cells, and are well into human clinical trials. Without doubt these recombinant derived biologicals will find wide scale commercial use as pharmaceuticals. Factor VIIIC represents the most genetically complex, biologically active protein to be produced by molecular biologists. The genetic organization of Factor VIIIC is illustrated in Figure 6. The DNA gene consists of 180,000 base pairs. The 26 exons comprise only about 5% of the DNA transcription followed by splicing and processing, gives rise to Factor VIIIC RNA of about 9000 bases (Figure 7). The native protein consists of 2,332 amino acids with a molecular weight of about 330,000 daltons after glycosylation. The glycosylated protein is further cloned to give active enzyme. It is not likely that recombinant derived Factor VIIIC will be any more or any less effective than plasma purified material. However, the risk of infectiousness will be removed. Commercialization of bioengineered Factor VIIIC will demand that the economics of the blood fractionation industry be

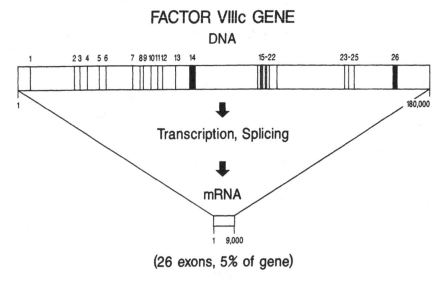

**FACTOR VIIIc GENE**

*Figure 6.*   Genetic organization of human Factor VIIIC.

considered. As biotechnology products replace the plasma-derived materials and fewer products are derived from plasma there will be an economic burden for the remaining plasma products.

## FACTOR VIIIc: mRNA TO ENZYME

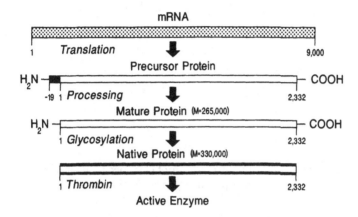

*Figure 7.* Expression and processing of Factor VIIIC protein to give biologically active enzyme.

*Plasminogen activators.* Therapeutic and preventive dissolution of fibrin blood clots with minimal effects on normal coagulation is needed in both arterial and venous vascular diseases. Urokinase (UK) and tissue plasminogen activator (TPA) are natural serine protease enzymes that convert plasminogen to plasmin, which in turn degrades fibrin (Figure 8). TPA may be more clot

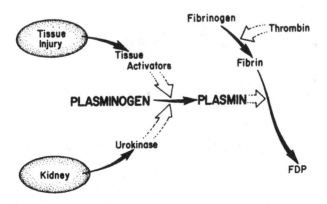

*Figure 8.* Illustration of activiation of plasminogen by urokinase and tissue plasminogen activator for degradation of fibrin.

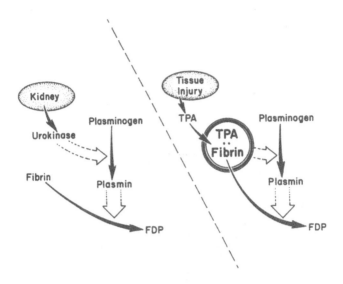

*Figure 9.* Illustration of possible mechanism of clot specific degradation of fibrin by tissue plasminogen activator.

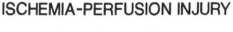

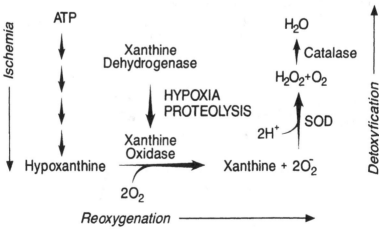

*Figure 10.* Summary of biochemical reactions that occur during ischemia (downward arrows), reperfusion (horizontal arrows), and destruction of free radicals by superoxide dismutase and catalase (upward arrows).

specific by binding directly to fibrin for activation. The complex then activates plasmin within the fibrin locale. The mechanism in theory, provides for clot specific degration of fibrin (Figure 9). Urokinase is conveniently available from urine or kidney cell culture. TPA has been produced conveniently from human genes cloned into heterologous cells, and the material is currently in clinical use. If these products significantly reduce thromboses and acute and chronic cardiovascular diseases that require surgical interventions, the demand for fresh blood for cardiopulmonary uses may decrease. This will allow vital supplies to go further and reach more patients.

## SUPEROXIDE DISMUTASE

```
                                10
Met Ala Thr Lys Ala Val Cys Val Leu Lys Gly Asp Gly Pro Val Gln
         20                                      30
Gly Ile Ile Asn Phe Glu Gln Lys Glu Ser Asn Gly Pro Val Lys Val
                                40
Trp Gly Ser Ile Lys Gly Leu Thr Glu Gly Leu His Gly Phe His Val
     50                                    60
His Glu Phe Gly Asp Asn Thr Ala Gly Cys Thr Ser Ala Gly Pro His
                     70                                      80
Phe Asn Pro Leu Ser Arg Lys His Gly Gly Pro Lys Asp Glu Glu Arg
                             90
His Val Gly Asp Leu Gly Asn Val Thr Ala Asp Lys Asp Gly Val Ala
             100                                    110
Asp Val Ser Ile Glu Asp Ser Val Ile Ser Leu Ser Gly Asp His Cys
                                 120
Ile Ile Gly Arg Thr Leu Val Val His Glu Lys Ala Asp Asp Leu Gly
     130                                    140
Lys Gly Gly Asn Glu Glu Ser Thr Lys Thr Gly Asn Ala Gly Ser Arg
                         150
Leu Ala Cys Gly Val Ile Gly Ile Ala Gln
```

*Figure 11.* Primary amino acid sequence of the subunit protein of human superoxide dismutase.

*Superoxide dismutase.* For decades the medical community has focused on restoring blood flow as fast as possible in treating heart attacks, strokes, and blood clots in other organs. As mentioned above new generations of bio-engineered fibrinolytic agents are projected to rapidly restore blood circulation to blocked tissues. The common belief that tissue and cells rapidly die when deprived of oxygen-carrying blood persisted until a few years ago. In fact cells can survive for substantial periods when deprived of oxygen. Animal studies have demonstrated that in many cases of temporary blockage of blood flow major damage occurs at the moment blood flow is resumed. The biochemical pathways have been elucidated whereby the sudden surge of oxygen-rich blood to oxygen-deprived cells instantly liberates oxygen free radicals (superoxide) and this sets up a reaction chain of various kinds of free radicals which is rapidly lethal to the cells and tissues (reperfusion injury). McCord has reviewed the mechanism for ischemia induced production of superoxide [14]. Figure 10 illustrates the biochemical reactions at ischemia and the production of free radicals when coupled to reoxygenation.

Normal injury to cells and organs by peroxides and superoxide is controlled by the enzyme superoxide dismutase (SOD) which is found in all living plant and animal tissues. Animal studies have clearly demonstrated that administration of superoxide dismutase at the time of reperfusion will dramatically prevent reperfusion injury by destroying oxygen free radicals (Figure 10) [15].

Human superoxide dismutase is currently available in large quantities via biotechnology processes. The cloned gene is readily produced in transformed yeast and other microorganisms [16]. The active enzyme is a dismer of the 153 amino acid subunit shown in Figure 11. Each molecule contains one Cu and one Zn molecule.

Recombinant derived human superoxide dismutase is currently undergoing clinical evaluations for safety and efficacy. The possible use of SOD in conjunction with fibrinolytic drugs to prevent reperfusion injury when blood again begins to flow may lead to fewer cardiovascular surgical procedures and consequently a shifting demand for blood transfusions (Table 4).

*Table 4.* Estimated uses of whole blood by clinical category

| Clinical category | Percentage of total blood |
|---|---|
| Malignant neoplasm | 20 |
| Cardiopulmonary | 17 |
| Gastrointestinal tract | 16 |
| Fractures, trauma | 13 |
| Organ transplantation, dialysis | 10 |
| Other procedures | 24 |

## New knowlegde affecting supply and use of blood and blood products

In looking to the future, we can predict that the era of biotechnology will continue to evolve and bring new knowledge about controlling malignant neoplasms, in-situ correction of genetic defects, specific controls of the immune system, and a more widescale use of organ transplantation. Practical success in any of these areas will shift the needs for hemotherapy. An estimate for the distribution of whole blood for various clinical categories is shown in Table 4. Knowledge breakthroughs leading to 'cure' or significant control in any area will shift the requirements for transfusion services. A few examples will illustrate.

*Constructing heritable characteristics.* The ability to reconstruct genes in living cells will provide the possibility for correcting defects. In situ correction of defects leading to hemophilia A or thalassemia would decrease the need for whole blood and antihemophilic factor (AHF) specific blood products.

*Cancer.* The future for bioengineered interferons, interleukins, tissue necrosis factors and other biological modulators plus an understanding and control of oncogenes will depend on continued progress in molecular and clinical investigations. Some of these bioengineering products may lead to additional controls for malignant neoplasms over the next decade. Hematologists will no doubt play major roles in identifying and assessing therapeutic and prophylactic applications for management of cancer may lead to fewer surgical procedures, and less demand for blood transfusions which now accounts for about 20% of total blood usage.

*Organ transplantation.* An understanding of immune tolerance at the molecular level could lead to bioengineered products enhancing organ transplantation successes. This will in turn increase the demand for blood and hemotherapy.

*Aging and chronic diseases.* An understanding of genes and gene functions at the molecular level has led to considerable knowledge about cell growth and development. It seems reasonable that reversal of these processes through loss of bioactive molecules by mutation or gene inactivity can result in aging and chronic diseases. Reactivation of genes or exogeneous supply of growth factors may limit aging and chronic diseases. The eventual sequencing of the human chromosome will provide knowledge and understanding of many basic life processes, including development and aging and chronicity. Although we don't envision a world of perpetual youth, some of the consequences of aging, such as muscle or bone wastage, may be minimized or corrected at the molecular level. In such an era we can expect that trauma and injuries will continue; new infectious agents may evolve; surgeries will continue; and blood and blood products will be required.

## Summary

We have at hand currently bioengineered products and molecular knowledge to improve the safety and efficacy of blood and blood products. Recombinant derived antigens for hepatitis B and AIDS diagnostics will soon be routine in blood banks. These transfusion transmitted diseases will be further minimized with use of the improved products. Hepatitis B vaccines represent the first commercial genetically engineered vaccines. As more immunized donors donate blood the risk for hepatitis B transfusion will decrease. AIDS and non-A non-B hepatitis are current major problems for transfusion medicine and both are major challenges for molecular biologists. Progress is substantial but breakthroughs do not appear to be near. New dimensions of knowledge will be needed to discover the non-A non-B viruses and to devise an immunization strategy for AIDS.

Bioengineered human Factor VIIIC and tissue plasminogen activator are now entering clinical use and may possibly affect both the economics and patterns of need for blood. Long term changing needs for hemotherapy can be expected as knowledge evolves about neoplasia, aging and organ transplantation.

Many of the predicted accomplishments for biotechnology have actually accrued over the past 10 years. Cloning and expression of genetic information is now simple, fast and routine. During the next decade human health care, including the blood transfusion segment, should expect and plan for the changes and breakthroughs that will surely come.

14

# References

1. Valenzuela P, Medina WJ, Amerer G, Hall BD. Synthesis and assembly of hepatitis B virus surface antigen in yeast. Nature 1982;298:347-50.
2. Stahl S, MacKay P, Magazine M, Bruce SA, Murray K. Hepatitis B virus core antigen: Synthesis in Escherichia coli and application in diagnosis. Proc Natl Acad Sci (USA) 1982;79:1606-10.
3. Stevens CE, Aach RD, Hollinger FB et al. Hepatitis B virus antibody in blood donors and the occurrence of non-A, non-B hepatitis in transfusion recipients: An analysis of the transfusion-transmitted viruses study. Ann Intern Med 1984; 101:733-8.
4. Alter HJ, Holland PV. Indirect tests to detect the non-A, non-B hepatitis carrier state. Ann Intern Med 1984;101:859-61.
5. Purcell RH, Rizzetto M, Gerin JL. Hepatitis delta virus infection of the liver. Semin Liver Dis 1984;4:340-6.
6. Rizzetto M, Verme G. Delta hepatitis: Present status. J Hepatol 1985;1:187-93.
7. Smuckler EA. Hepatitis, the delta agent and modern virology. Arch pathol Lab Med 1985;109:394.
8. Wang K-S, Choo Q-L, Weiner AJ et al. Structure sequence and expression of the hepatitis delta (δ) viral genome. Nature 1986;323:508-14.
9. Sanchez-Pescador R, Power MD, Barr PJ et al. Nucleotide sequence and expression of an AIDS-associated retrovirus (ARV-2). Science 1985;227:484-92.
10. Overby LR. Application of genetic engineering in blood banks and transfusion services. In: Edwards-Moulds JA, Tregellas WM (eds). Introductory molecular-genetics. Arlington: American Association of Blood Banks 1986:77-89.
11. Jönsson B. Cost-benefit analysis of hepatitis B vaccination. Postgrad Med J 1987;63(Suppl.):27-32.
12. Pennica D, Holmes WE, Kohr WJ et al. Cloning and expression of human tissue-type plasminogen activator cDNA in E. coli. Nature 1983;301:214-21.
13. Toole JJ, Knopf JL, Wozney JM et al. Molecular cloning of a cDNA encoding human antihemophilic factor. Nature 1984;312:342-7.
14. McCord JM. Oxygen-derived free radicals in postischemic tissue injury. N Engl J Med 1985;312:159-63.
15. Marklund SL. Clinical aspects of superoxide dismutase. Med Biol 1984;62:130-4.
16. Hallewell RA, Masiarz FR, Najarian RC et al. Human Cu/Zn superoxide dismutase cDNA: Isolation of clones synthesizing high levels of active or inactive enzyme from an expression library. Nucleic Acid Res 1985;13:2017-33.

# INTRODUCTION TO MOLECULAR GENETICS AND RECOMBINANT DNA TECHNOLOGY

E.J. Benz Jr

## Introduction

The basic repositories of biological information flow, called genes, consist of molecules of DNA. Molecular biologists attempt to understand the molecular basis for the flow and regulation of genetic information by using recombinant DNA methods to isolate and analyze genes. The ability of molecular biology to examine genes directly is revolutionizing the study of virtually all biological systems, including many areas relevant to transfusion medicine. This communication attempts to introduce the basic concepts of this field. For nearly two decades after the elucidation of the crystallographic structure of DNA, molecular geneticists were largely confined to the study of simple microorganisms. Complex genomes were beyond the capability of the limited repertoire of methods available for manipulating DNA molecules until a new approach, recombinant DNA technology, arose in the 1970's. Recombinant DNA methods combine advances in enzymology, nucleic acid biochemistry, and microbial genetics in ways that allow one to 'cut and paste' DNA molecules from diverse sources together to form novel DNA molecules and to introduce this DNA into new host cells, where it can be propagated and expressed. These capabilities permit one to physically isolate or 'clone' individual genes even if they originally represent only one part per million or less of a complex genome. Recombinant DNA technology thus provides a quantum increase in our capability to examine genes directly as individual physical entities. The real power of molecular genetic approaches resides in the universality with which these relatively simple methods can be productively applied. Thus, the basic approach one might use to study normal gene regulation during hematopoiesis is equally applicable to the analysis of abnormal gene expression occurring in inherited diseases of coagulation, or in situations of immune dysfunction. The principles described in this introduction are thus important to all areas of hematology.

## Principles of molecular genetics

The fundamental kernel of information storage in nature is the gene, which consists of deoxyribonucleic acid (DNA). DNA molecules are extremely long unbranched polymers consisting of nucleotide subunits. Each nucleotide contains a sugar moiety called deoxyribose, a phosphate group, and a purine or pyrimidine base (Figure 1). The linkages in the chain are formed by phosphoidester bonds between the 5' position and the 3' position of each sugar

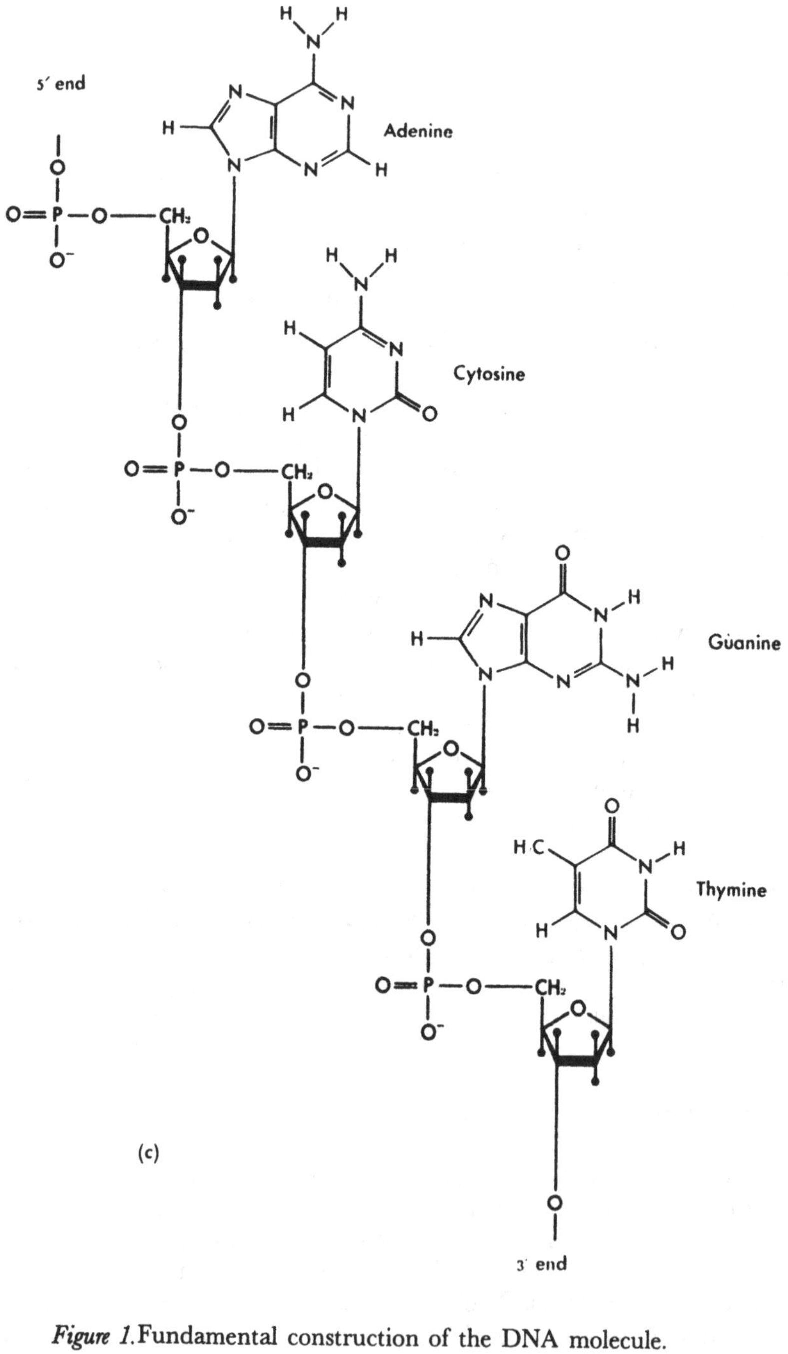

16

*Figure 1.*Fundamental construction of the DNA molecule.

residue in the chain (see Figure 1). These links form the backbone of the polymer, while the purine or pyrimidine bases project perpendicular to the chain.

The four nitrogenous bases in DNA are the purines: adenosine and the pyrimidines: thymine and cytosine. The basic chemical configuration of ribonucleic acid (RNA), is quite similar, except that the sugar is ribose, while the pyrimidine base uracil is used in place of thymine. The nitrogenous bases are commonly referred to by a short-hand notation: the letters A, C, T, G, and U are used to refer to adenosine, cytosine, thymine, guanosine, and uracil, respectively. The ends of DNA and RNA strands are chemically distinct. Because of the $3' \rightarrow 5'$ phosphodiester bond linkage that ties adjacent bases together (Figure 2), one end of the strand (3' end) will have an unlinked (free) 3' sugar position, and the other (the 5' end), a free 5' position. There is thus a 'polarity' to the sequence of bases in a DNA strand. The same sequence read a $3' \rightarrow 5'$ direction carries a different meaning than if read in a $5' \rightarrow 3'$ direction. Cellular enzymes can distinguish one end of a nucleic acid from the other; most enzymes that can 'read' along the DNA sequence tend to do so only in one direction ($3' \rightarrow 5'$ or $5' \rightarrow 3'$, but not both).

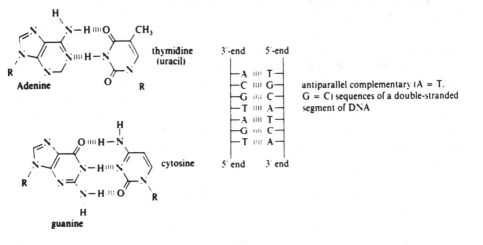

*Figure 2.* The four nitrogenous bases in DNA, which combine complementary in pairs: adenine-thymidine and guanine-cytosine.

The ability of DNA molecules to encode information resides in the sequence of nitrogenous bases. Under the conditions extant within living cells DNA is thermodynamically most stable when two strands coil around each other to form a double stranded helix. The strands are aligned in an 'antiparallel' direction. (That is, the strands have opposite $3' \rightarrow 5'$ polarity (see Figure 2)). This structure is stable only when the sugar phosphate backbones are arrayed on the outside of the helix with the nitrogenous bases stacked in the center (Figure 1). The two strands are held together (stabilized) by hydrogen bonds between the nitrogenous bases of each strand. Stereochemical considerations dictate that these hydrogen bonds can form only if adenine on one strand pairs with thymine on the opposite strand, and guanine with cytosine. In other words, an adenine occurring at a certain position along a DNA strand can only bind effectively to a DNA strand having a thymine at the analogous position along the opposite strand. These 'Watson-Crick' rules of base pairing are usually expressed by saying that only A-T and G-C base pairs can form. Two strands joined together in compliance with these rules are said to have 'complementary' base sequences.

The implications of these rules are apparent: The sequence of bases along one DNA strand immediately dictates the sequence of bases that must be present along the opposite or complementary strand in the double helix. For example, whenever an A occurs along one strand a T must be present on the opposite strand; a G must always be paired with C, a T with an A and a C with a G. This hydrogen bonding specificity confers on DNA strands their informational capacity. (Note: in RNA, U-A base pairs replace T-A base pairs). Enzymes that replicate or polymerize DNA and RNA molecules obey the base pairing rules. They utilize an existing strand of DNA or RNA as the 'template'. The new (daughter) strand is then transcribed or copied, by reading processively along the base sequence of the template strand and, at each position, adding to the growing strand only that nitrogenous base that is 'complementary' to the base in the template by the Watson-Crick rules. Thus, a DNA strand having the base sequence 5'-AATGGC-3' could only be copied by DNA polymerase into a daughter strand having the sequence, 3'-TTACCG-5'. Note that the sequence of the template strand immediately provides all the information needed to predict the nucleotide sequence of the 'complementary' daughter strand. Consider a double stranded DNA molecule that is separated into the two daughter strands. If each strand is then used as a template to synthesize a new daughter strand, what results in the creation of two double stranded daughter DNA molecules, each identical to the original parent molecule. This 'semiconservative' replication process is exactly what occurs during mitosis and meiosis as cell division proceeds. In this manner the rules of Watson-Crick base pairing provide for the ability of DNA molecules to transmit faithful copies of themselves to subsequent generations.

The information stored in a DNA base sequence achieves its impact on the structure, function, and behaviour of organisms by governing the structures and amounts of protein synthesized in the cells. The primary structure (amino acid sequence) of each protein determines its three dimensional conformation, and, therefore, its structural and functional properties (e.g. enzymatic activity, ability to interact with other molecules, stability, etc.). These proteins are the enzymes and structural elements that control cell structure and metabolism. Genes determine the structures of proteins that are synthesized, the timing of their production during development or differentiation, and the amounts produced in different cells or tissues. In this manner DNA sequences control the properties of the organism. The process by which DNA achieves its control of cells is called gene expression.

A schematic outlining the basic elements of gene expression is shown in Figure 3. The nucleotide base sequence in DNA is first copied into an RNA molecule, called messenger RNA, by mRNA polymerase. The mRNA has a base sequence complementary to the DNA coding strand. Genes in all species except certain micro-organisms consist of tandem arrays of sequences encoding

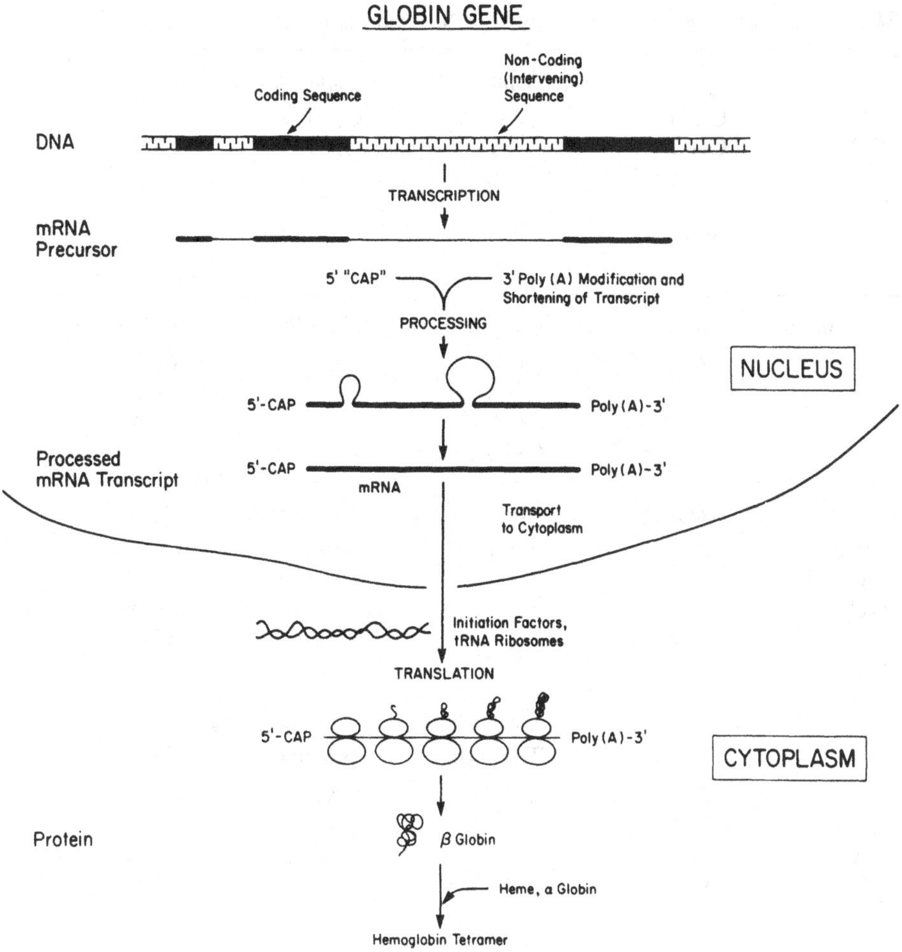

*Figure 3.* A schematic outlining of the basic elements of gene expression.

messenger RNA (exons) that alternate with sequences present in the initial mRNA transcript, or precursor, but absent from the mature mRNA (introns). The entire gene is transcribed into the large precursor, which is further processed ('spliced') in the nucleus so that the RNA regions complementary to the introns are excised and discarded. The mRNA is then exported to the cytoplasm, where it is decoded and translated into the amino acid sequence of the protein by association with a biochemically complex group of ribonucleoprotein structures called ribosomes.

Ribosomes read the mRNA sequence in a 'ticker tape' fashion *three bases at a time*, inserting the appropriate amino acid encoded by each three base code word, or codon, into the appropriate position of the growing protein chain. This process is called messenger RNA translation. Thus, DNA regulates the properties of organisms by expression in the form of protein synthesis. Genetic information flows in the direction DNA → mRNA→ protein. This polarity of information flow has been called the 'central dogma' of molecular biology.

*Table 1.* The genetic code. Messenger RNA codons for the amino acids.

| Alanine | Arginine | Asparagine | Aspartic acid | Cysteine |
| --- | --- | --- | --- | --- |
| GCU | CGU | AAU | GAU | UGU |
| GCC | CGC | AAG | GAC | UGC |
| GCA | CGA | | | |
| GCG | CGG | | | |
| | AGA | | | |
| | AGG | | | |

| Glutamic acid | Glutamine | Glycine | Histidine | Isoleucine |
| --- | --- | --- | --- | --- |
| GAA | CAA | GGU | CAU | AUU |
| GAG | CAG | GGC | CAC | AUC |
| | | GGA | | AUA |
| | | GGG | | |

| Leucine | Lysine | Methionine | Phenylalanine | Proline* |
| --- | --- | --- | --- | --- |
| UUA | AAA | AUG** | UUU | CCU |
| UUG | AAG | | UUC | CCC |
| CUU | | | | CCA |
| CUC | | | | CCG |
| CUA | | | | |
| CUG | | | | |

| Serine | Threonine | Tryptophan | Tyrosine | Valine |
| --- | --- | --- | --- | --- |
| UCU | ACU | UGG | UAU | GUU |
| UCC | ACC | | UAC | GUC |
| UCA | ACA | | | GUA |
| UCG | ACG | | | GUG |
| AGU | | | | |
| AGC | | | | |

Chain termination codons
UAA
UAG
UGA

* Hydroxyproline, the 21st amino acid, is generated by post-translational modification of proline.
** AUG is also used as the chain initiation codon.

The 'Rosetta stone' used by cells to know which amino acids are encoded by each DNA codon is called the genetic code (Table 1). The genetic code was deciphered by a series of elegant experiments conducted in several laboratories in the 1950's and 1960's. Each amino acid is encoded by a sequence of three successive bases, called a codon. Recall that a sequence read in the $5' \rightarrow 3'$ direction has a different biological meaning than a sequence read in the $3' \rightarrow 5'$ direction. Given this polarity, (and an alphabet of the four code letters, A, C, U, and G) there are $4^3$ or 64 possible three base codons.

There are 21 amino acids found in proteins, so that there are more codons available than there are amino acids to be encoded. As noted in Table 1, this redundancy or degeneracy of the genetic code results in the fact that some amino acids are encoded by more than one codon. For example, there are 6 possible codons that specify incorporation of leucine at a specific position in the amino acid chain, and 2 codons for glutamic acid, but only one each for methionine and tryptophan. However, in no case does a single codon encode more than one amino acid. Codons thus predict unambiguously the amino acid sequence they encode but one cannot easily read 'backward' from the amino acid sequence to decipher the encoding DNA sequence.

Some specialized codons serve as start and stop signals for an RNA translation. The initiator codon, AUG, not only codes for methionine but also serves as the signal to start protein synthesis when surrounded by the proper 'consensus' sequence of bases. Three codons, UAG, UAA, and UGA serve as terminators marking the end of translation. These codons do not specify incorporation of amino acid. Rather, they inform the ribosomal apparatus that the amino acid chain has been completed and that dissociation of the ribosomal subunits from the mRNA should occur.

The adaptor molecules which mediate individual decoding events during mRNA translation are called transfer RNA's. These are small RNA species, approximately 40 nucleotides long. When each tRNA is bound into a ribosome it exposes a 3 base segment, called the 'anticodon'. These 3 bases abut against the 3 base codon exposed on the mRNA that is also bound to the ribosome. Only transfer RNA's having a 3 base 'anticodon' complementary at mRNA codon will form a stable interaction among the mRNA, the ribosome, and the tRNA molecule. Within each tRNA is a separate region that is adapted for binding to an amino acid. The enzymes that catalyze the binding of the amino acid are constrained so that each tRNA species can only bind to a single amino acid. For example, tRNA molecules containing the anticodon 3'-TAG-5', which is complementary to a 5'-AUC-3' (isoleucine) codon in mRNA, can only be bound to or charged with methionine; tRNA containing the anticodon 3'-AAA-5' can only be charged with phenylalanine, etc. The properties of tRNA and amino acyl tRNA synthetase enzymes provide the specificity for translation of the genetic code. Ribosomes provide the reading apparatus by which tRNA anticodons and mRNA codons are brought together in an orderly linear and sequential fashion. As each new codon is exposed, the appropriate charged tRNA species is bound, and a peptide bond is formed between the amino acid carried by the tRNA and the existing nascent protein chain. The growing chain is transferred to the new tRNA in the process, so that it is held in place as the next tRNA is brought in.

Upon completion of translation, the polypeptide chain is released into the cytosol for further processing by other structures, such as endoplasmic reticulum and the Golgi apparatus. Some proteins associate chain with other subunits to form complex multimeric proteins (e.g. hemoglobin), for binding to cofactors, for processing (e.g. glycosylation) in microsomes, etc.

### Gene regulation

Virtually all cells of an organism receive a complete copy of the DNA genome transmitted to the organism at the time of its conception. In order to form distinct cell types and tissues, the genome must selectively express or repress different genes in each cell. Each cell must 'know' which genes to express, how actively to express them, and when to express them. This biologcial necessity has come to be known as 'gene regulation' or 'regulated gene expression'. An understanding of the ways that genes are selected for expression remains one of the major frontiers of biology and medicine. Although little is known about the mechanisms regulating gene expression, many of the molecular elements involved in regulation are becoming better understood as a result of the application of recombinant DNA technology.

Most of the DNA in living cells is inactivated by being bound into a nucleoprotein complex called chromatin. The histone and non-histone proteins in chromatin effectively 'hide' the majority of genes from enzymes needed for expression. It is now clear that there are DNA sequence regions, usually flanking the actual 'structural gene',* which serve as regulatory signals. These sequences do not usually encode RNA or protein molecules. Rather, they interact with nuclear proteins. These proteins alter conformation of the gene within chromatin in such a way as to facilitate or inhibit access to the apparatus that transcribes genes into mRNA.

Several types of DNA sequence elements have been defined according to the presumed consequences of their interaction with nuclear proteins.

*Promoters* are found just 'upstream' (to the 5′ side) of the start of mRNA transcription (the 'CAP') in almost every gene. Promoters appear to be the sequence loci at which mRNA polymerases bind and gain access to the structural gene sequences downstream. They appear to serve a dual function of binding the mRNA polymerase and 'marking' for the polymerase the point at which mRNA transcription should start.

*Enhancers* are DNA sequences that serve more complicated and less well understood functions. Enhancers can occur on either side of a gene, or even within the gene in introns. Enhancers appear to bind to nuclear proteins or 'transcription factors' and thereby stimulate expression of genes nearby. Some enhancers influence only the adjacent gene; others play a role in marking the boundaries of large multigene clusters (gene domains) whose co-ordinated expression is appropriate to a particular tissue type or a particular time. 'Silencer' sequences appear to serve a function that is the obverse of enhancers. When bound by the appropriate nuclear proteins, silencer sequences cause repression of gene expression.

---

* The structural gene is defined as the DNA sequence encoding the mRNA precursor.

## TYPES OF CUTS MADE BY RESTRICTION ENZYMES

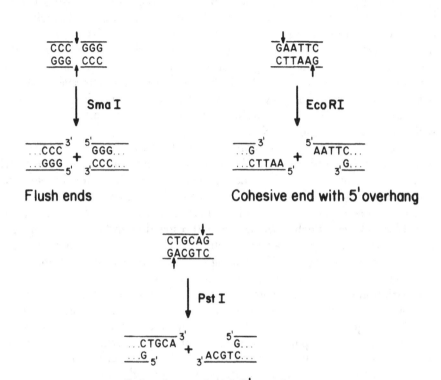

*Figure 4.*

### Basic tenets of recombinant DNA technology

The informational content of DNA molecules resides in the nucleotide sequence, rather than in the sugar phosphate backbone. Unfortunately, traditional biochemical methods do not provide straightforward ways to distinguish among nucleic acid molecules on the basis of their nucleotide sequences. In addition, genes do not exist in cells as discrete DNA molecules; rather, thousands of genes are linked together in tandem with very long stretches of intergenic DNA to form chromosomes. For example, in the human genome, the three billion base pairs of DNA exist as 23 chromosomes in the haploid genome. Each chromosome is thus about 100 million base pairs long. These facts render DNA an almost unworkable substance for direct physical purification of most genes. Recombinant DNA technology circumvents the biochemical problems inherent in the properties of DNA by combining enzymologic, microbiological, and genetic approaches.

**Restriction endonucleases**

A major advance in our ability to manipulate DNA molecules was the discovery of enzymes produced by bacteria called restriction endonucleases. Restriction endonucleases have the capacity to recognize short nucleotide base sequences (oligonucleotide sequences) and to cleave DNA within or near the recognition sequence. For example, EcoR1, a restriction endonuclease isolated from *Escherichia coli*, cuts DNA at the sequence 5'-GAATTC-3', but nowhere else (Figure 4). Thus, each DNA sample will be reduced reproducibly to an array of smaller sized fragments whose size ranges depend on the distribution with which 5'-GAATTC-3' is encountered. However, the DNA will not be degraded in any other way by the enzyme. Restriction endonucleases differ from other nucleases by the specificity and limited manner with which they degrade DNA.

Part of the 'jargon' that newcomers to the field of recombinant DNA technology often find difficult arises from the shorthand notation given to restriction endonucleases. These enzymes are generally named after the bacterium from which they were isolated. Thus, a restriction endonuclease activity purified from *Serratia marcescens* is called Sma1, that from *Bacillus amyliofaciens* is called BamH1, etc. Each of the nearly 500 restriction endonucleases that have been described recognizes a unique oligonucleotide sequence and cleaves the DNA only at those points. The biological function of restriction enzymes in their bacterial hosts remains poorly understood.

Restriction enzymes have proved to be extraordinarily useful gifts from the microbial world to molecular geneticists. They allow one to reduce the sizes of DNA fragments in a controlled and reproducible manner from several hundred million base pairs long to fragment arrays ranging from a few dozen to a few tens of thousands of bases long. These ranges are far more workable in the test tube. Moreover, by 'mixing and matching' combinations of restriction enzymes used to digest the same DNA sample, one can construct maps or 'fingerprints' of the restriction endonuclease sites in a genome. This strategy has made restriction endonuclease mapping as useful an approach for characterizing the fine structure of genomes as proteolytic digestion has been to protein chemists for peptide fingerprinting.. Some restriction endonucleases cut the DNA so as to leave short single stranded overhanging regions or 'sticky ends' at the 5' or 3' end of the cutting site, while cleavage by others leaves blunt or flush double stranded ends (Figure 4). Since many restriction endonucleases sites are palindromes (reading exactly the same in forward direction (5'→3') on one strand and the 'backward' (5'→3') direction on the opposite strand, (e.g. EcoR1: $\frac{5'\text{-GAATTC-}3'}{3'\text{-CTTAAG-}5'}$), enzymes leaving overhanging ends are particularly useful. If one digests DNA from two different sources, such as a bacteriophage DNA preparation and a human genomic DNA preparation, with a restriction endonuclease leaving overhanging or 'sticky ends', those ends will be complementary by Watson-Crick base pairing and can thus be annealed together by means of the single stranded overhangs. This is one popular method for generating recombinant DNA molecules.

## Enzymes useful for modifying DNA

Several other nucleic acid modifying enzymes have been critical to the development of recombinant DNA technology. Most notable among these are reverse transcriptase (RNA dependent DNA polymerase) and DNA ligase. Reverse transcriptase is the enzyme packaged inside retroviruses, which have an RNA genome. In order for retroviruses to reproduce themselves within their cellular hosts, their RNA genomes must be transcribed into DNA molecules (RNA→DNA) that can then be replicated (DNA→DNA) and expressed by host cell machinery (DNA→RNA).

Reverse transcriptase has the very useful property that, if provided with an appropriate 'primer' complementary to a messenger RNA molecule, it can read the mRNA strand in a 3'→5' direction and transcribe a single stranded DNA copy ('copy DNA', 'complementary DNA', or cDNA) of the RNA molecule. One can thus incubate reverse transcriptase with messenger RNA isolated from a cell or tissue of interest with reverse transcriptase, and generate thereby a family of single stranded DNA molecules representing the entire array of messenger RNA's expressed in that cell or tissue. Using additional enzymes that have been characterized and purified, for example *E. coli* DNA dependent DNA polymerase 1, (Klenow fragment), one can synthesize a complementary second strand of DNA (sDNA) from the single stranded cDNA template. This creates a double stranded DNA molecule containing the sequence information originally expressed in the form of mRNA. These DNA molecules can then be manipulated in essentially the same ways that native genomic DNA molecules can, by restriction endonuclease digestion, radioactive labelling, or insertion into microbial host vectors for cloning.

DNA ligase is an enzyme that can join two DNA molecules together to form a single novel DNA molecule. For example, one can join the aforementioned double stranded cDNA molecules with bacteriophage DNA molecules by incubating DNA from both sources together in the presence of DNA ligase. This ability to generate artificially recombined or 'recombinant' DNA molecules has given rise to the term recombinant DNA technology. A number of other enzymes beyond the scope of this review, have also been useful to the development of recombinant DNA technology.

## Microbial genetics and infectious DNA molecules

Enzymes that manipulate DNA would have had limited utility except for the discovery of certain small DNA molecules that possess remarkable biological properties. Many bacteria harbour DNA molecules that are not part of the single major bacterial chromosome. They are small (a few thousand to about 100 thousand bases long), circular, and endowed with sequences serving as independent origins of DNA replication. They can thus replicate in host cells independent of the host genome by utilizing cellular DNA replicating enzymes. These DNA molecules can be thought of as elemental commensal organisms, residing in the cell and capable of infecting other host bacteria. They have come to be called extra-chromosomal elements or episomes.

The forms of episomes most relevant to this discussion are the plasmid and bacteriophage. Plasmids useful in recombinant DNA technology usually carry one or more antibiotic resistance genes, an origin of DNA replication, and a limited but useful array of restriction endonuclease sites. Molecular biologists have engineered plasmids with a variety of desirable properties for customized recombinant DNA applications. Typically, these plasmids are only 3-10,000 bases long. They usually carry genes for ampicillin or tetracycline resistance, as well as a short DNA sequence, containing several thightly clustered restriction endonuclease sites, called a polylinker. The polylinker sequence is inserted into any one of several non-critical regions of the plasmid genome. Cells 'infected' with these plasmids can be detected and purified by their ability to grow in media containing the relevant antibiotic.

The most useful plasmids for recombinant DNA work are those in which the plasmid or its polylinker include several restriction endonuclease sites that occur only once in the plasmid genome. Digestion of a circular molecule with an enzyme that makes only a single cut in the circle will cause opening or linearization of the circle while leaving all of the biologically critical sequences intact. One can then insert a DNA molecule into the opening, reseal the circle with DNA ligase and thereby generate a recombinant DNA molecule retaining the biological activities of the parent plasmid.

Bacteriophages are viruses capable of infecting specific strains of bacteria. Their genomes are somewhat larger than plasmids and the DNA is covered during the extracellular part of the viral life span by a proteinaceous coat. However, bacterial genomes relevant to this discussion can also exist in the cell as episomes. The most useful bacteriophages for molecular genetics experiments have been bacteriophage $\lambda$, which can be used as a gene cloning vehicle, and the single stranded bacteriophage M13, which has proved to be useful for DNA sequencing applications. By analogy with plasmid genomes, bacteriophage genomes have been engineered to provide a number of useful DNA vectors.

The essential aspect of bacteriophages and plasmids important for this discussion is that they are biologically active even when they exist as simple free-standing DNA molecules. By combining the ability to recombine episomal DNA with DNA from mammalian sources (via restriction enzymes and ligase), with the capacity of the episomes for infection and phenotypic alteration of host cells, one can use these molecules to introduce 'foreign' DNA into host bacteria. Then, all of the useful properties of the vast array of microbial strains available become accessible for the study of genes from other species. Individual strains of bacteria can be readily isolated as single cell clones, grown in extremely large quantities for relatively little expense, and used as 'factories' for the production both of the foreign DNA 'passenger' and its protein products.

## Advances in nucleic acid chemistry

### 1. Synthetic oligonucleotides

During the past two decades, anhydrous methods for the synthesis of DNA molecules *in vitro* have been developed and automated. This has provided a capacity to synthesize short but useful DNA molecules even without the availability of a template or a DNA modifying enzyme. For example, the polylinker sequences used to introduce restriction endonuclease sites into plasmids can now be readily synthesized by machine and ligated into a plasmid in order to alter its restriction endonuclease map. Synthetic oligonucleotides can also be radiolabelled and used as customized molecular hybridization probes.

### 2. Molecular hybridization assays

The tendency of DNA and RNA molecules to prefer existence in double stranded forms in physiologic solution has been exploited by nucleic acid chemists for the development of 'molecular hybridization' assays. If DNA or RNA molecules are heated or exposed to certain denaturants, such as formamide, the hydrogen bonds holding two strands together are disrupted and the molecule is denatured into single stranded form. Temperature, salt and denaturing conditions that favour reannealing into the double stranded form can then be restored. This reannealing process is often called molecular hybridization: reannealing under a given set of conditions of temperature, salt, and denaturant is a function of the time of incubation and the concentrations of the two complementary strands.

When DNA and RNA strands are denatured into single stranded form, they will reanneal only with strands having a sequence complementary by the rules of Watson-Crick base pairing. Thus, one can denature a specimen of DNA or RNA (for example, messenger RNA from a human reticulocyte) and incubate it with a radioactively labelled, defined DNA or RNA sequence, for example, a cloned human $\beta$-globin gene. During the reannealing reaction, the labelled $\beta$-globin gene DNA probe will hybridize only to those mRNA molecules that are complementary by Watson-Crick base pairing, i.e., globin messenger RNA molecules. One can then utilize any one of several available techniques to recognize or separate the fraction of radioactively labelled DNA 'probe' molecules that have been bound into double stranded from form the unbound or unreacted single stranded molecules. For example, the enzyme $S_1$ nuclease degrades single stranded DNA molecules, leaving only the double stranded 'hybridized' molecules intact. The result is a convenient assay for detecting and quantitating the globin messenger RNA within the reticulocyte mRNA preparation. By extension of this reasoning, one can use molecular hybridization strategies to detect, quantitate, and map DNA sequences or RNA sequences derived from any tissue or source for which a complementary defined DNA probe is available.

Numerous variations of the basic molecular hybridization have been devised for a wide variety of applications, as will be apparent from the chapters in this volume. Detailed discussion is beyond the scope of this introduction.

However, the range of applications, theoretical rationale, and utility of most of these assays can be appreciated by their analogy to the use of antigen/antibody reactions in immunochemistry. The DNA probe serves the molecular geneticist in much the same way as a defined antibody probe serves the immunologist. The principles underlying the various molecular hybridization techniques used are very similar to those devised for using antibody probes to quantitate and detect defined antigens.

### 3. DNA and RNA blotting

Blot hybridization is a technique which permits the identification and characterization of a specific DNA or RNA species within a complex mixture of DNA or RNA fragments. Introduced in 1975 by E.M. Southern as a DNA analysis method, this general approach has been used extensively to map the coding and flanking regions of genes for which probes are available. Mapping by 'Southern' blotting has revealed polymorphisms in restriction sites within and adjacent to all genes studied so far; these polymorphic restriction sites have provided a new means for performing linkage analysis in the diagnosis of inherited disorders. Southern blotting has also been used to establish the absence of genes (e.g. in those thalassemias which are due to globin gene deletions), and for measurement of gene copy number.

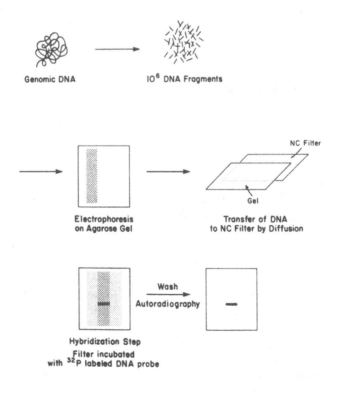

*Figure 5.* The Southern technique of blotting.

The 'Southern' technique is illustrated in Figure 5. First, total genomic DNA is extracted from the cells to be studied and digested with a restriction enzyme. The resulting mixture of fragments is separated by gel electrophoresis; due to the large number of fragments (in the range of one million for a human genome) generated by most endonucleases, the gel appears as a continuous 'smear' rather than as a series of discrete bands. After *in situ* denaturation of the fragments by incubation of the gel in alkali, transfer of the DNA fragments to a nitrocellulose filter is accomplised by diffusion (thus, the term 'blotting'). The nitrocellulose filter is incubated in buffer containing a cloned radiolabelled DNA probe for the gene of interest. The probe hybridizes only to the complementary DNA sequences on the filter; excess probe is then removed by washing. The bands indentified by autoradiography represent the fragment size(s) generated by that enzyme. Restriction mapping of the gene by blotting can then be achieved by comparing fragment sizes obtained with a variety of enzymes.

By means of simple modifications, blot hybridization has been adapted for analysis of RNA and proteins as well. 'Northern' blotting permits the identification of a specific mRNA species; in this procedure, a mixture of the cell's RNA (rather than DNA) is run on a gel and transferred to nitrocellulose. A DNA probe is used to identify the band of interest; hybridization conditions are controlled to favour formation of .pa DNA-RNA hybrids. In 'Western' blotting, *proteins* are run on the gel and transferred to a solid matrix; the probe used in this case is a labelled antibody.

## Coalescence of methodologies to produce and isolate recombinant DNA molecules

Advances in each of the areas just noted have been brought together for the purpose of physically isolating genes from complex genomes, such as a mammalian genome. DNA is isolated from, for example, a human lymphocyte and digested with restriction endonucleases to generate overhanging 'sticky ends'. (Alternatively, if one wishes to isolate only those DNA sequences encoding the specific array of genes expressed in a given tissue, one first isolates messenger RNA and converts it into cDNA by incubation with reverse transcriptase as a first step.) An infectious plasmid or bacteriophage DNA molecule is cut with the same restriction enzyme so that molecules from the two sources have complementary 'sticky' ends. The DNA's from the two sources are incubated together in the presence of DNA ligase under conditions that allow each plasmid or bacteriophage DNA molecule to ligate to only one lymphocyte DNA molecule. The recombinant DNA molecules are then 'sealed' with DNA ligase, so that each is now an infectious DNA species carrying a single DNA fragment from the lymphocyte as a 'passenger'.

The DNA molecules are then used to infect an excess number of host bacterial cells so that each cell acquires only a single recombinant DNA molecule. The host cells lack a property conferred by the infecting molecule, such as antibiotic resistance. The infected bacteria are then 'plated' on petri plates at a density allowing detection of individual colonies or bacteriophage plaques. Each colony or plaque represents the progeny of a single cell, and is thus a 'clone' of cells or phage carrying a single DNA fragment from the lymphocyte. Therefore, that DNA fragment, or gene, has been genetically isolated in its host cell from all other lymphocyte DNA fragments by the cloning process.

What remains is the need to identify the DNA fragment representing the specific gene one whishes to purify. One must locate within the array of plaques or colonies, called a recombinant DNA 'library', those cells or phages carrying the DNA sequence of interest. Numerous devices have been developed for screening these libraries for the presence of the occasional clone bearing the gene of interest. Different approaches are suitable depending on what information is available about the particular gene or its protein product. Discussion of these detailed area is beyond the scope of this review.

Once one has identified the colony or bacteriophage plaque containing the recombinant molecule of interest, that colony or plaque can be separated from the remainder of the library and harvested by growing in bacterial culture. In this manner, one can produce substantial quantities of recombinant DNA molecules from the cloned host cell. With respect to other DNA molecules derived from the lymphocyte, the recombinant DNA 'cloned' gene will be absolutely pure. The purified gene can then be used as hybridization probe, as the substrate for obtaining its DNA sequence, or as a template for controlled expression and production of its mRNA and protein products.

The elegance of recombinant DNA technology resides in the capacity it confers upon investigators to examine each gene as a discrete physical entity that can be purified, reduced to its basic building blocks for decoding of its primary structure, analyzed for its patterns of expression, and perturbed by alterations in sequence or molecular environment so that the effects of changes in each fine structural region of the gene can be assessed. Moreover, techniques have been developed whereby the purified genes can be deliberately modified or mutated to create novel genes not available in nature. These provide the potential to generate useful new biological entities, such as modified viruses that can serve as vaccines, modified proteins customized for specific therapeutic or industrial purposes, or altered combinations of regulatory and structural genes that allow for the assumption of new functions by specific gene systems. For example, it is now theoretically possible to utilize bone marrow cells (which can be readily removed from an individual, and later transplanted back into that individual or a compatible patient) as vehicles for gene therapy. It is theoretically possible to insert a gene for an important serum protein, such as a clotting factor, into the explanted cells than to and reimplant the bone marrow cells into the patient. The genetically engineered bone marrow cells will then serve as surrogate sources of a protein for which a patient may be deficient, even if the 'natural' cellular production of that protein in some other less accessible tissue, such as endothelial cells.

The specific ways by which purified genes greatly strengthen the arsenal used by molecular biologists to attack the mysteries of gene regulation can be summarized as follows:

First, the abundant and pure DNA fragments made available by molecular purification of a gene provide the characterized DNA sequences needed for use as hybridization probes in molecular hybridization assays. Thus, a purified gene is the source of molecular hybridization probes needed for the Northern or Southern blotting assays mentioned earlier.

Second, cloned genes allow one to accumulate sufficient amounts of a pure homogenous DNA sequence for determination of the exact nucleotide sequence of the gene. DNA sequencing techniques have become so reliable and efficient that it is often far easier to clone a gene encoding a protein of interest and determine its DNA sequence than it is to purify the protein and determine its amino acid sequence. As noted earlier, the DNA sequence of the gene will predict exactly what the amino acid sequence of the protein must be, since that amino acid sequence is encoded in the gene DNA.

By comparing normal gene sequences with the sequences of genes cloned from patients known to have abnormalities of a specific gene system, such as the globin genes in the thalassemia or sickle cell syndromes, one can compare the normal and pathologic 'anatomy' of genes critical to major hematologic processes. In this manner it has been possible to identify over 100 mutations responsible for various forms of thalassemia, hemophilia, red cell enzymopathies, porphyrias, etc.

Third, each purified cloned gene can be further manipulated by extension of the same types of 'cutting and pasting' techniques just described for studies of gene expression. Just as plasmid and bacteriophage vectors have been developed for the transfer of genes into microbial host cells, a variety of means for transfer of genes into eukaryotic cells have been devised. By judicious and adept application of these gene transfer technologies, one can place the gene into a controlled cellular environment and analyze its expression. These 'surrogate' or 'reverse' genetics systems permit one to analyze the normal physiology of expression of a particular gene, as well as the pathophysiology of abnormal gene expression resulting from mutations.

Fourth, detailed knowledge about the structure and expression of cloned genes greatly strengthens the opportunities investigators have to examine their protein products. By expressing the cloned genes in large amounts in micro-organisms or eukaryotic cells, one can produce proteins for use as immunogens, thereby allowing preparation of a variety of useful and powerful antibody probes for direct study of the protein products. Alternatively, one can prepare synthetic peptides deduced from the DNA sequence for use as immunogens. Controlled production of large amounts of the protein also allows one to conduct direct analysis of specific functions attributable to domains within that protein.

Finally, all of the above techniques can be extended greatly by taking advantage of methods available for mutating the genes and examining the effects of those mutations on the regulated expression of the genes and the properties of mRNA and proteins encoded by them. By 'swapping in' portions of one gene within another (chimeric genes), or abutting structural regions of one gene with regulatory sequences of another, one can investigate in previously inconceivable ways the complexities of gene regulation. These 'activist' approaches to modifying gene expression create the opportunity to generate new RNA and protein products of genes whose applications are limited only by the collective imagination of molecular biologists.

The most important impact of the genetic approach to the analysis of biological phenomena is presently the most indirect. Diligent and repeated application of the above algorithm to the study of many genes from diverse groups of organisms is beginning to reveal the basic strategies used by nature for the regulation of cell and tissue behaviour. As our knowledge of these 'rules of regulation' grows, our ability to understand, detect, and correct pathologic phenomena will increase massively. Similarly, our capacity to use biological strategies for production of useful substances is currently limited largely by our limited knowledge of the factors that constrain genes from maximal expression in various cell types. As our knowledge of these natural rules improves, so too will our opportunities to engineer useful biologicals.

# MOLECULAR GENETIC ANALYSIS OF HLA CLASS II POLYMORPHISM*

S.L. Holbeck, G.T. Nepom

HLA class II genes (termed DR, DQ, DO and DP) encode proteins which are important in generation of the immune response. These proteins are heterodimers, composed of an alpha and a beta chain. Each individual has at least 7 beta genes and 6 alpha genes (some of which are non-functional) clustered together on chromosome 6 (Fig. 1). These genes are highly related to one another. Most of these HLA class II genes are polymorphic, having multiple allelic forms. Thus the number of genes and the large number of alleles make this a complex system to study and provides a good example of the power of molecular genetic techniques.

Numerous studies have shown that certain HLA class II alleles are associated with increased risk of developing diseases believed to have an immune component. Our laboratory is particularly interested in two such diseases, rheumatoid arthritis (RA) and insulin dependent diabetis mellitus (IDDM) which have both been associated with HLA-DR4. DR4 is a specificity associated with the DR genes, but since DR genes are linked to other HLA class II genes this disease risk could also be due to any of these linked genes. We have approached this problem by asking the following questions. Can we identify DNA polymorphisms within DR4 individuals? If so, is there a subset of DR4 associated polymorphisms which gives a greater correlation with disease? Does the same subset of DR4 associated genes give increased risk for RA and IDDM? In this paper we review the results of our studies addressing these questions.

HLA CLASS II REGION

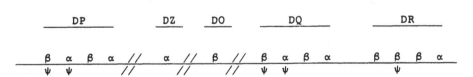

*Figure 1.* Map of the HLA class II region on chromosome six. Genes believed to be pseudogenes are indicated by a $\psi$. Protein products have been detected for the remaining genes.

* This work was supported by grants IM-450 from the American Cancer Society and AR37296 from the National Institutes of Health.

34

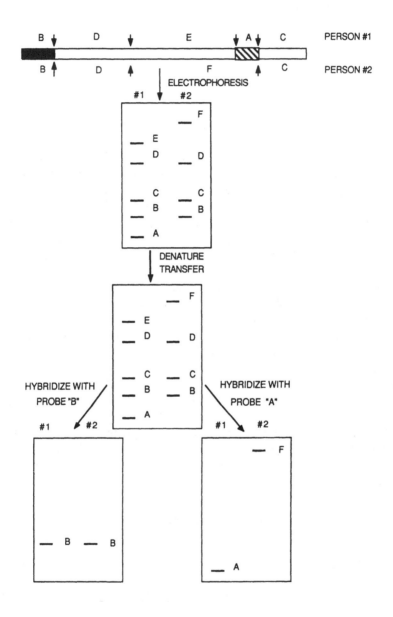

*Figure 2.* Schematic diagram of the Southern blotting procedure. DNA from person #1 and person #2 is cut with a restriction enzyme which cleaves at the arrows. The DNA of person #2 lacks one of these restriction endonuclease sites and thus gives fragment 'F' rather than the fragments 'A' and 'E' which person #1 produces. Fragments are separated and transferred to nitrocellulose as described in the text. When the blot is hybridized with probe 'B', indicated by the stippled box, DNA of both person #1 and person #2 display band 'B'. If an identical blot is hybridized with probe 'A', indicated by the slashed box, different bands are seen, demonstrating that the DNA of person #1 and person #2 differ in this region of the chromosome.

Molecular biology provides powerful tools to analyze a complex system such as HLA class II genes. Using Southern blots [1] one can determine how related different genes or alleles are. In this technique, illustrated in Figure 2, DNA is isolated from cells (PBLs are a convenient source). The DNA is cut into fragments with a restriction endonuclease. These enzymes recognize and cleave DNA at a particular sequence. For example, the enzyme Eco RI has the recognition sequence 5'GAATTC 3'. The fragments produced by this digestion are separated based on their size by agarose gel electrophoresis. The gel is soaked in alkali to denature the DNA, neutralized, and the DNA transferred to a nitrocellulose or nylon membrane. The immobilized DNA is hybridized with a cloned DNA probe specific for the gene of interest, then the blot is washed to remove non-specifically bound probe. The probe DNA is radiolabelled, so that upon exposure of the membrane to X-ray film fragments of DNA containing the gene of interest are visualized as dark bands. Thus one can detect a single gene over the background of the entire genome. If a particular gene from two individuals is very similar in sequence they are likely to produce identical Southern blot patterns. This is the case when DNA from different DR4 individuals is digested and hybridized with probes specific for DR beta genes [2]. Previous analysis of DR beta proteins [3,4] had shown that there were at least five variants of DR4. Since they all give identical Southern blot patterns these variants must be closely related. To reveal the fine structure differences between these DR4 variants Gregerson et al [5] sequenced DR beta cDNAs from these variants. This analysis showed that the DR4 variants differ from one another only by several nucleotides, and are closely related alleles. With this sequence data we designed allele specific oligonucleotide probes spanning the region where these alleles differ. These oligonucleotide probes are small (about 20 nucleotides long) and are single stranded. These probes can be used in Southern blots, with minor modifications to the protocol. Such oligonucleotides will hybridize only to an allele which is identical in sequence to the oligonucleotide and not to an allele which differs by a singel base pair. Using such allele specific probes we have determined the relative frequency of the DR4 associated DR beta alleles in RA and normal populations [6]. We find that two of these alleles, Dw4 and Dw14, are more prevalent in RA patients. Thus only a subset of DR4 individuals are at increased risk of developing RA.

We have applied similar analysis to the DQ beta genes among DR4 individuals. Since DQ beta is very near DR beta on the chromosome these genes tend to be co-inherited. Thus most individuals who are DR4 are also DQw3. When we look for DQw3 variants by Southern blot we find two variants which we have termed DQ$\beta$3.1 and DQ$\beta$3.2 [7]. These can be distinguished by Southern blots using many different restriction endonucleases [8]. This indicates that these alleles are quite different from one another. DNA sequence analysis of the genes [9,10, our unpublished observations] reveals that DQ$\beta$3.1 and DQ$\beta$3.2 differ substantially in both coding and non-coding regions. We have analyzed the DQ beta alleles present in DR4 IDDM patients by Southern blot [11]. All patients tested had the DQ$\beta$3.2 allele. Thus only a subset of DR4 individuals, those with the DQ$\beta$3.2 allele, are at increased risk of developing IDDM.

Table 1 summarizes the DR4 haplotypes (DQ beta and DR beta alleles on the same chromosome) we have identified. Some haplotypes carry increased risk for both RA and IDDM, some for only RA or only IDDM, and some of these haplotypes are not associated with risk for either of these diseases. The ability to more precisely define the HLA genes responsible for association with disease allows one to more accurately identify those at risk.

*Table 1.* HLA-DR4 associated haplotypes have different disease risks.

| | | At risk for: | |
| DQ beta allele | DR beta allele | RA | IDDM |
| --- | --- | --- | --- |
| DQβ3.2 | Dw4 | + | + |
| DQβ3.1 | Dw4 | + | – |
| DQβ3.2 | Dw14 | + | + |
| DQβ3.2 | Dw10 | – | + |
| DQβ3.2 | Dw13 | – | + |
| DQβ3.1 | Dw13 | – | – |

**References**
1. Southern E. Detection of specific sequences among DNA fragments separated by gel electrophoresis. J Mol Biol 1975;98:503-9.
2. Holbeck SL, Kim S-J, Silver J, Hansen JA, Nepom GT. HLA-DR4 associated haplotypes are genotypically diverse within HLA. J Immunol 1985;135:637-41.
3. Nepom BS, Nepom GT, Mickelson E, Antonelli P, Hansen JA. Electrophoretic analysis of human HLA-DR antigens from HLA-DR4 homozygous cell lines: Correlation between beta chain diversity and HLA-D. Proc Natl Acad Sci (USA) 1983;80:6962-6.
4. Groner JP, Watson AJ, Bach FH. Dw/LD-related molecular polymorphism of DR4 beta chains. J Exp Med 1983;157:1687-91.
5. Gregerson PK, Moriuchi T, Karr RW et al. Polymorphisms of HLA DR beta chains in DR-4, -7 and -9 haplotypes: Implications for the mechanisms of allelic variation. Proc Natl Acad Sci (USA) 1986;83:1949-53.
6. Nepom GT, Seyfried C, Holbeck SL, Wilske K, Nepom BS. identification of HLA Dw14 genes in DR4+ rheumatoid arthritis. Lancet 1986;ii:1002-5.
7. Kim S-J, Holbeck SL, Nisperos B, Hansen J, Maeda H, Nepom GT. Identification of a polymorphic variant associated with HLA-DQw3 characterized by specific restriction sites with DQ beta. Proc Natl Acad Sci (USA) 1985;82:8139-43.
8. Holbeck SL, Nepom GT. Exon specific oligonucleotide probes localize HLA-DQ beta allelic polymorphisms. Immunogenetics 1986;24:251-8.
9. Larhammar D, Hyldig-Nielsen J, Servenius B, Anderson G, Rask L, Peterson P. Exon intron organization and complete nucleotide sequence of a human major histocompatibility antigen DC beta gene. Proc Natl Acad Sci (USA) 1983;80:7313-7.
10. Michelsen B, Lernmark A. Molecular cloning of a polymorphic DNA endonuclease fragment associates insulin dependent diabetes mellitus with HLA DQ. J Clin Invest 1987;79:1144-52.
11. Nepom BS, Palmer J, Kim S-J, Hansen JA, Holbeck SL, Nepom GT. Specific genomic markers for the HLA-DQ subregion discriminate between DR4 positive IDDM and DR4 postive JRA. J Exp Med 1986;164:345-50.

# BIOENGINEERING IN BLOOD TRANSFUSION MEDICINE

G. Jacquin

For a relevant overview of the actual and future applications of 'bioengineering' in blood transfusion medicine, it is necessary to clearly separate between the field of diagnosis and the therapeutic area. In the first field laboratory applications such as blood group serology, HLA typing, diagnosis of viral diseases, advances in gene research, in cellular engineering and molecular biology have been very rapidly followed by technical, commercial and finally industrial applications. The very short period between the birth of the 'emerging biotechnologies' in the 1980's and these results is due to economical reasons and the relatively easy feasibility for the registration of these new reagents. In the field of therapeutic products, it often takes a long time between the cloning of the desired protein and the distribution of the new recombinant drug, which often tends to be the only replacement of the plasma protein. In spite of their drawbacks (purity, low yields) and the diseases which have been transmitted over recent years by conventionally produced clotting factors, it seems possible in the very near future to achieve tremendous advances in the preparation and the purification of many plasma proteins. They therefore will be available in larger amounts at lower prices, even if for some reason the blood and plasma collection all around the world remains at its actual level. Regarding safety, purity, availability, price and therapeutic efficacy, the comparison between the recombinant DNA produced proteins, or the monoclonal antibodies and the proteins extracted from human plasma can be expected more and more difficult, because the most efficient and elegant methods achieved with the tools of the 'new biotechnologies' can be successfully applied in some key areas of the fractionation industry, especially the use of monoclonal antibodies for the purification and the characterization of the most important proteins.

## Monoclonal antibodies: State of the art and perspective in immuno-hematology

Blood group serology has been the first field of applications which was touched by the revolutionary discovery in 1975 by Kohler and Milstein [1]. The first monoclonal antibodies to red cell antigens appeared before the 1980's. The CNTS in Paris proposed in 1981 a panel of MoAbs anti-A, anti-B and anti-A+B which was composed for each specificity of three different clones, in order to get the best avidity and specificity, as compared with the excellent polyclonal antibodies available in this area. Between 1981 and 1988, the replacement of the human or animal polyclonal antibodies has not been as

important and rapid as was predicted in the beginning of this decade. Several answers can be proposed:
- a long history with polyclonal antibodies, in an area where the new products must be more reliable and more specific than the conventional reagents;
- the immunological 'repertoire' of the mouse is limited; however, following the first results, especially in the ABO system, the technology of murine monoclonal antibodies did not permit the discovery of many specificities: The use and the development of human monoclonal antibodies was necessary;
- trends for the future are particularly focused in blood group serology in the development of automated procedures. These new methods do not demand large volumes of reagents: The need for large amounts of monoclonal antibodies, which was an industrial advantage, therefore, becomes less and less strategic.

It remains that monoclonal antibodies offer many important advantages from a technical, ethical and industrial point of view:
- specificity can be precisely characterized and biochemically defined;
- reproducibility in the results can be granted;
- culture in large amounts in industrial equipment is possible;
- immunization or boosting of blood donors can be stopped, which is a very significant progress.

Table 1 shows the available panel of MoAbs (murine and human) as presented in the recent 'Symposium on Monoclonal Antibodies Against Human Red Blood Cell and Related Antigens' held in Paris, September 23,24, 1987 [2] Step by step, specificity by specificity, progress in this field is achieved. Nevertheless, in spite of the efforts of many teams involved in this area, it is likely it will take still many years before total replacement of the polyclonal anti-

*Table 1.* Workshop in Paris, september 1987, Survey of the monoclonal antibodies available for blood typing.

| ABO | Anti-A | 29 | Anti-A$_1$ | 3 |
|---|---|---|---|---|
| | Anti-B | 26 | Anti-M | 8 |
| | Anti-A+B | 11 | | |
| Rhesus | Anti-D | 23 | Enti-E | 4 |
| | Anti-D+C | 2 | Anti-e | 4 |
| | Anti-c | 1 | | |
| KELL | Anti-Kell | 1 | | |
| M, N | Anti-M | 5 | | |
| | Anti-N | 8 | | |
| Others | Anti-C$_3$d | 3 | | |
| | Anti-Le$^a$ | 3 | | |
| | Anti-Le$^b$ | 2 | | |
| | Anti-P$_1$ | 2 | | |

bodies from immunized donors by monoclonal antibodies of good stability, of good specificity against weak antigens and capable to be used in automatic equipments, will be achieved.

## Diagnosis of infectious diseases: Trends and perspectives

Advances in molecular biology and improvements in equipment (synthesizers, sequencers, etc.) have led to a preindustrial and, in some cases, to an industrial feasibility for the synthesis of peptides of which the sequence is well characterized. Not only small peptides but increasingly larger ones as well. Closely related to the progress of cellular engineering and the development of viral cultures, the possibilities for diagnosing infectious diseases, a highly critical aspect of blood transfusion all around the world, has been deeply and very quickly changed in the recent three years. HIV-1 (and HIV-2), HTLV-I, HBV and NANB hepatitis virus are the most important viruses which can be transmitted by blood products. The screening and the safety of these products must be insured with reliable, rapid and low cost techniques.

### *HIV-1 and HIV-2: Screening for antibodies*

Since 1985, the screening of each donation for anti-HIV-1 is applied in the Blood Transfusion Organisations. Antibodies are not direct markers of the infection. The weakness of this strategy is well recognized, due to the absence of immune detectable response of the recipient during the first weeks of the viral infection, the so-called 'window phase'. Due to the significant remaining level of false positive results, this rapid screening (achieved with ELISA techniques) must be followed by confirmations obtained with Western blotting techniques. In order to improve the sensitivity, the rapidity and the specificity of these 'first generation' methods, the viral material obtained by purification of viral cultures and coupled to the solid phase of the kit was replaced by synthetic peptides. The cumbersome steps of the culture, the isolation, the inactivation and finally the purification of the virus are replaced by elegant procedures which lead to the production of well known, fully characterized and perfectly constant peptides. These peptides are used in 'second generation' tests, which probably will permit to avoid the use of the laborious confirmation techniques.

### *HIV-1 and HIV-2: Screening for antigens*

The screening is not yet available at an industrial scale. To further insure the safety of the blood supply and to allow early treatment of patients suspected from HIV infection (i.e. babies born from HIV positive mothers), HIV antigen screening could be very useful. Traditional techniques, using 'sandwiches' composed of polyclonal and/or murine monoclonal antibodies, must be replaced in the very near future by more sophisticated methods, based on the use of molecular hybridization and specific amplifications. Actually, these techniques are difficult, very often using isotope labelled probes and sofar only convenient for research purposes or clinical follow-up. With a panel of emerging new technologies (PCR amplification for example) it is likely that the progress in this area will be very rapid and will permit before 1990 the use of reliable and cheep methods for HIV antigen screening.

## HBV: A mature screening

Hepatitis B antigen was isolated in the 1970's, and the screening of the HBV antigen is routinely used since many years. Monoclonal antibodies (murine for the great majority of the reagents used in this area) have replaced polyclonal antibodies since 1980-1982, and actual trends in this technology are focused on new markers which could have clinical or practical applications:
-   HBe: Antibody and antigen;
-   Pre S2 antibodies;
-   screening for HBc: Antibody and antigen.

## Hepatitis NANB

A causative agent (or agents) has yet to be identified. This identification, and the subsequent isolation of antigen/antibody involved in the transfusion transmitted NANB hepatitis, were searched unsuccessfully over the last 15 years. The immunological response seems to be weak. The clinical follow-up of recipients infected by blood products is difficult and demands in general long term studies. Nevertheless, it appears that this problem could be solved as a result of the simultaneous progress in different fields, which must be integrated:
-   organization of epidemiological follow-up on a large number of recipients for a long term (2 or 3 years), transfused with red blood cell concentrates in large quantities;
-   progress in hepatocyte cultures, in order to set up new methods of characterization of the causative agent(s) on these cells;
-   progress in molecular biology, which could use viral cultures or biologicals to build the cloning and the sequencing of the suspected virus;
-   use of the method of characterization in hepatic cells to obtain monoclonal antibodies.

ALT screening and use of anti-HBc will be introduced in many countries in the next few years, in spite of the non specific character of these surrogate test techniques. A specific screening for NANB is in fact the most important need for the blood transfusion practice in the 1990's.

## HTLV-I: A rapid extension?

This retrovirus seems to be present in many countries, particularly in Japan, the Far East and America. For these countries the screening for this antigen in each blood donation appears to be an ethical and medical necessity. However, this is not the case in Europe. Technical developments for these tests will probably follow the example of HIV-1 and kits based on the same technologies are already available.

## Monoclonal antibodies: What is the future for their use in human therapy?

*Murine monoclonal antibodies*

These have been used since the early 1980's for therapy of various human B and T-cell lymphomas, leukemias, tumours and to treat graft rejections. Table 2 presents a recent survey of human clinical trials achieved with murine monoclonal antibodies (from Larrick and Bourla [3], 1986).

These trials have shown:
- murine MoAbs can be administered safely, due to the efficacy and the safety of the purifications employed;
- injected antibodies remain in circulation for a long period of time;
- in spite of immunosuppressive pretreatment of the patients, a human antimouse response has been reported.

The immunological response is a very important drawback of the agents, and a severe limiting factor for their use in repeated infusions. The use of immunosuppressive treatment is sometimes proposed and encouraged, but this has too many side effects to be a good alternative. A better alternative is the use of human/human monoclonal antibodies, or mouse/human antibodies, which were developed in the end of the 1970's.

*Human monoclonal antibodies*

The first human cell line secreting specific antibodies was described in 1977. During ten years, the development of the human monoclonal antibody technology has been a slow and often laborious excercise. Nevertheless, in spite of the many problems encountered, to date much work is done, supported by the belief that this technology could result in:
- improved diagnostics;
- therapeutics;
- a better knowledge of the immune system.

Table 3 presents the basic steps in the production of human monoclonal antibodies (from Keith James and Graham Thomas Bell [4]).

*Table 2.* Human trials with murine MoAbs.

| | | |
|---|---|---|
| Melanoma | 3 trials | Antimouse antibodies |
| Chronic lymphocytic leukemia (CLL) | 4 trials | 3/10 toxicity, no antimouse antibodies |
| Gastrointestinal | 1 trial | Immune response |
| Cutaneous T-cell lymphoma (CTCL) | 3 trials | Antimouse antibodies |
| Adult T-cell leukemia | 1 trial | Antimouse antibodies |
| Kidney transplant rejection | 4 trials | Antimouse antibodies |

The most critical points to consider in this technology appear to be the following:

*Lymphocyte enrichment* – Although it is apparent that the peripheral blood is not the best source of lymphocytes for human MoAbs, for practical and ethical considerations it will continue to be the main source in the future.

*Lymphocyte activation* – *In vivo* immunizations are difficult. *In vitro* immunization must be developed and optimized to circumvent this problem. Unfortunately, this step is very difficult too to achieve and not so easily realized as with murine lymphocytes.

*Lymphocyte immortalization* – Kohler and Milstein's technique [1] consists of a fusion of specific murine lymphocytes with a myeloma cell line. Since then fusion has remained the most popular immortalization strategy. The situation is quite different for human MoAbs. Due to the difficulty of the immortalization, many partners have been used but none has come to dominate. Several phenotypes are used currently:
- myelomas – very rare;
- lymphoblastoïd cell lines derived from an EBV transformation;
- heteromyelomas;
- human partners have been tried.

*Table 3.* Basic steps in the production of human monoclonal antibodies.

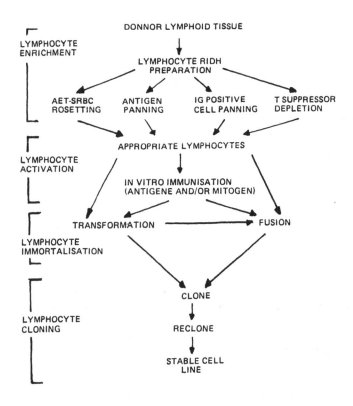

*The future: Trends and perspectives for therapeutics*

The next several years will see an increasing number of clinical studies using rodent or human MoAbs. The need for these MoAbs will be accelerated by an increasing concern with viral – known or suspected – contaminations from plasma proteins and the decreasing availability of immunized donors. In order to use the good specificity of murine MoAbs (easily obtained) and to avoid the immunogenicity of these cell lines, it seems very attractive to obtain 'humanized' monoclonal antibodies: The feasibility of generating chimeric murine/human antibodies has been demonstrated. These technologies must employ the most recent advances of molecular biology and fundamental immunology: Cloning, sequencing and expression of immune globulins are possible, and isolation and characterization in murine monoclonal antibodies of variable and specific regions involved in the efficacy and the specificity of the clones will lead to the construction of future therapeutic tools; more active and more specific, and less immunogenic.

### Blood derivatives and genetic engineering: Replacement or competition?

It is obvious that recent years have seen tremendous advances in gene-technology research and in the development of genetic engineered human plasma proteins. Between 1978 and 1985 the most important proteins identified in the human plasma have been cloned and expressed in various systems. On the other hand, in spite of repeated announcements, there is still in 1987 no plasma protein being produced on a large scale using genetic engineering. (The most advanced plasma protein is recombinant Factor VIII, which has been infused in two patients in the USA, as reported in these proceedings [5,6]).

*What are the reasons?*

- Practically without exception, plasma proteins have a high molecular weight (50,000 to 1,000,000).
- With the exception of albumin and a few other proteins, all human plasma proteins known sofar are glycosylated more or less in various ways (26 sites for example for Factor VIII!). If these carbohydrates and glycoproteins are split off, the biological activity often disappears, half life can be strongly shortened, and the degradation by proteinases can be highly accelerated.
- For this reason, post-translational modifications are necessary. Mammalian cell lines are practically the only system available today for producing these biologicals, whereas yeasts can provide a limited specific glycosylation, and *E. Coli* no modification at all.

*Mammalian cell lines offer many industrial and pharmaceutical difficulties*

- A very limited panel of cells is available, well known and accepted by the authorities.

- Yields are low, compared with *E. Coli* and yeast.
- Scaling-up is difficult, and culture in suspension not easily achieved.
- Plasma proteins are often very unstable and can be easily inactivated by proteases, which are always released when mammalian cells die. They must be specifically protected.
- Foreign proteins and contaminants (of the medium or the cell itself) must be drastically removed during the purification.

*What challenge for the purification?*

The requirements for the purity of genetically engineered plasma proteins will be very strong. The usual treatments are very often infusions of large quantities of proteins over long periods of time (a life time for hemophiliacs). Table 4 represents two examples, which do summarize the problem (Schwick/Biofutur, 1986 [7]).

If these 'foreign' proteins or contaminants are heterologous or undesirable, these requirements could be very difficult to be met. Viral validation must be added, in order to demonstrate the absence of viral particles in the final vial, if the chosen cell presents some risks related to viruses. The levels presented in Table 4, obtained with preprations of high purity (99,9%) could nevertheless lead to sensitization, and thus to side reactions. This problem is particularly acute for albumin, used actually in very large amounts (260 tons per year all around the world). Traditional methods must be employed in the first steps of the purification of the supernatants, and large scale chromatographic procedures (without using affinity chromatography) could lead to a success in this development, if some conditions are fulfilled:
- low cost of the medium (possible with yeast and *E. Coli*);
- simplicity of the medium (absence of foreign proteins);
- easy purification;
- problems of pyrogens avoided (difficult with *E. Coli*);
- low cost (overall).

These problems could be solved in 1990-1995, and it actually seems that an English company – Delta Biotechnology -, a subsidiary of the Bass Breweries is the leader in this competition which is focused on two key points:
- price/compared with human serum albumin;
- purity/related to the contaminants.

*Table 4.* Purity of recombinant proteins.

|  | Dosis patient | Purity | 'Foreign' protein |
|---|---|---|---|
| Albumin | 25 g | 99,90% | 25 mg |
|  | 100 g | 99,99% | 10 mg |
| Antihemophilic Factor VIII Acute treatment | 500 µg daily | 99,90% | 500 ng daily |

The situation for Factor VIII is different:
- from an industrial point of view: 2 to 3 kg of pure protein are necessary for the needs of the hemophiliacs, (compared with 260 tons for albumin);
- from a technological point of view: The expression of Factor VIII (2332 amino acids, 26 sites for glycosylation, high sensitivity to proteases) in mammalian cells is actually achieved; however, the yields remain low, if the entire molecule has to be expressed.

Simultaneously, monoclonal antibodies against Factor VIII and von Willebrand factor have been used in a first step for the complete characterization of the protein ('mapping' of the epitopes) and have led to a better understanding and knowledge of the behaviour of this complex protein (mechanisms for the activation of Factor VIII can be proposed now).

In 1981, monoclonal antibodies began to be used in affinity chromatography, and these immunoaffinity procedures are now ready to be used on a large scale for the purification of plasma Factor VIII. The purity of these plasma products is very high and could be very useful in the treatment of seropositive hemophiliacs, who present very often immunological disorders.

The outcome of the competition between these plasma ultrapure products and the future recombinant proteins remains very uncertain. It could take many years more before the total replacement by bioengineered material of the two current leader plasma proteins Factor VIII and albumin, will be achieved.

As a conclusion, it seems very likely to foresee in the next decade the following events, which could lead to a gentle transition from the 20th century Blood Transfusion to the Blood Transfusion era of the 21st century:

1. Partial decrease of the use of red blood cells, and replacement in certain applications by new products (recombinant Epo, polymerized or recombinant hemoglobin, chemicals...).
2. Development of the large scale culture of stem cells.
3. Distribution on a large scale of recombinant Factor VIII which will compete with improved ultrapure plasma Factor VIII (1990/1992).
4. Distribution on a large scale of recombinant albumin, at low cost, which could be competitive with a plasma albumin, of which the price could increase due to the presence of recombinant Factor VIII (1992/1995).
5. Increase of the use of intravenous immunoglobulins, which cannot be produced by genetic engineering.
6. Other plasma proteins will be replaced step by step, if research and development expanses can be justified by new or increasing therapeutic needs.

## References

1. Kohler G, Milstein C. Continuous cultures of fixed cells secreting antibody of predefined specificity. Nature 1975;256:495-7.
2. Symposium on Monoclonal Antibodies Against Human Red Blood Cells and Related Antigens. International Society of Blood Transfusion, September 21-22, 1987, Paris, France. Proceedings in press.

3.   Larrick JW, Bourla JM. Journal of Biological Response Modifiers 1986;5:379-93.
4.   James K, Bell T. Human monoclonal antibody production, current status and future prospects. J Immunol Meth 1987;100:5-40.
5.   Roberts HR, Macik BG. Factor VIII and IX concentrates: Clinical efficacy as related to purity. In: Verstraete M, Vermylen J, Lijnen HR, Arnout J (eds). Thrombosis and haemostasis 1987. Leuven University Press, Leuven, 1987:563-81.
6.   High KA, White II GC, McMillan CW, Macik BG, Roberts HR. *In vivo* characteristics of rDNA factor VIII: the impact for the future in hemophilia care. In: Smit Sibinga CTh, Das PC, Overby LR (eds). Biotechnology in blood transfusion. Martinus Nijhoff Publ., Boston/Dordrecht/Lancaster, 1988:223-230.
7.   Schwick HG. How far is the development of blood products by genetic engineering. Biofutur 1987;Jan:61-4.

# DISCUSSION

L.R. Overby, C.Th. Smit Sibinga

*T.J. Hamblin (Bournemouth):* I wonder if I could just make some comments about the therapeutic use of monoclonal antibodies, which Dr Jacquin referred to in his last presentation, because I think what has been surprising is how little monoclonal antibody has been used therapeutically despite the fact that it is available now for 7 or 8 years. People do not appreciated to what extent one has to pay for the specificity that you get with monoclonal antibody. For a start most mouse monoclonals are incapable of fixing human complement. This is a great drawback in their use. Secondly, as you have already said they are immunogenic. However, antimouse antibodies are uncommon. Thirdly, a point which is really not appreciated is that most mouse monoclonals are totally unable to react with human K-cells. The human K-cell does not have a receptor for mouse Fc, therefore people have blindly given monoclonals hoping that they were going to get ADCC killing and that in fact does not happen. They do react with monocytes, but the monocyte reaction is prob ably unimportant *in vivo.* It is very unlikely that we are going to get human monoclonal antibodies against most tumour types to use. So your suggestion that chimeric antibodies, which are part human part mouse, are useful, is a very good one. However, it is a very long and difficult pathway to genetically engineer even one chimeric antibody. It is much simpler to do this chemically. You can obtain human Fc very easily from donor plasma and it is usually available without problems. You can also obtain mouse Fab' fragment very easily and link these molecules together to produce a univalent antibody with mouse Fab' and human Fc, which does not cause antigenic modulation.It has a long survival in circulation (21 days like a human molecule compared to three days with a mouse). It is much less immunogenic, because the most immunogenic part of the molecule is the Fc portion. We have done this in our laboratory for a number of specificities now and I reckon this might be a much easier way of producing these chimeric antibodies then try to genetic ally engineer them.

*G. Jacquin (Paris):* Quite attractive I agree. I wanted to outline that chimeric mouse human antibodies could be one response to the different problems encountered today with monoclonal antibodies.

*T.J. Hamblin:* Dr Benz, one of the things I found difficult when I was beginning to learn about molecular biology were all these geographical terms. I am sure that many of the audience are confused between Southern, Northern, and Western blotting. Could you just explain the difference?

*E.J Benz, Jr (New Haven):* Southern blotting applies to analysis of DNA or DNA fragments. It is not really a geographical term. In fact, it is named after a person Dr Ed Southern, who invented the blotting method. When people who studied RNA found that an analogous blotting technology could be used to analyse RNA, they chose the name Northern blotting, as a subtle complement to Ed Southern. Western blotting, of course, is quite familiar to most of you, because it is used so effectively for immunologcial types of studies. It is an analogous blotting procedure that is used to see proteins on a nitrocellulose support by means of antibodies. So, Northern blotting is for RNA, Southern blotting is for DNA and Western blotting is for protein. Recently, 'Southwestern' blotting has been developed. Nuclear proteins are run on a gel, and probed with a radioactive DNA fragment in an effort to locate regulatory proteins that bind to specific DNA promoter or enhancer regions.

*J.Ph.H.B. Sybesma (Dordrecht):* Dr Jacquin, I want to know when to use monoclonal antibodies and when not, because I can imagine that when you use monoclonal antibodies you may find antigens that you could not find with polyclonal ones.

*G. Jacquin:* The application of murine monoclonal antibodies for example in immunohematology was discussed 2 or 3 years ago. If you recognize just one epitope, you can have perhaps a less good reaction with monoclonal antibodies than with polyclonal antibodies. But progress has been achieved and we can say that with one specificity the application in immunohematology is as good as with polyclonal antibodies. For example in the National Blood Centre some 4 years ago, we were obliged to mix 2 or 3 specificities of monoclonal antibodies in order to have a good specificity. But it can be predicted perhaps that in the future a mix of monoclonal antibodies might be necessary in order to have an optimal efficacy in that field.

*C.Th. Smit Sibinga (Groningen):* Dr Susan Holbeck has givena marvellous presentation on the HLA DR sequencing in relation to disease. It is known that organ transplant rejection very much depends on the matching. Specifically the acceptance of the organ seems to be very much related to a match on the DR. Could it be so that by sequencing the DR from donors we could much better predict which sequence would be the favourable one and which would be the less favourable one in the acceptance of the organ?

*S. Holbeck (Seattle):* I think that when people are matched by specificity and the graft is rejected, it is not that they themselves actually have different alleles. As we have seen in the case of DR4 there are actually 5 different alleles that have the typing specificity DR4 on them. So, different molecules that all have a common epitope. The other thing that can happen is that although they have the same allele DR, they can have other different alleles and other class II genes. We have seen that in fact in bone marrow transplant patients in a study we did at the Puget Sound Blood Center that there are cases of unexplained Graft-versus-Host disease. In those cases, although the siblings were matched, they have had a crossover within the HLA-region. So they were matched at DR and had identical alleles at DR, but in fact had different alleles at DP and so a sort of hidden-in within the typing date. Although I think that sequencing techniques have become a lot more rapid, probably the use of allele nuclear type probes for more defined typing will be the future. There are several companies working on such allele nuclear type typing kits.

*L.E. Overby (Emmeryville):* Dr Benz we hear a lot about DNA typing and RFLP's to get a unique identity. Do you think that those procedures in due time become simple enough, so that they can be practized on a wide enough scale to really serve as a substitute for finger printing or matching of individuals. Now I understand it is still fairly complicated, and it takes a sophisticated laboratory to really run RFLP on blood.

*E.J. Benz, Jr:* This is an area I did not cover for two reasons. One is there was insufficient time and the other is I do not think I understand the technology very well. There are two existing ways that one can obtain some individualized profile of DNA in a single person. One is by looking at the pattern of restriction endonuclease sites that surround specific genes or specific parts of DNA for which DNA probes are available. These methods have been the kind that have lead people to identify the region of DNA that is involved in diseases such as Huntington's chorea or manic depressive illness. They lead to the kinds of breakthroughs that you hear about periodically as providing clues to the causes of genetic disease. The practicality of using those for forensic purposes I think is limited by the fact that one will have to do a very large number to get a unique profile for an individual and in many cases one has to get the profile from very suboptimal specimens. But there is a variation or an enhancement of that technology that has been pioneered by Dr Alec Jeffreys which does hold more promise. I think within the not too distant future perhaps within the next few years this will find its place in practical use for identifying individuals. This is called DNA fingerprinting and refers to the fact that there are many parts of the human genome in which there are repeated sequences that occur next to a gene. So, for instance in mygene the sequence may occur two times. Next to another person's gene it might occur four or five or even three dozen times. These are called hypervariable regions. Therefore, there will be a great deal of variability amongst individuals; a handful of those markers, perhaps ten or twelve could be studied in one or two blotting experiments. This many markers has good sufficient uniqueness for diagnostic or legal purposes. However, the impediment is how to develop the multiplicity of analyses in a simple test fast enough to be of;use.

*T.J. Hamblin:* Dr Jeffreys' technique actually is in current use by the British Government to check on immigrants who claim to be related to people who are already in the country and is now being marketed as a way of testing for paternity in Britain. So, I am sure that is going to be available very quickly. Dr Holbeck, the concept of suballeles at the alleles on DR is new to me today – I am interested in it. The differences of about four amino acids in these various suballeles are very tiny. Can you give us some sort of idea of how the differences between DR4, DR3 and DR2 relate to that. Are they of similar size or much larger size?

*S. Holbeck:* They are of much larger size. I do not know out of my head the differences. I think that the differences between DR2 and DR4 are in the order of 70 or 80% homology. In addition you can distinguish them by Southern blotting which indicates that they have a lot of differences in the surrounding DNA sequence. So the DR4 suballeles as you have called them are not actually suballeles, they are alleles themselves which serve a common element which has been recognized by the antibodies that were used fotyping in the past.

*T.J. Hamblin:* The question is how stable is this area genetically. Is it subject to somatic mutation like immunoglobulin genes are or to rearrange in some ways, so you get these minor differences occurring in such a wide variety.

*S. Holbeck:* It is not subject to somatic mutation, but it is a group of very close genes. There has been quite some suggestive evidence that gene conversion goes on generate diversity between generations and that you can find little cassettes of information that have been transferred for one generation on to another. So, it is certain that evolution is taking bits of one gene making a new gene out of it.

*T.J. Hamblin:* Does that mean that within families these alleles do not in fact always breed through and that you may get a change from one generation to the next?

*S. Holbeck:* No, one has found to my knowledge an example of gene conversion happening with a single generation in man. I think it has definitely been shown to happen in mice though.

*T.J. Hamblin:* But I mean it must happen during one generation if it happens at all.

*S. Holbeck:* It does. But it is an issue of whether those individuals have been typed or not and whether you catch it in the act of doing.

*T.J. Hamblin:* Because one is aware that rheumatoid arthritis and diabetes for instance do tend to occur in families, but that is by no means a general affair. I mean it often skips generations and I wonder whether it has a genetic explanation or an environmental.

*S. Holbeck:* I think that it is probably a combination of things, because certainly all individuals who have the risk at the allele that we might have to find, do not have for instance diabetes. Even in families where there are multiple individuals with diabetes it is not always the case that every member of that family who has that risk really develops diabetes. It is a fairly high percentage but it is certainly a complex system and there are many factors that are influencing development of disease.

*E.J. Benz, Jr:* Just a quick comment to amplify what Dr Holbeck has said about variation in genes that are relevant to clinical purposes. One of the challenges that has to be faced is determining which of the changes that are encountered and studied are either involved in the pathophysiology of the disease or the determinant of a relevant clinical phenotype and which changes are really polymorphic. Many of the genetic changes that have been linked to human diseases are in fact not at all related to the mechanism causing the disease, but are simply located nearly in the genome. These changes are very similar to the saying that people with bloodgroup A have a propensity to get peptic ulcer. They simply are associated findings that are coinherited and frequently are not at all involved in the pathophysiology.

*S. Holbeck:* I might make a comment on that as far as it relates to HLA. I think that the feeling is that these molecules are actually involved in the disease process, because HLA class II antigens are the molecules which present antigen to the immune system. Both of these diseases that I have discussed have an immune component. So the idea is that if something is going wrong with the immune system, either a failure to suppress an abberant response or presentation of an antigen that should not be presented, that that is somehow involved in causing disease. But that has not been definitely shown.

# II. Laboratory application of biotechnology

# BIOTECHNOLOGY IN BLOOD GROUP SEROLOGY – APPLICATION AND TRENDS FOR THE FUTURE

D. Voak

## Introduction

The monoclonal technology of Kohler and Milstein [1] has enabled selected stable cloned cell lines to be developed that produce high yields of useful monoclonal antibodies by specialized tissue culture technology, although ascitic fluid production may have an economic advantage if the reagent can be produced at high dilution. Selected monoclonal antibodies offer considerable advantages to reagent manufacturers by providing unlimited quantities of high quality reagents.

Monoclonal antibodies have now been produced to many red cell antigens [2], but the aims of this paper are to describe mainly those monoclonal antibodies that can meet the large volume i.e. thousands of litres/year requirements of routine blood transfusion reagents; and only to briefly discuss the use of monoclonal antibodies in paternity testing and forensic serology as that has been described elsewhere [3].

High volume reagent requirements fall into three groups:
1. *Anti-A, anti-B and anti-A,B* produced from selected murine monoclonal antibodies [4,5].
2. *Anti-Rh(D)* from Epstein Barr Virus (EBV) treated human B lymphocytes secreting anti-D [6] and stabilized by a fusion with a mouse myeloma [7] or hybrid myeloma [8].
3. *Polyspecific anti-human globulin reagents* produced by blending mainly murine monoclonal anti-C3c/C3d or just anti-C3d with rabbit anti-IgG.

## ABO monoclonal antibody reagents

ABO grouping reagents should meet FDA standards [9] for speed of reaction and titre, and they must be stable and specific. Selected mouse monoclonal anti-As, anti-Bs and anti-A,B antibodies achieve these criteria and are in widespread use as blood grouping reagents [4,5]. These IgM anti-A/anti-B antibodies are potent red cell hemolysins in the presence of the complement of fresh serum. Therefore, the reagents must be formulated with EDTA (0.01m) at pH 7.1-7.3 for use as typing reagents.

*Avidity characteristics*

The results of avidity tests given in Table 1 show the avidity (time in seconds to produce a macroscopic reaction) and the critical tests are with $A_2B$ for anti-A and $A_1B$ for anti-B reagents [4] as these red cells have relatively low antigen site densities, and avidity times of less than 10 seconds are considered adequate. However, our experience with monoclonal antibodies raised new problems as the most avid anti-A and anti-B antibodies with an adequate or even excellent avidity time can give a poor clump size (or intensity) of agglutination with strong antigen red cell types. For example, 3D3 and MHO4 anti-As may be blended to make a reagent, as 3D3 gives better clump size with $A_1$ cells than MHO4, which is a high avidity anti-A that sees $A_x$. Also, NB1/19, 5A5 and/or 3B4 may be blended to make a reagent as NG1/19 has a better slide reaction with B and $A_2B$ cells than 5A5 or 3B4 that are of higher avidity and agglutinate subgroups of B that are missed by NB1/19. The avid anti-B (5B2) cannot be blended to make a good slide anti-B reagent as it even ruins the excellent slide characteristics of the anti-B NB1/19. Thus each monoclonal anti-A or anti-B must be evaluated on its own merits and in trial blends before making bulk reagent.

*Table 1.* Avidity (potency) FDA slide tests* with supernatant anti-A and anti-B monoclonal antibodies and control reagents.
1 volume of antibody reagent = 1 volume of 35% cells in plasma.
Avidity is time in seconds to give agglutination.

| Anti-A | $A_1$ | $A_2$ | $A_1B$ | $A_2B$ |
|---|---|---|---|---|
| Commercial X (USA) | 2 | 3 | 2 | 5 |
| 3D3 neat | 2 | 3 | 3 | 4 |
| MHO4 neat | 1 | 1 | 1 | 2 |

| Anti-B | $A_1B$ | $A_2B$ | B |
|---|---|---|---|
| Commercial X (USA) | 4 | 3 | 3 |
| NB1/19 neat | 4 | 4 | 4 |
| 5A5 neat | 3 | 3 | |
| 3B4 | 5 | 4 | 3 |
| 5B2 | 4 | 3 | 4 |

* After two minutes all gave agglutination >1mm, except 5B2.

*Saline titres by spin-tube tests*

The saline titres of some excellent monoclonal anti-A/anti-B antibodies are shown in Tables 2 and 3. The anti-A MHO4 is an example of a superior anti-A that exceeds conventional anti-A reagent specifications, by reacting with $A_x$, and it is also better with weak $A_2B$ ('$A_3B$') and cord AB bloods [4,5,10].

The anti-A (3D3) reacts about as well as a polyclonal FDA licensed serum anti-A reagent, and makes a good blending partner for good slide test reactions (see above).

*Table 2.* Saline titres of tissue culture supernatant monoclonal anti-A reagents.

| 3% cells saline RT | Anti-A reagents | | |
|---|---|---|---|
| | 3D3 neat | MHO4 neat | Group B serum commercial X (USA) |
| $A_1$ | 1024 | 1024 | 512 |
| $A_2$ | 512 | 512 | 256 |
| $A_1B$ | 512 | 512 | 512 |
| $A_2B$ | 64 | 256 | 64 |
| $A_2B$ weak | 4 | 256 | 8 |
| $A_3B$ | 0 | 256 | 1 |
| $A_3$ | 4 | 256 | 4 |
| $A_x$ | 0 | 64 | 0 |
| B(A)+ + + | 0 | 32 | 0 |

Saline tests negative x B, O, $A_m$ and A $_{end}$ RBC.

*Table 3.* Saline titres of tissue culture supernatant monoclonal anti-B reagents.

| 3% cells saline RT | Anti-B reagents | | | | |
|---|---|---|---|---|---|
| | NB1/19 | 3B4 | 5A5 | 5B2 | Group A serum commercial X (USA) |
| $A_1B$ | 256 | 64 | 256 | 128 | 64 |
| $A_2B$ | 512 | 128 | 512 | 256 | 64 |
| B | 512 | 128 | 512 | 256 | 128 |
| B cord | 256 | 64 | 256 | 128 | 64 |
| B weak* | 0 | 32 | 64 | 32 | 64 |
| $A_1$ | 0 | 0 | 0 | 0 | 0 |
| O | 0 | 0 | 0 | 0 | 0 |

*Similar results obtained with 25 additional subgroups of B.

Selected blends of monoclonal anti-Bs are at least equal to good conventional FDA licensed reagents. The examples described here do not detect acquired B and they are very useful in forensic work in which acquired B is a frequent source of difficulty in the determination of the ABO group.

*Special characteristics of anti-A MHO4*

MHO4 is the most powerful anti-A we have examined and it gave macroscopic reactions with 20 out of 24 examples of $A_x$ [4,5]. Absorption and heat (56°C) elution studies with MHO4 confirmed it was an anti-A and not some form of anti-A,B antibody as it was not absorbed or eluted from B or control O cells. The strength of binding of MHO4 absorbed by $A_1$ red cells is so strong that it is not eluted from $A_1$ cells, although it does elute from $A_2$, $A_2B$ and $A_x$ red cells. Thus the selection of monoclonal antibodies for blood grouping based on high avidity criteria produces reagents unsuitable for use by classical forensic elution techniques.

We suggest that forensic workers use these avid reagents by ELISA method or select monoclonal antibodies to lower avidity criteria.

MHO4 anti-A was used in thousands of automated and manual blood grouping tests using the UK sedimentation tube technique read after pipette transfer of the cell button to microscope slide and no reactions were observed with B or O red cells. However, later in 1985 MHO4 and 3D3 anti-As from Celltech were blended to produce Ortho's Bioclone anti-A, and after some months it became apparent that this reagent reacted weakly with a low incidence of 'normal' group B red cells. Samples of some of these reactive group B bloods were referred to D. Voak by D. Davies (Ortho) and M. Beck (Kansas City) and we demonstrated that the reactive B red cells were reacting with the MHO4 anti-A.

We called these anti-A reactions with B red cells the B(A) phenomenon and the reactive B cells were called B(A) as the reactions were proved to be with an A antigen and specifically inhibitable by A substance [11].

*Characteristics of the B(A) phenomenon [12] are:*
1. Shown by certain monoclonal anti-A that see $A_x$ (e.g. MHO4. Table 2).
2. Also shown by anti-A of anti-A,B sera that see $A_x$ (anti-B and anti-A,B removed by absorption).
3. B(A) agglutination is verry fragile almost soft aggregation rather than agglutination destroyed by quite gentle agitation.
4. Method sensitive, best detected by gently read spin-tube technique.
5. Inhibited by group A but not group B secretor salivas, which confirm it is an A reaction.
6. Due to the B transferase enzymes making a little A [13] and the serum of people with B(A) reactive red cells have elevated B transferase levels.
7. Low incidence in saline tests (mainly in Negros) but the red cells of all group Bs can be shown to have a little A if the spin-tube tests are enhanced by enzyme treatment.
   Careful reading of tests has revealed B(A) with Ortho's Bioclone anti-A in 0.1-0.3% of group Bs. Only Beck has reported a higher incidence of 1.0% in Kansas (only one third could be confirmed by the FDA (personal communication A. Hoppe, C. Santos), which reflects on the exquisite sensitivity of his reading method.
8. Mainly a problem in North America, where difficulties in interpretation are due to failure to carry out reverse serum grouping.

*Quality control of superior monoclonal anti-A reagents*

The Paris Monoclonal Antibody Workshop [2] revealed numerous mono-clonal anti-As that can detect $A_x$ [15]. Some showed B(A) reactions and it is clear that there are now sufficient of these superior anti-A antibodies available for use by most major manufacturers in their future anti-A reagents.

Therefore it is important to realize that this type of reagent development is not prevented by the B(A) phenomenon, as B(A) reactions are a function of anti-A concentration that can be quality controlled with B(A) or papainised B red cells. The MHO4 anti-A diluted at 1/90 is still a superior anti-A reagent negative with the B(A) papainised B and O control cells by carefully read spin-tube tests (Table 3). The ability to detect weak $A_x$ red cells is reduced, but the 1/90 MHO4 reagent still detects more examples of $A_x$ than the excellent BRIC-131 anti-A of Dr. Anstee and the FDA licensed conventional anti-A,B control reagent (Table 4).

*Table 4.* MHO4 anti-A dilution not detecting A in group B(A) red cells detects many weak A variants.

| Spin tests | | | Number of variants detected | | |
|---|---|---|---|---|---|
| | | Anti-A reagents | | | Anti-A,B |
| Subgroup | Number tested | Bioclone Ortho | MHO4 1/90 | BRIC-131 supernatant | Conventional |
| $A_x$ | 24 | 17 | 14 | 9 | 7 |
| $A_3$ | 6 | 6 | 6 | 6 | 6 (1 weak) |
| '$A_3B$' | 8 | 8 | 8 | 8 | 8 |
| $A_xB$ | 1 | 1 | 1 | 1 | 1 |
| Control-A in B | B(A)++ | ++ | 0 | 0 | |
| | BA+ | + | 0 | 0 | |
| Papain | B | 1+ | 0 | 1+weak | ++++ |

## Anti-A,B reagents for the detection of weak subgroups of A and B

Several monoclonal anti-A,B antibodies have now been described [10,16,17], but a single anti-A,B antibody will not make an anti-A,B reagent e.g. one anti-A,B, [16] reacts well with all group A types down to and including $A_x$, but only reacts weakly with even strong group B cells. Thus it must be blended with a potent monoclonal anti-B to make an anti-A,B reagent. Anti-A,B reagents can also be made by blending a monoclonal anti-A (MHO4) that sees $A_x$ with a monoclonal anti-B (5A5) that sees weak B variants, as shown in Table 5.

*Table 5.* Anti-A MHO4 is superior to conventional anti-A and detects weak A variants, as well as an anti-A,B serum.

| | Anti-A reagents | | | | Anti-A,B reagents | | | |
|---|---|---|---|---|---|---|---|---|
| | Monoclonal MHO4 neat supernatant | | Serum commercial X | | Monoclonal A +B MHO4 +5A5 | | Serum (group O) commercial X | |
| Cells | spin | slide | spin | slide | spin | slide | spin | slide |
| $A_x$ | ++ | +++ | W | − | ++ | +++ | ++ | ++ |
| $A_x$ | + | ++ | − | − | + | ++ | + | + |
| $A_3$ | +++ | ++ | + | + | ++ | '++ | +++ | +++ |
| $A_3B$ | +++ | C | ++ | ++ | C | C | C | C |
| $A_2B$ | C | C | +++ | +++ | C | C | C | C |
| B | − | − | − | − | C | C | C | C |
| O | − | − | − | − | − | − | − | − |

Note: Immediate spin-tube tests, 1 volume antibody = 1 volume 3% red cells in saline.
　　　Slide tests, two minute tests, 1 volume antibody to 1 volume 35% red cells in plasma.

The supernatant of the superior anti-A e.g. MHO4 can detect 20 out of 24 examples of $A_x$ [4,5] and it can be used at this concentration in an anti-A,B blend, whereas it must be used diluted in anti-A reagent blends to minimize B(A) reactions and thus is less effective for $A_x$ detection than the optimum anti-A,B reagent. However, the weakest link in ABO grouping is with the weak A of cord AB bloods that cannot be checked by anti-A,B reagents because of the masking anti-B reactions, and thus have often been mistyped (personal experience), especially in very warm weather in non air-conditioned laboratories.

Superior monoclonal anti-A and anti-B reagent blends are more reliable than conventional reagents for the detection of weak A and weak B in adult and cord bloods, especially of $A_3$, $A_x$ and weak A in cord AB bloods. Thus the continued use of anti-A,B reagents is questionable. Admittedly they do confirm that anti-A or B reagents were added to tubes, but only for A or B and not for AB samples; and surely the reverse serum grouping is an adequate check for the cell typing, with the exception of cord bloods. Furthermore, the detection of weak $A_x$ is only of research interest and of no clinical significance while examples of clinically significant $A_h$ with very weak A are more reliably detected by their anti-H reaction with group O cells than by detection of their weak A antigen.

*Economy of automated ABO grouping (Technicon Autogrouper 16C)*

MHO4 anti-A at a 1:500 dilution of the supernatant detects all A subtypes down to '$A_3B$' (weak $A_3B$) but not $A_x$. A more concentrated 1:50 dilution of MHO4 anti-A was used in an anti-A,B blend with a 1:50 dilution of monoclonal anti-B (5B2) to detect weak subgroups of A and B. This anti-A,B and reverse grouping also confirms the ABO groups. This procedure enables us to identify $A_x$ donors for research purposes as we did not want them to be labelled as group A donors. The monoclonal anti-B (5A5) was used at a 1:100 dilution.

Accurate results were obtained with these reagents and no false results were obtained in 113,703 tests with the anti-A, 135,039 tests with the anti-B and 47,259 tests with the anti-A,B. The economy of these selected monoclonal anti-A/B antibodies, enhanced by methyl cellulose (0.6-1.0%) and bromelin (0.25%) is at least five times better than with conventional reagents and offers complete reliability of donor or patient blood typing by automated systems and microplate techniques using manual or semi-automated procedures.

## RhD monoclonal antibody reagents [3,5]

The first monoclonal IgG anti-D was an IgG antibody [17] and most workers experienced difficulties in stabilizing the anti-D secreting cell lines which were Epstein Barr Virus (EBV) transformed human B lymphocytes. Monoclonal IgG anti-D antibodies have not yet offered advantages over polyclonal anti-D reagents, as the yields are not economic and they miss weak $D(D^u)$ and some D variants [6 and Tippett personal communications].

However, progress has been made on stabilising anti-D secreting cell lines by fusing them with a human-mouse heteromyeloma [8] or a mouse myeloma [7] and excellent IgM anti-Ds suitable for reagent use have been produced. Therefore, routine RhD typing can now be performed by simple saline tests and several examples of high titre IgM monoclonal anti-Ds are in routine use. The tissue culture supernatant of the MAD-2 cell line [7] has a saline spin-tube titre of 1,024 with red cells of the $R_1r$ phenotype (pool of 4) and that of a French CNRGS reagent was nearly as potent with a titre of 512.

These reagents are sufficiently potent for use by slide or immediate spin-tube tests and completely reliable for typing all normal RhD positive phenotypes, but IgM anti-D antibodies are unreliable for the detection of weak $D(D^u)$ by saline tests (18,20 and see Table 6). The French reagent's better activity with the weak D samples is probably due to potentiation of the IgM antibody activity by enhancers, but has the disadvantage of requiring a diluent control that increases reagent costs and for patient typing the detection of weaker forms of $D^u$ is unnecessary [18,19] because as potential recipients we prefer to regard them as RhD negative.

Table 6. Saline test reactions of IgM monoclonal anti-Ds with weak $D(D^u)$ samples (all weak D samples positive with papain treated RBC).

| | Weak D samples | | | | | | |
| anti-D | 1 $R_2{}^ur$ | 2 $R_1{}^ur$ | 3 $R_1{}^ur$ | 4 $R_1{}^ur$ | 5 $R_1{}^ur$ | 6 $R_1{}^ur$ | 7 $R_2{}^ur$ |
|---|---|---|---|---|---|---|---|
| MAD-2 neat supernatant | WK | 0 | + + | + + | 0 | WK | + |
| 86121 CNRGS* | + + + | + | + + + | + + | + + | + | + + |

* Diluent control tests negative.

In the case of RhD typing donor bloods it is desirable to detect at least high grade $D^u$ and D variants [21]. In this case improved sensitivity can be achieved by potentiation of the reagents (e.g. Ficoll, dextran, pvp), but has the diluent control cost penalty for all tests, and simple one-stage mixture tests with enzymes cannot be used as the enzymes destroy the in-line antibody [18,20]. Two-stage enzyme tests do enhance the reactions with $D^u$ red cells, but some D variants (Category VI) are still undetected and in any case the method is impractical.

Fortunately there is a simple answer to this problem as the high titre IgM monoclonal anti-D reactions are not blocked by levels of selected IgG anti-Ds that can detect $D^u$ and D variants by antiglobulin tests. Therefore a single D typing reagent can be made by a blend of IgM monoclonal anti-D (titre of $1,024 \times R_1r$ red cells) with conventional IgG anti-D. Thus normal RhD positives can all be detected by simple saline tests and any negative or weak reactions can be converted to antiglobulin tests for the detection of weak D types, as seen in Table 7. This procedure will also resolve any discrepancies between saline tests with these monoclonal IgG anti-Ds and conventional albumin or enzyme anti-D reagents that may give strong reactions with weak D types.

*Table 7.* Tests for weak D(Dᵘ) with an IgM (MAD-2) + IgG anti-D blend.*

| Method | 1:1 vols – spin-tube tests × 3% RBC weak D(Dᵘ) samples | | | | | | | |
| | 1 $R_1^u r$ | 2 $R_2^u r$ | 3 $R_2^u r$ | 4 $R_2^u r$ | 5** $R_1^u r$ | $R_1^u r$ | $R_2^u r$ | rr |
|---|---|---|---|---|---|---|---|---|
| IMM spin saline | WK | + | WK | + + + | (+) | + + + + | + + + + | 0 |
| 15 min 37°C saline | 0 | + | 0 | + + + | WK | + + + + | + + + + | 0 |
| AGH | + + + | + + + | + + + | N/T | + + + | N/T | N/T | 0 |

* Saline titre 1024×$R_1^u r$ (pool of 4).
** Previously grouped as $R_1^u r$ with an albumin anti-D.

Currently available IgG monoclonal anti-Ds are not suitable for blending with the IgM anti-Ds for reagent use as they are unreliable with some weak D and D variant types, especially Category VI [3, 18, and P. Tippett, personal communication].

However, one potentially useful IgG monoclonal anti-D was revealed at the recent workshop in Paris [2]. Thus in the future monoclonal IgG anti-Ds, probably as blends, may replace conventional IgG anti-D for reagent use. Although this may only become an economic reality if and when monoclonal IgG anti-D antibodies can replace the large supplies of conventional IgG anti-D needed for *in vivo* prophylactic treatment for the prevention of anti-D immunization in RhD-negative women.

## Monoclonal anti-complement (C3c/C3d) for use in polyspecific anti-human globulin reagents (AHG)

Monoclonal anti-complement antibodies [22,23,34] are much easier to standardise than conventional (rabbit) anti-C3c/C3d reagents, which are also difficult and expensive to make. However, monoclonal anti-IgG antibodies are unlikely to replace conventional rabbit anti-IgG reagents as these are excellent and easy to make [22,23].

The main difficulty in the standardisation of polyspecific AHG reagents is the adjustment of the anti-C3d level to avoid false positives with the C3d levels on normal red cells. A state of the art problem existed for manufacturers as some reagents that passed FDA false positives with just washed red cells still gave troublesome 'false' positives in routine work (see Table 8). This problem was due to the failure to appreciate that the incubation of fresh sera with red cells increases their C3d level and that the reagents must be standardised to this level of C3d coated cell. The ISBT/ICSH joint Working Party on AHG Reagents recommends simulated crossmatch tests using both standard (NISS) and low ionic strength (LISS) tests for the standardisation and quality control of antiglobulin reagents [23]. The FDA has now also adopted this procedure as their false positive test procedure and this should help to improve the quality of AHG reagents. Generally anti-C3c is used as the major anti-complement component with a less amount of anti-C3d. The former is the main component for the detection of complement bound in *in vitro* tests and

*Table 8.* 'False' positives with C3d complement on normal donor's RBC.

| Commercial USA polyclonal AHG | Simulated crossmatch tests −37°C Fresh sera* × RBC from CPD-A segments (5-30 D) | | | | | C3d titres × E3d | |
|---|---|---|---|---|---|---|---|
| | 1 | 2 | 3 | 4 | 5 | immediate spin | 5 min |
| A | − | − | − | − | − | <1 | 4 |
| B | − | WK | − | − | − | 2 | 4 |
| C** | + | − | WK | + | WK | 4 | 8 |

* ISBT/ISH procedure – adopted by the FDA April 1986.
** This reagent is clean with washed RBC not incubated with serum.

the latter is used to detect *in vivo* bound complement. The ISBT/ICSH Working Party has selected both a conventional polyspecific AHG (R3P) and a polyspecific AHG (RIIIM) that contains monoclonal anti-C3c and anti-C3d, and these clean, potent, reference preparations [23] represent the state of the art and can be obtained from Professor C.P. Engelfriet (Amsterdam).

Several new types of polyspecific anti-complement blends have been made and there are four possible types of polyspecific reagent, as shown in Table 9.

*Table 9.* Four types of AHG free of 'false' positives in crossmatch tests.

| Various types of anti-C3 blended with rabbit serum anti-IgG | Spin type titres × EC3d indicator RBC | | | | 5 minute delay* |
|---|---|---|---|---|---|
| | immediate (15-30 sec) tests | | | | |
| | C3c | C3g | C3d | | C3d |
| 1. Conventional (rabbit) −C3d −C3d** | 16 | 0 | <1 | | 4-8 |
| 2. Monoclonal −C3c −C3d e.g. RIIM | 64 | 0 | 2 | increased | 8 |
| 3. Monoclonal −C3d (BRIC 8) *NO* C3c | 0 | 0 | 8 | | 8-16 |
| 4. Monoclonal −C3g (HL9) + rabbit −C3c | 16 | 32 | 0 | | 0 |

* 5 minute tests are essential to measure low levels of anti-C3d.
** Also contains some anti-C4c (titre 2-4).

In the case of the IgM anti-C3d BRIC-8 [24], experience in the UK has shown that this anti-C3d, suitably standardised, makes an excellent clean anti-complement without the need for anti-C3c. It is also interesting that BRIC-8 anti-C3d produced in a tissue culture supernatant is cleaner than the ascitic fluid material allowing the potency titre to be increased from 8-16 to 32. Also, we have a monoclonal anti-C3g that can be blended with an anti-C3c (monoclonal or polyclonal) which detects *in vivo* as well as 'in vitro' bound complement, as well as a good anti-C3d. However, this anti-C3g [22] is still unique and needs to be used at neat supernatant strength, so it remains to be seen if future anti-C3g monoclonal antibodies are sufficiently economic for reagent use, or whether this antibody will simply remain as a valuable research tool to characterise C3 components on various types of red cells [22,25].

62

## Other monoclonal antibodies for blood group serology

Many other monoclonal antibody specificities have been found. Monoclonal anti-M, anti-N, anti-Le$^a$ and anti-Le$^b$ are in routine use and others, including e, E, c, K and k, are under evaluation [2].

In conclusion, monoclonal antibodies have already made an impact in blood group serology. The most important final comment to be made is that each monoclonal antibody should be evaluated on its own merit as some have demonstrated idiosyncrasies not seen with polyclonal reagents e.g. the B(A) phenomenon and the extreme dependency of anti-M/N reagents on a critical pH.

## References

1. Kohler G, Milstein C. Continuous cultures of fused cells secreting antibody of predefined specificity. Nature 1975;256:495-7.
2. First ISBT Workshop on Monoclonal Antibodies to Red Cell and Related Antigens. Paris, 1987. Rouger P, Salmon Ch (eds). In press.
3. Voak D, Davies D, Sonneborn H, Moulds J, Fletcher A, Downie DM. The application of monoclonal antibodies for the detection of genetic markers of human red cells. 12th Int. Congress Soc. Forensic Haemogenetics, 1987. In press.
4. Voak D, Lennox E. Monoclonal antibodies for laboratory aspects of transfusion practice. In: Cash J (ed). Progress in transfusion medicine 1. Edingburgh: Churchill Livingstone, 1986:1-18.
5. Voak D. Monoclonal antibodies: Application to blood group serology. Labmedica 1986 August/September:27-31.
6. Crawford DH, Barlow MJ, Harrison JF, Winger L, Huehns ER. Production of human antibody to Rhesus D antigen. Lancet 1983;i:386-8.
7. Thompson KM, Melamed MD, Eagle K et al. Production of human monoclonal IgG and IgM antibodies with anti-D rhesus specificity using heterohybridomas. Immunology 1986;58:157-60.
8. Nelson N, Teng H, Lum SH, Riera FC, Kaplan HS. Construction and testing of mouse-human heteromyelomas for human monoclonal antibody production. Proc Natl Acad Sci (USA) 1983;80:7308-12.
9. Hoppe AH. The role of the bureau of biologics in assuring reagent reliability. In: Considerations in the selection of reagents. Technical Workshop. Washington DC: American Association of Blood Banks, 1979:1-24.
10. Messeter L, Brodin T, Chester MA et al. Mouse monoclonal antibodies with anti-A, anti-B and anti-A,B specificities; some superior to human polyclonal ABO reagents. Vox Sang 1984;46:185-94.
11. Voak D. In: A scientific forum on blood grouping anti-A (murine monoclonal blend) Bioclone. Stroup M, Treacy M (eds). Raritan NJ: Ortho Diagnostic Systems Inc, 1987:9-12.
12. Stroup M, Treacy M (eds). A scientific forum on blood grouping anti-A (murine monoclonal blend) Bioclone. Raritan NJ: Ortho Diagnostic Systems Inc, 1987.
13. Greenwell P, Yates AD, Watkins WM. Blood group A synthesizing activity of the blood-group B gene specified $\alpha$-3-galactosyl transferase. In: Schaur R, Boer P, Buddecke E, Kramer MF, Vliengenthart JCF, Wiegendt H (eds). Glycoconjugates. Stuttgard: Thieme, 1979:268-9.

14. Yates A. In: A scientific forum on blood grouping anti-A (murine monoclonal blend) Bioclone. Raritan NJ: Ortho Diagnostic Systems Inc, 1987:4-7.
15. Voak D. The evaluation of monoclonal anti-A antibodies for use as blood grouping reagents. In: Roger P, Salmon Ch (eds). Proceedings 1st ISBT International Workshop on Monoclonal Antibodies to Red Cells and Related Antigens. Paris: 1987. In press.
16. Voak D, Lowe AD, Lennox E. Monoclonal antibodies : ABO serology. Biotest Bulletin 1983;4:291-9.
17. Moore S, Chirnside A, Micklem LR et al. A mouse monoclonal antibody with anti-A(B) specificity which agglutinates $A_x$ cells. Vox Sang 1984;47:427-34.
18. Voak D. Monoclonal anti-D antibodies: Trends for reagents and research. BBTS Newsletter 1986;10:1-2.
19. Moore BPL. Does knowledge of $D^u$ status serve a useful purpose. Vox Sang 1984;46:95-102.
20. Lowe AD, Green SM, Voak D et al. A human-human monocloanl anti-D by direct fusion with a lymphoblastoid line. Vox Sang 1986;51:212-6.
21. Tippett P, Sanger R. Observations on subdivision of the Rh antigen D. Vox Sang 1962;7:9-13.
22. Voak D, Downie DM, Moore BPL, Engelfriet CP. Anti-human globulin reagent specification: The European and ISBT/ICSH view. Biotest Bulletin 1986;1:7-22.
23. Engelfriet CP, Voak D. International reference polyspecific anti-human globulin reagents. Vox Sang 1987;53:241-7.
24. Holt PDJ, Donaldson C, Judson PA et al. NBTS BRIC-8: A monoclonal anti-C3d antibody. Transfusion 1986;25:267-9.
25. Lachmann PJ, Voak D, Oldroyd RG, Downie DM, Bevan PC. Use of monoclonal anti-C3 antibodies to characterise the fragments of C3 that are found on erythrocytes. Vox Sang 1983;45:367-72.

# THE CHARACTERIZATION OF MONOCLONAL ANTIBODIES DIRECTED AGAINST CARBOHYDRATE EPITOPES BY IMMUNOCHEMICAL MEANS; THE IMPORTANCE OF SUCH MONOCLONAL ANTIBODIES FOR THE RECOGNITION OF BLOOD GROUP ANTIGENS

L. Messeter, K. Löw, A. Lundblad

## Introduction

A number of monoclonal antibodies (MABs) raised against blood group active carbohydrate antigens have proved to be useful as blood grouping reagents [1]. The possibility to determine the fine specificity of these antibodies and the increasing knowledge about the importance of carbohycrate antigens as markers in cell differentiation and in carcinogenesis [2,3] have made many of these MABs even more important as diagnostic tools in immuno-histology and immuno-pathology. Since a blood group active carbohydrate antigen may have different chain structures and can be attached to lipids or polypeptides the presentation of the antigen may differ in different tissues even if the immuno-dominant structure is the same [4,5]. On the other hand, cell surface antigens which seemingly are identical might show fine qualitative differences when studied with specific reagents [6]. Thus it might be possible that weak ABO variants which can be demonstrated on red cells of rare individuals may contain epitopes which differ also qualitatively from those of 'standard' red cell phenotypes.

For these reasons it is not selfevident that an antibody which performs well in red cell grouping is equally useful in other applications and it is therefore of great importance to elucidate which epitope an antibody does recognize.

In this paper we will give a few examples of how antibodies against H and Lewis antigens can be evaluated, starting from the serological reaction pattern.

## Materials and methods

H and Lewis antigens occur e.g. on human red cells and in blood group substances from human ovarian cyst material. Lewis active sugars also occur in human milk. Antigens from these sources were used for immunization of Balb/c mice (Table 1). The Lewis active milk sugars LNF II (Lacto-N-fucopentaose II, Le$^a$ active) and LND I (Lacto-N-difucohexaose I, Le$^b$ active) were coupled to edestin or KLH before use. The immunization protocol has been described earlier [7]. MABs were produced by the mouse-mouse hybridoma technique as described earlier [7]. Tissue culture supernatants from growing hybridomas were screened against selected human red cells using manual hemagglutination tests. Promising antibodies were further

*Table 1.* Antigens used and resulting antibodies.

| Antigen used | Blood group activity | Serological reaction pattern of produced antibodies |
|---|---|---|
| LND I-edestin/KLH | Le$^b$ | anti-Le$^b$, anti-H |
| LNF II-edestin/KLH | Le$^a$ | anti-Le$^a$ |
| H, Le$^b$ substance | H, Le$^b$ | anti-H |
| Le$^a$ substance | Le$^a$ | anti-Le$^a$ |
| Human red cells | B, Le$^a$, Le$^b$, H and others | anti-H, anti-B and others |

*Table 2.* Antigens used in ELISA testing.

| Name | Structure |
|---|---|
| Lacto-N-tetraose LNT | Gal$\beta$-3GlcNAc$\beta$-3Gal$\beta$-4Glc—BSA* |
| Lacto-N-fucopentaose I LNF I, H I antigen | Gal$\beta$-3GlcNac$\beta$-3Gal$\beta$-4Glc ╱ BSA* <br> 12 ╲ Cer** <br> Fuc$\alpha$ |
| Lacto-N-fucopentaose II LNF II, Le$^a$ antigen | Gal$\beta$-3GlcNac$\beta$-3Gal$\beta$-4Glc ╱ BSA* <br> 14 ╲ Cer** <br> Fuc$\alpha$ |
| Lacto-N-difucohexaose I LND I, Le$^b$ antigen | Gal$\beta$-3GlcNac$\beta$-4Gal$\beta$-4Glc ╱ BSA* <br> 12　　14 ╲ Cer** <br> Fuc$\alpha$　Fuc$\alpha$ |
| Lacto-N-neofucopentaose I LNnF I, H II antigen | Gal$\beta$-3GlcNac$\beta$-3Gal$\beta$-4Glc ╱ BSA* <br> 12 ╲ Cer** <br> Fuc$\alpha$ |
| Lacto-N-neofucopentaose III LNnF III, X antigen | Gal$\beta$-3GlcNac$\beta$-3Gal$\beta$-4Glc ╱ BSA* <br> 13 ╲ Cer** <br> Fuc$\alpha$ |
| Lacto-N-neodifucohexaose I LNnD I, Y antigen | Gal$\beta$-3GlcNac$\beta$-3Gal$\beta$-4Glc ╱ BSA* <br> 12　　13 ╲ Cer** <br> Fuc$\alpha$　Fuc$\alpha$ |

* Antigen coupled to BSA; ** Glycolipid.

evaluated in hemagglutination against a large number of red cells of different phenotypes.

Antibodies which were considered useful as reagents for blood grouping were selected for immunochemical studies.

These comprised solid phase ELISA tests [8] in microtiter trays coated with a number of representative oligosaccharides (coupled to BSA), or glycolipids (Table 2).

## Results and discussion

One of the goals was to produce MABs against H and Lewis antigens with sufficient potency to be useful for routine phenotyping.

Table 1 gives a summary of the antibodies obtained, classified according to their serological reaction pattern. Interestingly, neither red cells nor blood group substance provoked formation of Le$^b$ antibodies in any of the fusions performed whereas both red cells, H, Le$^b$ blood group substance and LND I gave rise to antibodies reacting as anti-H in hemagglutination.

### Anti-H

After immunization with H, Le$^b$ blood group substance, red cells or LND I-edestin, a number of antibodies were obtained which preferentially agglutinated group O red cells. Most of these antibodies were quite weak and did not distinguish well between A1 and A2 cells but a few antibodies from fusions with either of the used antigens gave reactions similar to those expected of a *Ulex europaeus* extract (Table 3). Ulex lectin recognizes a $\alpha$-fucosyl residue and reacts well with H type 1 and 2 [9].

However, when the binding characteristics to the glycoconjugate panel were studied in ELISA test, these antibodies showed varying reaction patterns (Figure 1). It is quite clear that even if the serological results show good specificity only one of these antibodies has a binding pattern which is similar to that of the Ulex lectin. This antibody, 647/9 A2, therefore is a true anti-H which in the hemagglutination test recognizes H structures that occur on human red cells.

All the other three antibodies show a more or less pronounced cross reactivity with the difucosylated type 2 structure, the Y antigen, which so far has not been isolated from human red cells [10]. In fact, the MAB 672/7 E3 which behaves as a rather satisfactory anti-H in hemagglutination is in the ELISA a pure anti-Y. The antibody might therefore recognize H type 3 which occurs on red cells.

The antibody 64/4 D8 shows another binding pattern: it binds equally well to type 1 and 2 difucosylated structures i.e. Le$^b$ and Y antigens, and also shows some cross reactions with H type 1 and 2. Since the antibody was raised against the Le$^b$ active milk sugar LND I, the cross reactions in ELISA with this antigen are not astonishing. It might be expected, however, that in hemagglutination, Lewis negative cells, particularly those from non secretors would react less well. This was also the case but the reactions were

*Table 3.*  Hemagglutination titers of some MABs.

**647/9 A2**  (mice immunized with group B human red cells)
Antibody dilution

| Red cell | 1:1 | 1:2 | 1:4 | 1:8 | 1:16 | 1:32 | 1:64 | 1:128 | 1:256 |
|---|---|---|---|---|---|---|---|---|---|
| A1 | – | – | – | – | – | – | – | – | – |
| A1B | 1 | 1w | – | – | – | – | – | – | – |
| A2 | 4 | 4 | 4w | 4w | 3 | 3w | 1 | – | – |
| A2B | 2 | 2 | 2 | 1 | 1w | – | – | – | – |
| O | 4 | 4 | 4w | 4w | 3 | 3w | 2 | 1 | – |

**672/7 E3**  (mice immunized with H, Le^b blood group substance)
Antibody dilution

| Red cell | 1:1 | 1:2 | 1:4 | 1:8 | 1:16 | 1:32 | 1:64 | 1:128 | 1:256 | 1:512 |
|---|---|---|---|---|---|---|---|---|---|---|
| A1 | 1w | – | – | – | – | – | – | – | – | – |
| A1B | – | – | – | – | – | – | – | – | – | – |
| A2B | 4 | 4 | 4 | 4 | 4w | 4w | 3 | 2 | 2 | 1 |
| A2B | 2 | 2 | 2w | 1 | 1 | 1w | – | – | – | – |
| O | 4 | 4 | 4 | 4 | 4w | 4w | 3 | 3w | 2 | 2w |

**64/4 D8**  (mice immunized with LND I-edestin)
Antibody dilution

| Red cell | 1:1 | 1:2 | 1:4 | 1:8 | 1:16 | 1:32 | 1:64 | 1:128 | 1:256 |
|---|---|---|---|---|---|---|---|---|---|
| A1 | – | – | – | – | – | – | – | – | – |
| A1B | – | – | – | – | – | – | – | – | – |
| A2 | 4 | 4w | 3 | 3w | 1 | 1w | – | – | – |
| A2B | 2 | 1 | 1 | 1w | – | – | – | – | – |
| O | 4 | 4 | 4 | 3 | 3 | 3 | 2 | 1w | – |

still strong and the difference in titer only 1-2 steps if compared to other Lewis phenotypes. One explanation could be that the Lewis antigens occur only in minute amounts on human red cells [11] and therefore the cross reactions with H type 2 or H type 3 are more important for the agglutination reaction.

## Anti-Le^a

When the milk sugar LNF II or Le^a active ovarian cyst material was used for antigen in a couple of fusions, only one antibody was worthwhile to study further. This antibody, 318/2 B3 was raised against cyst material and agglutinated Le^a red cells of all ABO groups. Le^b cells were not agglutinated even after enzyme treatment of the cells. In the ELISA, however, the antibody bound equally strongly to the Le^a active sugar and to the non-fucosylated type 1 chain (LNT), whereas cross reactions with H type 1 and X were not so pronounced. LNT is not expressed on red cells.

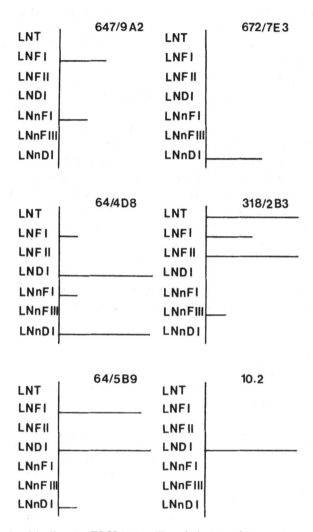

*Figure 1.* Relative binding in ELISA (undiluted tissue culture supernatant) to oligosaccharides coupled to BSA, or to glycolipids. Abbreviations, see Table 2).

## Anti-Le$^b$

After immunization with LND I a number of antibodies showing anti-Le$^b$ specificity were obtained. Most of these had serological characteristics as anti-Le$^{bh}$ but some also reacted with A1, Le$^b$ red cells. 10.2 has been described before [7] and binds to LND I and to the Le$^b$ glycolipid. It also binds to some degree to lactodifucotetraose, a milk oligosaccharide which does not occur on red cells, but not to Le$^a$, X or Y glycolipids. Another anti-Le$^b$, 64/5 B9 obtained in another fusion, gave the same serological reactions as 10.2 but the binding pattern was broader. Cross reactions with H I and Y could be demonstrated, whereas non specific agglutination of Le$^a$ or Lewis negative cells were never observed.

These examples illustrate nicely how difficult it is to produce a specific antibody against antigens of this type which probably is due mainly to the structural similarity. Even if purified antigens are used for immunization, the possibility of cross reactions is very large.

From these examples it is also quite evident that the serological specificity not always corresponds to the pattern which can be demonstrated by immunochemical means. This was also well illustrated in the recent workshop on monoclonal antibodies against human red cell and related antigens [12].

Several laboratories had studied the fine specificity of many different antibodies against carbohydrate antigens and their suitability in different applications. Many antibodies which are excellent blood grouping reagents do not give conclusive or even correct information if used in histology according to the stated serological specificity. The antibodies discussed in this paper further corroborate this fact. If an antibody which in hemagglutination seemingly is an anti-H, but in reality is an anti-Y should be used uncritically, very misleading information might be obtained. Therefore, all these MABs should be thoroughly characterized and it should be clearly stated that the reactions obtained in hemagglutination tests do not necessarily reflect exactly the same specificity if the antibody is used in other applications.

## References

1. Hakomori S. Monoclonal antibodies directed to cell-surface carbohydrates. In: Monoclonal antibodies and functional cell lines. New York: Plenum Press 1984: 67-100.
2. Hakomori S. Philip Levine Award Lecture: Blood group glycolipid antigens and their modifications as human cancer antigens. Am J Clin Pathol 1984;45:635-48.
3. Feizi T. Demonstration by monoclonal antibodies that carbohydrate structures of glycoproteins and glycolipids are onco-developmental antigens. Nature 1985; 314:53-7.
4. Hakomori S. Blood group ABH and Ii antigens of human erythrocytes: Chemistry, polymorphism, and their developmental change. Seminars in Hematology 1981;48:39-62.
5. Watkins WM. Biochemistry and genetics of the ABO, Lewis and P blood group systems. In: Harris H, Hirschhorn K (eds). Advances in human genetics. New York: Plenum Press, 1980:1-137.
6. Gane P, Vellayoudom J, Mollicone R et al. Heterogeneity of anti-A and anti-B monoclonal reagents. Vox Sang 1987;53:117-25.
7. Messeter L, Brodin T, Chester MA, Karlsson K-A, Zopf D, Lundblad A. Immunochemical characterization of a monoclonal anti-Le$^b$ blood grouping reagent. Vox Sang 1984;46:66-74.
8. Engvall E, Perlmann P. Enzyme-linked immunosorbent assay, ELISA. III. Quantitation of specific antibodies by enzyme-labelled anti-immunoglobulin in antigen-coated tubes. J Immunol 1972;109:129-35.
9. Pereira MEA, Kisailus EC, Gruezo F, Kabat E. Immunochemical studies on combining site of the blood group H-specific lectin 1 from Ulex europaeus seeds. Arch Biochem Biophys 1978;185:108-15.

10. Kannagi R, Levery SB, Hakomori S. Le[a]-active heptaglycosylceramide, a hybrid type 1 and type 2 chain, and the pattern of glycolipids with Le[a], Le[b], X (Le[x]), and Y (Le[y]) determinants in human blood cell membranes (ghosts). J Biol Chemistry 1985;260:6410-5.

11. Hanfland P. Isolation and purification of Lewis blood-group active glycosphingolipids from the plasma of human O Le[b] individuals. Eur J Biochem 1978;87: 161-70.

12. First ISBT Workshop on Monoclonal Antibodies to Red Cell and Related Antigens. Paris, 1987. Rouger P, Salmon Ch (eds). In press.

# BIOCHEMISTRY OF HLA-B27 IN TRANSFECTED CELLS AND TRANSGENIC MICE

H.L. Ploegh, E.J. Baas, P.J.F.M. Derhaag

To study the functional properties of HLA Class I molecules (Figure 1), genes encoding these proteins have been isolated and used to transfect mouse cells. We have isolated the genes encoding the HLA-B27k and -B27w proteins [1]. A number of diseases are associated with certain HLA alleles. Of these associations, the one linking the HLA-B27 alleles with ankylosing spondylitis is the most pronounced. Several models have been presented over the past few years to explain this fact. However, the lack of a proper model system to study this HLA disease association has restricted the experimental basis for these theories. Transgenic mice may provide us with a better defined model system to study the immunobiology of HLA-B27 and – together with biochemical analysis of the HLA-B27 gene product – may give us better insight in HLA disease association.

In the analysis of transfection experiments involving human Class I genes we have developed reagents that are capable of reacting with Class I heavy chain even after full denaturation and hence they can be used in Western blots [2,4]. Moreover these reagents possess excellent locus specificity [4, Stam & Ploegh, unpublished). Because Western blotting performed in IEF gels will resolve most of the commonly occurring HLA Class I heavy chains, application of this technology to clinical or forensic problems deserves consideration.

Transfection of mouse cells with the HLA-B27k or -B27w gene does not result in any surface expression of the HLA heavy chain as detected by FACS analysis using the monoclonal antibody W6/32, reactive with human heavy chain associated with the HLA light chain, $\beta$-2-microglobulin [5]. This is in contrast to transfection experiments with the genes for HLA-B7 or -A2, where HLA-B7 or -A2 heavy chains are expressed on the cell surface of the transfected mouse cells associated with murine $\beta$2M (m$\beta$2M) as detected with W6/32 [6]. The level of expression of HLA on these transfectants is comparable to the level of expression on human B lymphoblastoid cell lines. The HLA-B27 transfectants do express HLA heavy chain intracellulary, as indicated by immunoprecipitations of metabolically labelled proteins with monoclonal antibody HC-10, reactive with the human free heavy chain [4]. This pool of free HLA-B27 heavy chain is not sialylated and is endo-H sensitive, indicative of accumulation of the protein in the pre-Golgi stage of biosynthesis. Transfected cells having received both the HLA-B27k and the -A2 gene further confirmed this clear difference in biochemical behaviour of both proteins: HLA-A2 is expressed at the cell surface, HLA-B27k is arrested intracellularly. HLA-B7 and -B27 are identical in aminoacid sequence of their $\alpha$3 domain down to their carboxy terminus. Differences in m$\beta$2M binding capacity therefore must be contributed by the $\alpha$2 domain. Exon shuffling

74

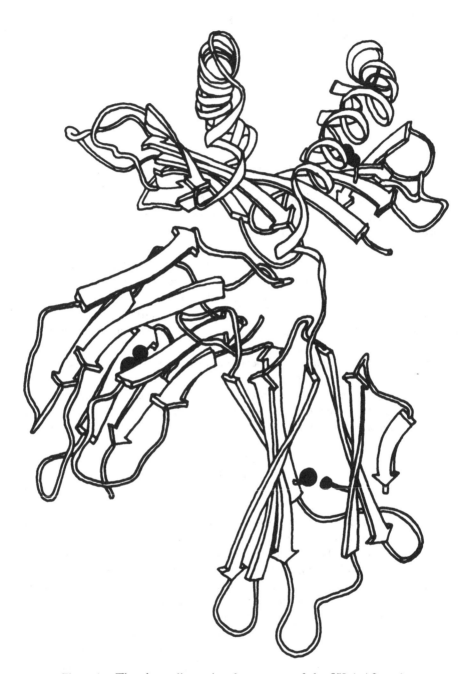

*Figure 1.*   The three-dimensional structure of the HLA-A2 antigen.

*Figure 1A.*   The three-dimensional structure of HLA-A2 as determined by X-ray crystallography [7].
The folding pattern of the polypeptide backbone reveals the heavy and light chains, where the light chain (beta₂-microglobulin) is visible in the lower left. At the top of the molecule the two alpha-helices that are crucial for the presentation of antigen to cytotoxic T cells are visible.

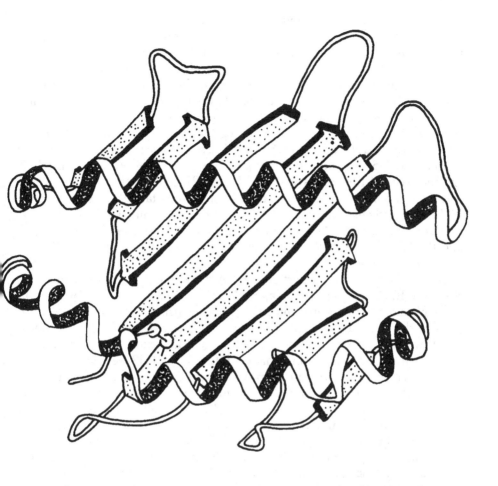

*Figure 1.* The three-dimensional structure of the HLA-A2 antigen.

*Figure 1B.* A top view of the antigen-binding site on HLA-A2.
The two alpha-helices present in the HLA-A2 structure are more clearly visible in this top view. The two alpha helices are contributed by the alpha-1 and alpha-2 domains. They are supported by eight strands of beta sheet, likewise contributed by the alpha-1 and -2 domains. Antigen is thought to bind in the cleft formed by the alpha-helices. From the structure it may be deduced that T cells will recognize short peptides that fit in the cleft, rather than the intact antigen from which they are derived.
These figures have been redrawn from [7].

experiments have confirmed this notion [Hochstenbach et al, personal communication), in agreement with the recently published 3-D structure of the HLA-A2 protein [7] (Figure 1).

To overcome the lack of surface expression of HLA-B27 in mouse transfected cell lines, we have cloned the gene encoding the human $\beta$-2-microglobulin (h$\beta$2M) as well and used this gene in a second round of transfection on the HLA-B27 transfected mouse cells [8]. Normal surface expression of HLA-B27 is the result, with human $\beta$2M as light chain. There is thus a striking resemblance with the situation in the human line DAUDI, where no heavy chain is detectable on the cell surface due to a mutation in the $\beta2M$ gene, resulting in a defective mRNA and the inability to synthesize $h\beta2M$ protein. Association of the heavy chain with a light chain (human or murine) thus appears necessary for cell surface expression. Inability to form the complex results in absence of surface expression of human class I antigens. The double transfected cells (having received both HLA-B27 and $h\beta2M$) express a correctly assembled protein, having $h\beta2M$ as light chain as shown by immunoprecipitations with W6/32. The heavy chain is sialylated and endo-H resistant. FACS data fully substantiate the surface expression of HLA-B27. On the basis of the results with the HLA-B27 gene in transfection experiments we can make a clear prediction: in order to obtain expression of HLA-B27 in a transgenic mouse model, both human subunits will be required to produce authentic HLA-B27. Only by introducing both the HLA-B27 gene and the $h\beta2M$ gene in the germline can we expect to obtain HLA-B27 expressing transgenic mice.

To study the in-vivo properties of HLA-B27k, the pI6 plasmid containing the HLA-B27k gene was microinjected into fertilized eggs of (CBA×C57Bl/LiA) mice to generate transgenic mice [8]. The offspring shown to have incorporated the gene, as indicated by Southern blot analysis of genomic mouse DNA, was analyzed for transcription of the gene and expression of the human heavy chain. Of 12 mice transgenic for HLA-B27k all 12 were shown to produce the correct mRNA and, intracellulary, the heavy chain protein.

In addition a second set of transgenic mice was generated, with an identical murine background, using the human $\beta$-2-microglobulin gene containing plasmid $p\beta2m$-13. Southern blot analysis indicated 12 mice to have incorporated the $h\beta2M$ gene [9] in their genome. However, only 2 of these appeared to produce the appropriate mRNA and to express the $h\beta2M$ protein, probably due to the presence of bacterial vector sequences flanking the microinjected gene. These sequences are not present in the microinjected HLA-B27k gene.

On crossing an HLA-B27k positive mouse with a transgenic expressing $h\beta2M$, offspring was produced of which some individuals were positive for both human genes. Immunoprecipitations and FACS analysis show the obligatory requirement of $h\beta2M$ for HLA-B27k expression, in concordance with the data of the transfection experiments. Mice transgenic for $h\beta2M$ *only* do express the human light chain on splenocytes, associated with certain murine H-2 heavy chains. These H-2 class I heavy chains were not characterized further. On splenocytes of mice transgenic for both HLA-B27k and $h\beta2M$ (double transgenic mice, dTGM) a level of HLA class I expression comparable with the level of expression found on human EBV transformed B cell lines was seen.

Human alloreactive CTL raised against human HLA-B27k expressing cells are able to specifically lyse dTGM splenocytes, indicating the expressed human class I molecule indeed to be conformationally identical to the HLA-B27k molecule as expressed on human cells. In order to analyse the *in vivo* function of the HLA-B27k/$h\beta2M$ complex, the ability of the dTGM to raise HLA-B27k restricted CTL was studied. After *in vivo* priming with either

Sendai virus or influenza A/X79, the ability of dTGM splenocytes to lyse virus coated (Sendai) or virus infected (influenza) autologous cells or human HLA-B27k or -B27w positive cells was measured in a chromium release assay. HLA-B27 negative human lymphocytes served as control [10]. The results indicate that the murine T cell repertoire is capable of specifying HLA-B27k restricted CTL, and antigen can be presented in the context of HLA-B27k in these transgenic mice. This antigen restriction is HLA-B27k specific: HLA-B27w, another HLA-B27 subtype, does not serve as restriction element. This ability to discriminate between HLA-B27 subtypes differing in only 3 aminoacids accurately reflects the situation observed in the human system.

In conclusion, the HLA-B27k transgenic mice offer a suitable model system for *in vivo* HLA studies. Association of the HLA-B27 heavy chain with murine $\beta$2M appears insignificant, and in dTGM the presence of h$\beta$2M prevents the formation of such hybrid molecules: none were detectable with the w6/32 antibody. The use of these transgenics in disease association studies now focusses on the immunological effects of expression of HLA-B27k: dTGM are tolerant for HLA-B27k and h$\beta$2M, thereby possibly also creating other 'holes' in the T cell repertoire, as well as the mode of presentation of specific antigen by HLA-B27k molecules, resulting in a HLA-B27k restricted murine T cell response. It remains to be seen whether a challenge with arthritogenic micro-organisms will result in ankylosing spondylitis-like symptoms in HLA-B27 transgenic mice.

# References

1. Seemann GHA, Rein RS, Brown CS, Ploegh HL. Gene conversion-like mechanisms may generate polymorphism in human Class I genes. EMBO J 1986;5:547-52.
2. Neefjes JJ, Breur-Vriesendorp BS, van Seventer GA, Ivanyi P, Ploegh HL. An improved biochemical method for the analysis of HLA-Class I antigens. Definition of new HLA-Class I subtypes. Human Immun 1986;16:169-81.
3. Neefjes JJ, Doxiadis I, Stam NJ, Beckers CJ, Ploegh HL. An analysis of Class I antigens of Man and other species by one-dimensional IEF and immunoblotting. Immunogen 1986;23:164-71.
4. Stam NJ, Spits H, Ploegh HL. Monoclonal antibodies raised against denatured HLA-B locus heavy chains permit biochemical characterization of certain HLA-C locus products. J Immunol 1986;137:2299-306.
5. Parham PR, Barnstable CJ, Bodmer WF. Use of a monoclonal antibody (W6/32) in structural studies of HLA-A, B, C, antigens. J Immunol 1979;123:342-9.
6. Rein RS, Seemann GHA, Neefjes JJ, Hochstenbach FMH, Stam NJ, Ploegh HL. Association with $\beta$2-microblobulin controls the expression of transfected human class I genes. J Immunol 1987;138:1178-83.
7. Bjorkman PJ, Saper MA, Samraoui B, Bennet WS, Strominger JL, Wiley DC. Structure of the human class I histocompatibility antigen, HLA-A2. Nature 1987;329:506-12.
8. Krimpenfort P, Rudenko G, Hochstenbach F, Guessow D, Berns A, Ploegh HL. Crosses of two independently derived transgenic mice demonstrate functional complementation of the genes encoding heavy (HLA-B27) and light ($\beta$2-microglobulin) chains of HLA Class I antigens. EMBO J 1987;6:1673-6.

78

9. Guessow D, Rein R, Ginjaar I, Hochstenbach F, Seemann G, Ploegh HL. The human β2-microglobulin gene, primairy structure and definition of the transcription unit. J Immunol 1987;139:3132-8.
10. Kievits F, Ivanyi P, Krimpenfort P, Berns A, Ploegh HL. HLA restricted recognition of viral antigens in HLA transgenic mice. Nature 1987;329:447-9.

# BIOTECHNOLOGY IN THE DEVELOPMENT OF
# HIV DIAGNOSTIC PROCEDURES

Ch. Rouzioux

Since the discovery of HIV as the etiological agent of AIDS, a large number of diagnostic procedures has been developed to detect the different markers of HIV infection. The severity of the disease and the psychological consequences for the patient explain the absolute need of high reliability for antibody detection procedures, i.e. good specificity and sensitivity.

The screening for HIV positive subjects in done by ELISA (enzyme-linked-immunosorbent-assay). In the first generation tests, the viral antigens are prepared from supernatants of HIV infected cells. This raises the problem of contamination with cellular proteins, and false positive results should be avoided by including a cellular control antigen. The second generation ELISA tests are performed with rDNA proteins corresponding to *core* and *env* antigens of the virus. Some of the tests are built as competitive assay and the antigen is fixed by means of prefixed monoclonal antibodies. These tests present a very good sensitivity and are useful for the detection of HIV low positive sera, particularly to detect low antibody titers during the development of AIDS. They are also necessary for the detection of low positive sera during HIV seroconversion [1,2].

Although those 2nd generation ELISA tests are very sensitive but not entirely specific, the Western blot analysis appears to be essential to confirm all true positive results. This technology is highly sensitive and specific, allowing the characterization of antibodies specifically directed against various viral proteins. All sera containing antibodies against envelope proteins must be considered positive. That is the reason why it is crucial that the nitrocellulose sheets contain a good variety of those envelope proteins (GP41, GP110, GP160).

In France, different evaluations of HIV-Ab techniques have been conducted by the retrovirus group of the French National Society of Blood Transfusion. The specificity of the tests has been studied by evaluating the number of false positive results (which are not confirmed by Western blot or radioimmunoprecipitation) in a large group of negative blood donors. The sensitivity has been studied by means of a panel of 13 selected sera (seroconversion, low HIV-1 positive sera, HIV-2 positive sera and tricky sera: P-25 or P-18. The results show not only increased sensitivity and specificity for some of the kits, but also show the capacity to detect specific antibodies for HIV-2 [3-5].

## HIV-2

HIV-2 is the second AIDS retrovirus. It was isolated in France in November 1985. It belongs to the same family, presents all the same biological and pathological properties, but the proteins of HIV-2 differ from those of HIV-1 with 58% of homology for gag genes and 60% for pol genes. This virus is clearly related to West Africa. Seroprevalence in France among blood donors seems very low but the problem of HIV-2 exists. By means of HIV-1 serology, it has been possible to detect HIV-2 positive sera confirmed with specific HIV-2 Western blot: 12 HIV-2 blood donors have been detected in different parts fo France since January 1986. For all of them a link with West Africa has been clearly demonstrated [6].

HIV-2 epidemiology presents a different pattern from that of HIV-1. A study has started in France in order to evaluate the prevalence of HIV-2 among blood donors and eventually to determine whether or not it is necessary to systematically screen for HIV-2 antibodies.

### HIV-1 antigen detection

Another concern for blood banks appears with the development of the technology of HIV-1 antigen detection. In those tests HIV-1 antigens are detected by immunocapture assay using monoclonal or polyclonal antibodies. This test is able to detect viral antigens before the appearance of antibodies. So it could be possible to detect infectious persons among negative blood donors. This test seems to be a good marker for viral replication and may be very useful for therapeutic evaluations of antiviral drugs.

The techniques of detection of HIV markers have gained the benefit from recent developments in biotechnology. Moreover they have been developed in a very short time with good sensitivity and specificity [7].

In conclusion a large panel of biotechnology for HIV diagnostics is available: ELISA tests are very useful to quantify HIV antibodies; Western blot analysis permits to characterize them and HIV-1 antigen detection is important for thereapeutic follow-up and detection of seroconversion.

For blood banks, the risk of transfusion is not entirely solved with HIV-1 screening. The problems of HIV-1 Ag, HIV-2 and even of HTLV-1 remain, if blood donors are not well selected or well informed. This raises the question of the development of new biotechnologies in order to detect infected patients and 'putative' infectious blood donors (window phase). These methods would improve the safety of blood products. However, at the present time information about AIDS is most essential to prevent HIV dissemination.

## References

1.  Ranki A, Valle SL, Krohn M et al. Long latency precedes overt seroconversion in sexually transmitted human-immunodeficiency-virus infection. Lancet 1987; ii:589-93.

2.  Courouce AM. Latency preceding seroconversion in sexually transmitted HIV infection. Lancet 1987;ii:1025.
3.  Courouce AM, Barin F, Baudelot J et al. Evaluation de 3 trousses immuno-enzymatiques de dépistage des anticorps anti-LAV. Comparaison avec des tests de confirmation. Rev Franç Transf 1985;28:325.
4.  Courouce AM, Barin F, Baudelot J et al. Nouvelle évaluation de 3 trousses immunoenzymatiques de dépistage des anticorps anti-LAV (par le groupe d'étude de la Société Nationale de Transfusion Sanguine). Rev Franç Transf 1986;29.
5.  Courouce AM, Barin F, Barre F et al. Conduite et difficultés de la sérologie HIV: Groupe de travail 'Rétrovirus' de la Société Nationale de Transfusion Sanguine. Spectra Biologie, 1987 (in press).
6.  Courouce AM, Rouzioux C, Barin F, Chamaret S. LAV2/HTLV IV. Infection among blood donors, multitransfused patients and different AIDS risk groups, in France. Abstracts Volume III. International Conference on Acquired Immunodeficiency Syndrome (AIDS), Washington, DC 1987:211.
7.  Backer U, Weinauer F, Gathof G, Eberle J. HIV antigen screening in blood donors. Lancet 1987;ii:1213.

# BIOTECHNOLOGY AND THE DEVELOPMENT OF HBV DIAGNOSTIC PROCEDURES

P.E. Highfield

This presentation describes how biotechnology has been applied to the diagnosis of hepatitis B virus (HBV) infection. Infection with HBV usually leads to an acute liver disease followed by clearance of the virus and the establishment of immunity during the subsequent convalescent phase. Occasionally the acute infection can be asymptomatic. In a proportion of cases (about 10% in the West, higher in certain ethnic groups) the infection does not resolve and the individual may become a virus carrier with or without chronic symptoms. Carriers may suffer from progressive liver damage and go on to develop hepatocellular carcinoma. It is thought that there are 200 million such HBV carriers in the world [1]. Clearly, this important public health problem needs good diagnostic tests for a number of reasons. Firstly, blood donations must be screened to identify those which are potentially infectious and so prevent transfusion associated infection. Secondly the proper management of a patient can depend upon correct diagnosis of the course of infection. Finally it is becoming increasingly important to assess both the effect of chemotherapy on HBV carriers and also the efficacy of vaccination programmes.

The infectious virus particle was first described by Dane and colleagues [2] and is known as the Dane particle. This virion is 42nm in diameter and consists of a lipid envelope surrounding a nucleoprotein core which contains the genetic information of the virus, a partially double-stranded DNA molecule. The envelope contains the viral surface antigen (HBsAg) embedded in a lipid membrane derived from the host cell. The nucleocapsid is a regular array of multiple copies of a single polypeptide, encoded by the core gene, and this structure has the core antigen (HBcAg) activity. Another important viral antigen is the so-called e-antigen (HBeAg) which can be derived by disaggregation of the core particles by proteolysis or detergent treatment. The viral polymerase is attached to the DNA within the core and is used to replicate the viral genome in the infected cell.

The major markers of HBV infection are HBsAg/anti-HBs, HBeAg/anti-HBe and anti-HBc (both IgG and IgM). It is HBsAg which is important for blood screening and any HBsAg-positive units are rejected. In clinical diagnosis the wider pattern of markers is used to determine the status and prognosis of a patient.

So far, an *in vitro* culture system has not been developed for HBV and this is the overwhelming reason why biotechnology has had such an impact not only on the study of HBV but also on the diagnostic tests available. HBV infects only man and chimpanzees and the latter are neither a convenient nor economically-viable animal model. This has greatly hampered research and also limited the reagents available for diagnostic testing because infected, and possibly infectious, body tissues and fluids are the starting points for preparing antigens and antibodies. This is obviously unsatisfactory because the supply of reagents is unreliable and batch-to-batch variation occurs, in addition to the containment required for handling large amounts of potentially infectious material. The discovery of human retroviruses, which affect predominantly the same risk groups as HBV, only highlights the problem.

It is not the intention to describe the techniques of gene cloning or monoclonal antiboy production because they are dealt with in other chapters. Given the problems of using conventional techniques to study HBV it is not surprising that this was one of the first virus sequences to be cloned [3-7]. The genomes of a number of different HBV serotypes have been cloned, sequenced and various gene products expressed [8-11]. Monoclonal antibodies to particular HBV antigens have been produced by immunization with whole virus preparations, purified virion proteins or recombinant proteins. High-titre polyclonal antibodies have been produced using purified proteins. How have these reagents been used in diagnostic testing for HBV infection?

The primary screening test for HBV infection is to measure the HBsAg present in serum. Since their introduction in the early 1960s, when the marker was called Australia Antigen, HBsAg tests have developed from a relatively insensitive immunodiffusion assay through hemagglutination and on to radioimmunoassays (RIA) of great sensitivity. Enzyme-linked immunoassays are now available which are equally as sensitive but are more convenient than the RIAs.

In all honesty the improvements made to the speed, sensitivity and convenience of HBsAg tests have not depended upon the biotechnological techniques mentioned above. There are a number of reasons for this. Firstly the need to reduce transfusion associated hepatitis provided a tremendous impetus for the development of improved HBsAg tests. Secondly, high-titre HBsAg and anti-HBs positive individuals can be found and these provide an accessible source of reagents. Purified HBsAg can be used to raise high-titre anti-HBs antisera in a variety of animals. It is the availability of these reagents combined with continuing technical developments which have improved the HBsAg immunoassay. A point has been reached where any increase in sensitivity would not noticeably increase the detection of positive samples because so few donors present with HBsAg levels below the detection limit of current assays (about 1 ng/ml). Future developments will be concerned with improved specificity, speed and convenience. For example monoclonal antibodies are used in current HBsAg assays because the solid phase, sample and conjugate can be incubated simultaneously which reduces the total assay time.

For other markers such as anti-HBc and HBeAg/anti-HBe the situation is rather different. The reagents needed for these tests are much harder to obtain conventionally; e.g. HBeAg is a marker for highly-infectious serum and HBcAg is obtained from infected livers. The production of monoclonal antibodies (MAB) specific for HBcAg and HBeAg and the expression of these antigens by recombinant techniques has changed the situation entirely. New types of assays for these markers are now possible.

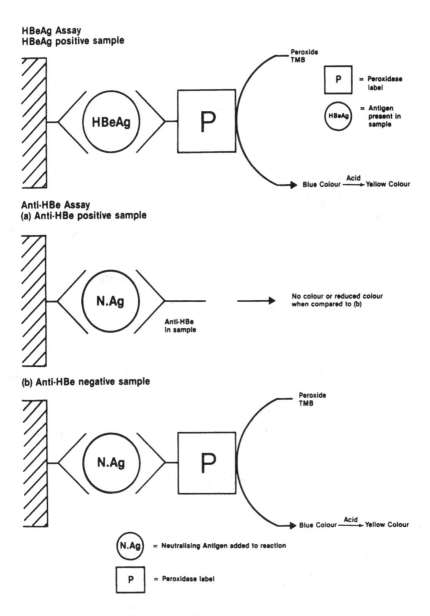

*Figure 1.* HBeAg/anti-HBe assays. HBeAg: Monoclonal antibody is coated onto a solid support and incubated with the samples in the presence of a second monoclonal antibody which is conjugated with horseradish peroxidase. If HBeAg is present in the sample then the conjugate will be bound to the solid support and a coloured reaction product will result when TMB (3,3',5,5'-tetramethylbenzidine) substrate is added. If the sample is HBeAg-negative then the conjugate will be removed at the washing step and no colour will be produced. Anti-HBe: The solid phase is incubated with the sample in the presence of both conjugate and recombinant HBeAg (neutralizing antigen). If the sample is anti-HBe-positive then there will be competition for binding to the added HBeAg and there will be little to no colour development. For an anti-HBe-negative sample the conjugate will bind to the HBeAg and colour will develope.

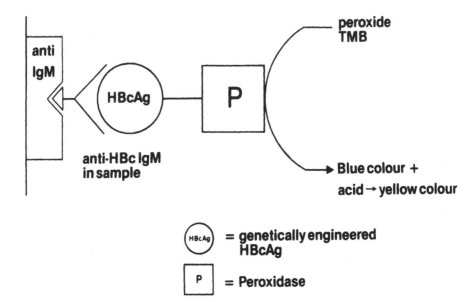

*Figure 2.* Anti-Hbc IgM assay. Monoclonal anti-human IgM is coated onto a solid support and incubated with the sample. The sample IgM is captured onto the support and washed to remove other Ig. Recombinant HBcAg, conjugated with horseradish peroxidase, is added and anti-HBc IgM-positive samples will capture the conjugate onto the solid phase. Colour will develop when TMB substrate is added.

Figure 1 outlines assays for HBeAg and anti-HBe which use monoclonals specific for different epitopes on HBeAg and HBeAg purified from a recombinant *E. coli* strain. The solid phase is coated with MAB and any HBeAg present is bound to the surface. A different MAB, conjugated with horseradish peroxidase, can react with the captured HBeAg to give a positive signal. If the same reaction contains a fixed amount of added recombinant HBeAg then anti-HBe antibodies are detected by competition with the conjugated MAB for binding to the HBeAg. These assays can be completed in as little as 2-2.5 hours especially if elevated incubation temperatures are used.

Figure 2 outlines an assay for anti-HBc IgM which uses monoclonal anti-human IgM and recombinant HBcAg conjugated with horseradish peroxidase. IgM in the sample is captured onto the solid phase and any anti-HBc specific antibody is detected by binding the conjugated HBeAg. This type of assay can be completed in 2.5 hours at room temperature.

Now that many of the constraints have been removed, our understanding of HBV has expanded greatly in the last few years. In particular the discovery of similar viruses (hepadna viruses) in ground squirrels, woodchucks and Pekin ducks (GSHV, WHV and DHV respectively) has lead to the development of alternative animal model systems which now allow us to study the biology of hepadna virus infection. Diagnostically, the most significant observations to come out of the work on both the human and animal viruses are that the viral proteins expressed during infection are more varied than at first thought and that all these proteins can provoke an immune response in at least some individuals. The importance of these markers will become clear in the next few years as their significance is assessed. Figure 3 mentions the more important ones.

## NEW HBV MARKERS

| | |
|---|---|
| pre–$S_1$/$S_2$ | Antibodies may be significant for virus neutralization and clearance |
| gene X | Unknown significance |
| DNA | Marker for the HBV genome |

*Figure 3.* The pre-S1 and pre-S2 antigens are the protein coding regions found preceding the part of the surface antigen gene which encodes HBsAg. It has been shown that these sequences can be expressed during infection and can be found on HBsAg particles. The X gene is an open reading frame found in all HBV serotypes and which has an equivalent region in other hepadna viruses but has no known function in the virus life-cycle. Antibodies to the potential gene product have been detected in some individuals. The use of DNA probes permits the direct detection of the viral genome rather than using inferential markers (HBsAg or HBeAg).

Responsiveness to the pre-S1 and pre-S2 regions of HBsAg may determine the outcome of an infection, so anti-pre-S1/2 could become an important clinical marker(s). Indeed a great deal of effort is going into the development of vaccines which contain these immunogens. Whilst it is clear that vaccines containing only HBsAg can induce protective immunity in the majority of recipients, there are a number of so-called non-responders. Work in mice suggests that pre-S epitopes improve the response to HBsAg epitopes, so these non-responders might need a vaccine formulation which contains both pre-S and S epitopes. So measurement of the anti-pre-S response could also be important in assessing the efficacy of a vaccination regime.

The use of DNA probes to detect HBV DNA in serum samples has been widely used in research over the last few years [12-14]. It has been shown that the usual markers for infectivity such as HBsAg and HBeAg do not always correlate with the presence of HBV DNA and, by implication, infectious virus [15-17]. However I do not envisage a DNA probe test becoming a screening assay for HBV infection. In part this is because, with the methodology currently available, the assays would take too long to perform. However the major reason is that the current screening tests have been effective in protecting the blood supply and it is difficult to see what advantage it would be to know that a donation was HBV DNA-positive rather than HBsAg-positive.

DNA probe assays will find, indeed have already found, a niche in monitoring the effect of chemotherapy on chronic carriers [18,19]. The more, indirect markers (HBsAg, HBeAg) often show a delayed response to antiviral treatment and active viral replication can be eliminated before these markers are reduced. In an even more specialised approach, probes can be used to examine the state of the HBV DNA in the infected hepatocytes, or other cell types, by Southern blotting. This technique can determine whether or not the viral sequences are integrated into the genome and whether active replication is occurring.

The importance of other markers such as the X protein is more speculative. This protein may be involved in regulation of HBV DNA expression in infected cells and so measuring the amount of HBxAg or anti-HBx *may* prove to be a marker for progression to liver damage and long-term prognosis [20,21].

Developing tests for all these new markers would have been very difficult if not impossible using conventional techniques. Indeed the pre-S and X antigens were unknown before the cloning, sequencing and expression of the HBV genome. These new findings have confirmed that HBV is a complex entity and it uses its rather frugal genetic information to produce a variety of proteins. It is possible to glimpse how the virus can be responsible for a range of disease conditions depending upon the interaction of these various proteins with the host.

The delta agent has been shown to be a defective virus (hepatitis delta virus, HDV) which uses HBV as its helper. Co-infection with HDV increases the severity of HBV associated disease in either the chronic or acute phases. As with HBV, the lack of a suitable culture system has hampered basic research on the virus and the development of good diagnostic tests. Recently the HDV genome has been cloned and it is now known that it consists of a single-stranded circular RNA approximately 1700 bases long [22]. Examination of the genomic sequence shows that there are a number of potential open reading frames (ORFs) which might code for the proteins of HDV. In particular, at least one ORF has been shown to encode a protein which can be recognised by sera from HDV-infected individuals. Clearly there will soon be one or more HDV-specific antigens available which could form the basis of diagnostic tests for HDV infection. This will represent a much more satisfactory source of material than infected serum.

To sum up then, the use of monoclonal antibodies, recombinant antigens and cloned DNA has changed the nature of the assays for viral hepatitis markers and increased the range of markers which can be monitored. This has been less noticeable for HBsAg testing because in this test conventional techniques have already been pushed to the limit. The major impact of these new tests will be for clinical diagnosis rather than blood screening except for HDV where improved screening tests should soon be available.

# References

1. Deinhardt F, Zuckerman AJ. Immunization against hepatitis B: Report on a WHO meeting on viral hepatitis in Europe. J Med Virol 1985;17:209-17.
2. Dane DS, Cameron CH, Briggs M. Virus-like particles in the serum of patients with Australia antigen associated hepatitis. Lancet 1970;i:695-700.
3. Burrell CJ, MacKay P, Greenaway PJ, Hofschneider PH, Murray K. Expression in *Escherichia coli* of hepatitis B virus DNA sequences cloned in plasmid pBR322. Nature (London) 1979;279:43-7.
4. Pasek M, Goto T, Gilbert W et al. Hepatitis B virus genes and their expression in *E. coli*. Nature (London) 1979;282:575-9.
5. Sninsky JJ, Siddiqui A, Robinson WS, Cohen SN. Cloning and endonuclease mapping of the hepatitis B viral genome. Nature (London) 1979;279:346-8.
6. Charnay P, Pourcel C, Louise A, Fritsch A, Tiollais P. Cloning in *Escherichia coli* and physical structure of hepatitis B virion DNA. Proc Natl Acad Sci (USA) 1979;76:2222-6.
7. Galibert F, Mandart E, Fitoussi F, Tiollais P, Charnay P. Nucleotide sequence of the hepatitis B virus genome (subtype ayw) cloned in *E. coli*. Nature (London) 1979;281:646-50.
8. Hardy K, Stahl S, Kupper H. Production in *B. subtilis* of hepatitis B core antigen and of major antigen of foot and mouth disease virus. Nature (London) 1981; 293:481-3.
9. Stahl S, MacKay P, Magazin M, Bruce SA, Murray K. Hepatitis B virus core antigen: Synthesis in *Escherichia coli* and application in diagnosis. Proc Natl Acad Sci (USA) 1982;79:1606-10.
10. MacKay P, Pasek M, Magazin M et al. Production of immunologically active surface antigens of hepatitis B virus by *Escherichia coli*. Proc Natl Acad Sci (USA) 1981;78:4510-4.
11. Valenzuela P, Medina A, Rutter WJ, Ammerer G, Hall BD. Synthesis and assembly of hepatitis B virus surface antigen particles in yeast. Nature (London) 1982;298:347-50.
12. Kam W, Rall LB, Smuckler EA, Schmid R, Rutter WJ. Hepatitis B viral DNA in liver and serum of asymptomatic carriers. Proc Natl Acad Sci (USA) 1982;79: 7522-6.
13. Berninger M, Hammer M, Hoyer B, Gerin JL. An assay for the detection of the DNA genome of hepatitis B virus in serum. J Med Virol 1982;9:57-68.
14. Weller IVD, Fowler MJF, Monjardino J, Thomas HC. The detection of HBV-DNA in serum by molecular hybridisation: A more sensitive method for the detection of complete HBV particles. J Med Virol 1982;9:273-80.
15. Harrison TJ, Bal V, Wheeler EG, Meacock TJ, Harrison JF, Zuckerman AJ. Hepatitis B virus DNA and e antigen in serum from blood donors in the United Kingdom positive for hepatitis B surface antigen. Br Med J 1985;290:663-4.
16. Scotto J, Hadchouel M, Hery C, Yvart J, Tiollais P, Brechot C. Detection of hepatitis B virus DNA in serum by a simple spot hybridisation technique: Comparison with results for other viral markers. Hepatology 1983;3:279-84.
17. Lieberman HM, LaBrecque DR, Kew MC, Hadziyannis SJ, Shafritz DA. Detection of hepatitis B virus DNA directly in human serum by a simplified molecular hybridisation test: Comparison to HBeAg/anti-HBe status in HBsAg carriers. Hepatology 1983;3:285-91.
18. Moestrup T, Hansson BG, Widell A, Blomberg J, Nordenfelt E. Hepatitis B virus-DNA in the serum of patients followed-up longitudinally with acute and chronic hepatitis B. J Med Virol 1985;17:337-44.

19. Bonino F, Recchia S, Farci P et al. Hepatitis B virus replication and clinical outcome in carriers of HBsAg. Perspectives of treatment with DNA inhibitors. Liver 1983;3:30-5.
20. Meyers ML, Trepo LV, Nath N, Sninsky JJ. Hepatitis B virus polypeptide X: Expression in *Escherichia coli* and identification of specific antibodies in sera from hepatitis B virus-infected humans. J Virol 1986;57:101-9.
21. Siddiqui A, Jameel S, Mapoles J. Expression of the hepatitis B virus X gene in mammalian cells. Proc Natl Acad Sci (USA) 1987;84:2513-7.
22. Wang KS, Choo QL, Weiner AJ et al. Structure, sequence and expression of the hepatitis delta viral genome. Nature (London) 1986;323:508-13.

# MONOCLONAL ANTIBODIES IN BLOOD COAGULATION

C.V. Prowse

In the last eight years, a considerable investment of time and money has led to the development of monoclonal antibodies (MAB) to most of the proteins involved in hemostasis. Table I lists some of these together with selected references. In the main, these reagents were developed in research laboratories as tools for the investigation of molecular structure and function. The availability of commercial reagents or MAB-based assay kits is still in its infancy compared, for example, to the situation in the field of hormone assays.

*Table 1.* Specificity of some monoclonal antibodies to hemostatic proteins.

| | |
|---|---|
| Factor XII [3,4] | Protein C [29,30] |
| Factor XI [5,6] | Protein S [31] |
| High molecular weight kininogen [7] | Protein Z [32]; |
| | Thrombomodulin [33] |
| Factor IX [8,9,10,11] | C4-binding protein [34] |
| Factor VIII [1]; | |
| Von Willebrand factor [1] | Antithrombin III [35] |
| Factor X [12] | Antiplasmin [36,37,38] |
| Factor V [13,14] | Antitrypsin [39] |
| Prothrombin [15,16] | Plasminogen activator inhibitors [40,41] |
| Fibrinogen [17,18] | Tissue plasminogen activator [42,43] |
| Tissue factor [19] | Urokinase [44,45] |
| Factor VII [20] | Plasminogen [37,46,47,48] |
| Fibrin [21,22,23] | Fibrin degradation products [49,50,51] |
| Factor XIII [24] | C1-inhibitor [52] |
| Fibronectin [25,26,27] | Thrombospondin [53,54] |
| Thrombin [28] | Platelet factor 4 [55] |

Antibodies or antisera have been used for many years in the study of hemostasis. MAB offer the potential advantage of precise specificity and the ability to repeatedly make large quantities of the reagent. Given these properties, a number of applications of MAB in the study of hemostasis may be considered apart from the fundamental investigation of structure and function mentioned above. These include their use in various forms of immunoassay and chromatographic procedures designed to purify or remove materials from complex mixtures, as well as their potential use as direct inhibitors of molecular function or as therapeutic agents. In this survey, which is not a comprehensive review, examples will be given for each of these potential applications in the field of human hemostasis. Where the appropriate

92

reagents are commercially available, this will be indicated. It should be noted that, while MAB offer advantages for some applications, polyclonal reagents may be preferable for others.

## Structure – function relationships

Perhaps best the example of this has been the investigations performed on Von Willebrand factor (vWf). There are a large number of MAB described that react with this protein [1]. Amongst these are ones that inhibit the reaction between platelet glycoprotein Ib (GP.Ib) and vWf in the presence of ristocetin, between collagen and vWf, between GP.IIb/IIIa on activated platelets and vWf and between the adhesion of platelets to sub-endothelial components at high shear as well as MAB that prolong the bleeding time when given to animals. Use of MAB unequivocally demonstrates that such activities are due to vWf and further allow the assignment of functional sites within the molecule. This has been done for vWf and other molecules by assessing the binding of molecular fragments to MAB with defined inhibitory activities. Figure 1 summarizes the results of such studies for vWf. Furthermore, by performing competition-binding studies between such MAB, an epitope map giving some idea of the three-dimensional relationships between various binding/activity sites may be obtained [2].

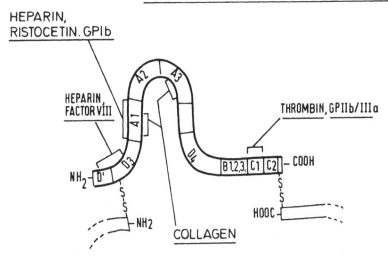

*Figure 1.* Structure-function of Von Willebrand factor.
A, B, C and D refer to internal sequence homologies within the vWf subunit. The multimeric, antiparallel arrangement of subunits is denoted by fragments of the adjacent subunits. Functional sites within the subunit for interaction with Factor VIII, heparin, GP.Ib, collagen and GP.IIb/IIIa are indicated.

Other examples of such studies include the confirmation of platelet membrane glycoprotein involvement in congenital [56,57] or acquired immune deficiency diseases [58] as well as attempts to demonstrate their involvement in the storage defect of platelets which develops during blood component storage [59]. While such studies are fundamental to our understanding of the mechanics of hemostasis, their routine application is likely to be indirect and to involve one of the following techniques.

## Immunoassays

Classically, most immunoassays using animal antisera have used limiting amounts of antibody and relied on competition between the antigen of interest and small amounts of pure labelled antigen e.g. radioimmunoassay. This has recently become less true with the increasing use of enzyme-linked immunoassays (ELISA). While competitive assays have been described [38,60] in view of their availability in large amounts as pure preparations MAB are usually better suited to assays in which excess labelled antibody is used e.g. ELISA or immunoradiometric assays (IRMA).

Currently most such assays are performed in multiwell microtitre trays or plastic beads are employed and the sandwich principle is used in which one antibody is used to capture the antigen and a second (labelled) non-crossreactive antibody is used to detect the antigen. If the antigen exhibits polymorphism, the use of MAB may be disadvantageous if the antibody does not bind all forms of the molecule and if the assay is designed to detect the total amount of antigen present. This has been observed, for example, by Thompson, when comparing the use of polyclonal and monoclonal antibodies in the assay of Factor IX [61] and has led to the use of cocktails of MABs e.g. in IRMAs for Factor VIIIC:Ag [62] and urokinase (u-PA) [45] and in the Western blotting of partially degraded vWf [63]. Such restricted specificity can be turned to advantage; it is in such applications that MAB have a true advantage over conventional reagents.

Figure 2 schematically represents some of these applications. For total antigen assays, MAB really only have an advantage where it is very difficult to obtain pure antigen. With the increasing difficulty of obtaining human antibody to Factor VIIIC:Ag that can be guaranteed non-infective and given the low immunogenicity of this protein in animals, a MAB based assay for Factor VIIIC:Ag may represent one such application. Such assays have been described by Vermeer et al [62] and Rotblat et al [64] but they have yet to be developed for or assessed in routine use.

Assays which detect only certain forms of an antigen (Figure 2B) are exemplified by ones detecting Factor IX types that do or do not bind calcium [65] or discriminate between the position 148 threonine and alanine molecular forms [11,66,67] and assays that only detect the active form of tissue-type plasminogen activator (t-PA) [43,68]. These have potential applciations in determining the extent of Factor IX carboxylation e.g. during coumarin therapy or in monitoring cell cultures, as an alternative to gene probing in the diagnosis of hemophilia B and in monitoring fibrinolytic therapy.

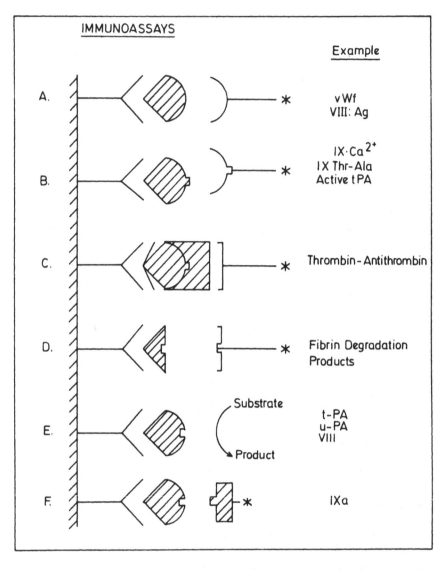

*Figure 2.* Possible variants of 2-site antibody assays.

A. Total antigen assay.

B. Assay to detect only one form of a polymorphic antigen.

C. Detection of bimolecular complex.

D. Assay to detect neoantigens.

E. Bioimmunoassay.

F. Probing of active site with labelled inhibitor.

A somewhat different application is in detecting antigens that are only formed during the activation, degradation or complexing of the parent molecule (neoantigens, Figure 2D). Assays developed on this basis, such as that described by Whitaker et al [69], which allows detection of the fibrin degradation product D-dimer in plasma since it is insensitive to the parent fibrinogen, represent one of the few applications for which a commercially MAB-based kit is available. An alternative approach for the assays of complexes, e.g. between enzyme and inhibitor, is to use a sandwich in which the two antibodies are directed to the two separate components of the complex (Figure 2C). Holvoet et al [47] have described such an assay for plasmin-antiplasmin complexes.

Lastly, MAB which are not inhibitory may be used to remove proteins from complex mixtures without affecting their activity. The bound active molecule may then be detected directly by the addition of the appropriate substrate as in the bioimmunoassays described for t-PA [70], u-PA [71] or Factor VIII [72] (Figure 2E). Alternatively, the active moiety may be detected indirectly (Figure 2F) as in the IRMA for vWf, which corresponds to the ristocetin cofactor activity [73] or the assay of Factor IXa, which makes use of radiolabelled antithrombin as an active site probe [74]. Combination assays are also possible, such as that described by Wotja et al [75], in which t-PA is captured and its activity and antigen contents determined sequentially, thereby allowing the determination of active and inactive forms of t-PA in the same sample.

Few of the assays described above have been used on a routine basis; nor is the development of more sensitive and faster assays, based on the use of fluorescent labels, fluid phase reactions or immobilization on latex particles [20] in place of plastic microtrays or large beads, likely to improve this situation. However other assays which make use of MAB for probing, such as the blotting of electrophoretically separated proteins or the immuno histological staining of tissues, may be more readily adopted in routine diagnostic and laboratory procedures. Examples of these include the staining of electrophoretically separated vWf multimers or protein degradation products in the diagnosis of Von Willebrand's disease [63,76], the staining of t-PA, vWf and Factor VIII in cultured cells or tissue sections [44,77,78] and the Western blotting Factor VIII as part of the characterization of therapeutic Factor VIII concentrates [79].

While MAB-based immunoassay kits for hemostatic proteins have yet to be developed commercially in any number (assays for fibrin D-dimer and plasminogen activator inhibitor 1 are available), a range of MAB is available, either as ascites or purified immunoglobulins, from most of the established immunological reagent suppliers (e.g. Atlantic Antibodies, American Diagnostics, Cappel Laboratories, Dako, Hybritech, Seralab, Serotec, etc.) as well as a number of more specialized suppliers (e.g. Australian Monoclonal Antibody Development, Bioclone Australia, Biopool, Bioscot, MAbCo, Monozyme, Porton Products, Scottish Antibody Production Unit, etc.).

## Purification and depletion

The use of MAB to purify human Factors VIII [80,81] and V [82] has been an essential step in the isolation and subsequent sequencing and cloning of these two labile proteins. Corresponding processes have been described for other hemostatic proteins (Table 2), one of the more interesting being that from Dr. Mann's group, in which sequential chromatography on 5 distinct MAB columns allows the isolation of the whole range of vitamin K-dependent coagulation factors from the barium citrate eluate of human plasma [83].

*Table 2.* Some hemostatic proteins purified by monoclonal antibody immunochromatography.

Factor VIII [80,81,84,85,86,87]
Factor V [82]
Vitamin K dependent Factors (II, VII, IX, X, C, S)
[12,20,30,31,83,88,89,90,91,92]
Plasminogen activators (t-PA and u-PA) [93,94,95,96]
Factor XI [5,97]
Factor XII [3,4]
C.1.inhibitor [52]
Plasminogen activator inhibitor [40,98,99]
Factor IX [83,88,100,101]
Tissue factor [19]
Factor XIII [24]
Plasminogen [48]

In most instances, elution requires chaotropic eluants or buffers of extreme pH. Ethylene glycol is often a constituent of elution buffers. Elution under milder conditions is obviously preferable, but it requires either a large amount of luck or a great deal of forward planning in MAB selection. Furthermore, the choice of coupling chemistry and support gel type may be critical [87]. Calcium-dependent MAB allow purification (e.g. of Factor IX [100]) by elution with EDTA, while the development of a pH-dependent antibody to vWf has enabled the isolation of both vWf and Factor VIII from human plasma [86]. Alternatively, MAB to proteins which complex the protein of interest may be used to purify the latter by elution for the chromatographic gel with buffers which disrupt either the antibody complex or the internal protein: protein bonding within the complex. Thus, 0.25 M calcium may be used to elute Factor VIII from an anti-vWf gel loaded with vWf-Factor VIII complex [80] or PA inhibitor complexed to t-PA purified using anti-t-PA

*Table 3.* Actual and potential therapeutic products obtained using monoclonal antibodies.

| Process | Contains | Antibody to | Elution buffer |
|---|---|---|---|
| Hemofil M (Hyland)* | Factor VIII | Factor VIII | 50% ethylene glycol |
| Monoclate (Armour)* [80] | Factor VIII | vWf | 0.25 M calcium |
| Immunotech [86] | Factor VIII/vWf | vWf | Triethanolamine pH 8.5 |
| K Smith [100] | Factor IX | Factor IX (Ca$^{2+}$ dependent) | EDTA |
| H Bessos [88] | Factor IX | Factor IX | Ethylene glycol pH 10 or 7 M urea pH 7 |
| M Einarrson [96] | t-PA | t-PA | 3 M KSCN |

* At clinical trial.

[99]. Immobilized MAB have also been used to separate or concentrate protein C [102] and vWf [79] from interfering substances to allow their assay in situations where this is not directly possible in plasma.

Some of these processes are now being applied to the production of therapeutic products, two Factor VIII preparations being at clinical trial at present (Table 3). Other processes that are potentially applicable to the production of therapeutic products (Factor VIII, IX, t-PA) are also listed in Table 3. Such products, which may be highly purified, have been claimed to have clinical benefits in patient management e.g. in reducing the immunosuppressive effect of therapy in hemophiliacs [106], although the evidence for this must at best be regarded as preliminary. More immediately, it seems likely that many of the recombinant products that are currently being developed in the area of hemostasis will be purified, at least initially, by MAB immunoaffinity chromatography.

Depletion of human plasma by MAB immunoaffinity chromatography has been described for a range of coagulation factors (Table 4); and plasmas depleted of Factors VIII (±vWf), IX or VII are commercially available (Table 5).

*Table 4.* Protein depletion of normal plasma using monoclonal antibodies.

Factor VIII [103]
Factor IX [8]
Factor VII [89]
Fibronectin [104]
Factor XI [5]
Factor XII [3,4]
Protein C [105]

*Table 5.* Commercially available immunodepleted plasmas.

**Factor VIII and vWf depleted**
Diagen/Porton products [103]
Mertz and Dade
Stago

**Factor VIII depleted**
Organon-Teknika

**Factor IX**
Diagen/Porton products [8]
Organon-Teknika

**Factor VII**
Diagen/Porton products

*Figure 3.* Comparison of congenitally deficient and monoclonal antibody depleted plasma in one-stage assays of coagulation factors.

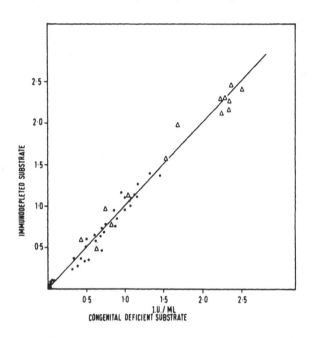

*Figure 3A.* Factor VIII/vWf depleted plasma (depleted with immobilised MAB to vWf, ESvWf 8 and Factor VIII, ESH5 and ESH8). ● plasma samples, △ Factor VIII concentrates (plotted on one fifth scale). r = 0.99, regression; slope = 1.000.

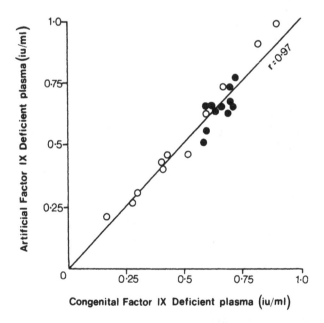

*Figure 3B.* Factor IX depleted plasma (depleted with MAB ESN3). ● normal plasmas, ○ plasma from coumarin treated patients. r = 0.97; slope = 0.998.

Such products are intended for use as substrates in the one-stage assay of the corresponding factors and, as such, represent products based on MAB technology that are available now and have an advantage (potentially less infective and cheaper) than the established reagents. Comparison of congenitally deficient plasma with such depleted plasmas shows that they may be used for assays of normal and patient plasmas and of therapeutic concentrates [3,4,8,88,103]. Figure 3 shows some results from such a comparison of Factor VIII/vWf and Factor IX depleted plasmas obtained in the author's laboratory. One preliminary report has indicated that congenitally deficient and Factor VIII/vWf depleted plasmas might yield discrepant results for Factor VIII concentrates of very high purity and that this could be minimized by the addition of pure vWf [107]. These observations require further study.

## Miscellaneous and therapeutic applications

High affinity MAB to the active site region of enzymes or the active regions of cofactors can rapidly inhibit their activity. Where simpler specific inhibitors are unavailable, such MAB may be used to quench activity. This can be useful in establishing the identity of proteins, such as those produced by recombinant technology, and in removing single proteins without interfering in the assays of other hemostatic proteins. Thus MAB to the active site of t-PA have been used in the anticoagulant for blood sampling during thrombolytic therapy to quench t-PA without interference in the assay of other fibrinolytic parameters [67,108].

An area of increasing interest in which MAB should prove useful tools is the interaction between hemostatic proteins and cells. MAB have already been used in the study of platelets by the technique of fluorescence-activated cell sorting to show an increased exposure of alpha-granule membrane glycoprotein during thrombin activation, but not during extracorporeal circulation, which results in decreased surface exposure of GP.IIb/IIIa [109,110]. Direct MAB binding assays show a decreased exposure of platelet GP.IIb/IIIa during passage through bubble oxygenators [111], an increased exposure of Mr 53,000 platelet granule protein during bypass operations [121] and no change in GP.Ib exposure during platelet concentrate storage [59]. Use of MAB to hemostatic proteins in similar studies should provide useful data on the distribution of coagulation factors on cells during the process of hemostasis.

In the therapeutic arena, MAB may be of direct therapeutic benefit or be used to target other therapeutic agents. Both approaches have been extensively studied in the cancer field, but only a few examples exist in hemostasis, and these have yet to be applied in man. MAB, or their Fab fragments, have been used to promote the binding of plasminogen activators to fibrin clots *in vitro* [112,113] as well as to allow the location (imaging, after radiolabelling) of thrombin in animal models [114]. Recent experiments by Coller et al [115] suggest that, in animals, certain MAB to GP.IIb/IIIa may have a direct antithrombotic effect, while the development of anti-idiotypic antibodies to Factor VIII MAB has potential applications in the treatment of hemophiliacs who have developed inhibitors to Factor VIII [116].

Use of recombinant techniques has recently been used to locate the binding site of MAB within the t-PA and Factor IX molecules by assessment of their binding to fragments of the Factor IX molecule [117] or deletion mutants of t-PA [118]. Inversion of this procedure to demonstrate the presence of selected epitopes within recombinant or plasma-derived heat-treated proteins by their ability to bind MAB [60,119,120] should prove useful in the characterization of such products.

## Conclusions

Since the author last reviewed this field [119], the main developments have been in the development of bioimmunoassays, the MAB purification of therapeutic products and in the availablility of immunodepleted plasmas. While these latter products are now a reality in the field of immunoassay, there has been little development of commercial kits, although many more assay examples have been described, and hence of the possibility of their widespread use. For the future, it seems likely that, in addition to further developments in the above areas, the major new areas of MAB application will be in the study of cellular interactions and recombinant products and, possibly, in the development of direct therapeutic products.

## References

1. Goodall AH, Meyer D. Registry of monoclonal antibodies to factor VIII and von Willebrand factor. Thromb Haemost 1985;54:878-91.
2. Meyer D, Baumgartner HD, Edington TS. Relative role of intramolecular loci in mediation of platelet adhesion to the subendothelium. Br J Haematol 1984;57: 602-20.
3. Saito H, Ishihara T, Suzuki H, Watanabe T. Production and characterization of a murine monoclonal antibody against heavy chain of Hageman factor (factor XII). Blood 1985;65:1263-8.
4. Small EJ, Katzmann JA, Tracy RP, Ratnoff OD, Goldsmith GH, Everson B. A monoclonal antibody that inhibits activation of human Hageman factor (factor XII). Blood 1985;65:202-10.
5. Sinha D, Koshy A, Seamen FS, Walsh PN. Functional characterization of human blood coagulation factor XIa using hybridoma antibodies. J Biol Chem 1985;260:10714-9.
6. Akiyama H, Sinha AD, Seamen FS, Kirby EP, Walsh PN. Mechanism of activation of coagulation factor XI by factor XIIa studied with monoclonal antibodies. J Clin Invest 1986;78:1631-7.
7. Berrettini M, Lammle B, White T et al. Detection of in vitro and in vivo cleavage of high molecular weight kininogen in human plasma by immunoblotting with monoclonal antibodies. Blood 1986;68:455-62.
8. Goodall AH, Kemble G, O'Brien DP et al. Preparation of factor IX-deficient human plasma by immunoaffinity chromatography using a monoclonal antibody. Blood 1982;59:664-70.
9. Bajaj SP, Rapaport SI, Maki SL. A monoclonal antibody to factor IX that inhibits the factor VIII: Ca potentiation of factor X activation. J Biol Chem 1985;260:11574-80.

10. Bessos H, Micklem LR, McCann M et al. The characterisation of a panel of monoclonal antibodies to human coagulation factor IX. Thromb Res 1985;40: 863-8.
11. Smith KJ. Monoclonal antibodies to coagulation factor IX define a high frequency polymorphism by immunoassays. Am J Hum Genet 1985;37:668-79.
12. Church WR, Mann KG. A simple purification of human factor X using a high affinity monoclonal antibody immunoadsorbant. Thromb Res 1985;38:417-24.
13. Katzmann JA. Isolation of functional human coagulation factor V by using a hybridoma antibody. Proc Natl Acad Sci (USA) 1978;78:162-6.
14. Annamalai AE, Rao AK, Chiu HC et al. Epitope mapping of functional domains of human factor Va with human and murine monoclonal antibodies: evidence for the interaction of heavy chain with factor Xa and calcium. Blood 1987;70:139-46.
15. Malhotra OP, Sudilovsky O. Monoclonal antibodies to prothrombin. Thromb Res 1987;47:501-10.
16. Owens J, Lewis RM, Cantor A, Furie BC, Furie B. Monoclonal antibodies against human abnormal (des-gamma-carboxy) prothrombin specific for the calicum-free conformer of prothrombin. J Biol Chem 1984;259:13800-5.
17. Sola B, Avner PR, Zilber MT, Connan F, Levy D. Isolation and characterisation of a monoclonal antibody specific for fibrinogen & fibrin of human origin. Thromb Res 1983;29:643-53.
18. Francis SE, Joshua DE, Exner T, Kronenberg H. Some studies with a monoclonal antibody directed against human fibrinogen. Am J Hematol 1985;18:111-9.
19. Carson SD, Ross SE, Bach R, Guha A. An inhibitory monoclonal antibody against human tissue factor. Blood 1987;70:490-3.
20. Broze GJ, Hickman S, Miletich JP. Monoclonal anti-human factor VII antibodies: detection in plasma of a second protein antigenically & genetically related to factor VII. J Clin Invest 1985;76:937-46.
21. Kudryk B, Rohova A, Ahadi M, Chin J, Wiebe ME. Specificity of a monoclonal antibody for the $NH_2$-terminal region of fibrin. Mol Immunol 1984;21: 89-94.
22. Muller-Berghaus G, Scheevers-Borchel U, Fuhge P, Eberle R, Heimburger N. Detection of fibrin in plasma by a monoclonal antibody against the amino terminus of the alpha chain of fibrin. Sc J Clin Lab Invest 1985;45(suppl 178):145-51.
23. Hui KY, Haber E, Matsueda GR. Monoclonal antibodies of predetermined specificity for fibrin – a rational approach to monoclonal antibody production. Hybridoma 1986;5:215-22.
24. Gniewek RA, Kurosky A. Immunological characterization of human plasma factor XIII including monoclonal antibodies. Fed Proc 1987;46:2244.
25. Dziadek M, Richter H, Schachner M, Timpl R. Monoclonal antibodies used as probes for the structural organisation of the central region of fibronectin. FEBS Lett 1983;155:321-5.
26. Reinders JH, de Groot PG, Dawes J et al. Comparison of secretion & subcellular localisation of von Willebrand protein with that of thrombospondin and fibronectin in cultured human vascular endothelial cells. Biochim Biophys Acta 1985; 844:306-13.
27. Dixit VM, Haverstik DM, O'Rourke K et al. Inhibition of platelet aggregation by a monoclonal antibody against human fibronectin. Proc Natl Acad Sc 1985; 82:3844-8.
28. Dawes J, James K, Micklem L, McClelland DBL, Pepper DS, Prowse CV. Monoclonal antibodies directed against human $\alpha$-thrombin and the thrombin-

102

antithrombin complex. Thromb Res 1985;36:397-409.
29. Suzuki K, Matsuda Y, Kasumoto H et al. Monoclonal antibodies to human protein C: Effects on the biological activity of activated protein C & the thrombin-catalysed activation of protein C. J Biochem 1985;97:127-38.
30. Laurell M, Ikeda K, Lindgren S, Stenflo J. Characterization of monoclonal antibodies against human protein C specific for the calcium ion-induced conformation or for the activation peptide region. FEBS Lett 1985;191:75-81.
31. Litwiller RD, Jenny RJ, Katzmann JA, Miller RS, Mann KG. Monoclonal antibodies to human vitamin K-dependent protein S. Blood 1986;67:1583-90.
32. Miletich JP, Broze GJ. Human plasma protein Z antigen: Range in normal subjects & effect of warfarin therapy. Blood 1987;69:1580-6.
33. Maruyama I, Majerus PW. The turnover of thrombin-thrombomodulin complex in cultured human umbilical vein endothelial cells and A549 lung cancer cells: Endocytosis and degradation of thrombin. J Biol Chem 1985;260:15432-8.
34. Comp PC, Thurnau GR, Welsh J, Esmon C. Functional and immunological protein S levels are decreased during pregnancy. Blood 1986;68:881-5.
35. Herion P, Francott M, Siberdt D, Soto GG, Urbain J, Bollen A. Monoclonal antibodies against plasma protease inhibitors – production & characterisation of 15 monoclonal antibodies against human antithrombin III – relation between antigen determined and functional sites of antithrombin III. Blood 1985;65:1201-7.
36. Herion P, Siberdt D, Soto GG, Urbain J, Bollen A. Monoclonal antibodies against plasma protease inhibitors:. I: Production and characterisation of 23 monoclonal antibodies against alpha -2-antiplasmin. Biosc Rep 1984;4:39-48.
37. Hattey E, Wojta J, Binder BR. Monoclonal antibodies against plasminogen and alpha-2-antiplasmin: Binding to native and modified antigens. Thromb Res 1987;45:485-95.
38. Wotja J, Korninger C, Kirchheim J, Hattey E, Turcu L, Binder BR. Practical applications of monoclonal antibodies to the diagnosis of disturbances of fibrinolysis. Wien Klin Wochenschr 1985;97:244-8.
39. Herion P, Siberdt D, Francotte M, Urbain J, Bollen A. Monoclonal antibodies against plasma protease inhibitors. II: Production and characterisation of 25 monoclonal antibodies against hman $\alpha_1$-antitrypsin: Correlation between antigen structure and functional sites. Biosc Rep 1984;4:139-47.
40. Lecander I, Astedt B. Isolation of a new specific plasminogen activator inhibitor from pregnancy plasma. Br J Haematol 1986;62:221-8.
41. Nielsen LS, Lecander I, Andreasan PA, Henschen A, Astedt B, Dano K. Plasminogen activator inhibitors from placenta and fibrosarcoma cells are antigenically different as evaluated with monoclonal and polyclonal antibodies. Thromb Res 1987;46:411-23.
42. Wallen P, Bergsdorf N, Pohl G, Stigbrand T. Differentiation of one-chain and two-chain tissue type plasminogen activation by monoclonal antibodies. Haemostasis 1984;14:42(ab).
43. Mac Gregor IR, Micklem LR, James K, Pepper DS. Characterisation of epitopes on human tissue plasminogen activator recognised by a group of monoclonal antibodies. Thromb Haemost 1985;53:45-51.
44. Dano K, Dabelste E, Nielsen LS, Kaltoft K, Wilson EL, Zeuthen J. Plasminogen activating enzyme in cultured glioblastoma cells – an immunofluorescence study with monoclonal antibody. J Histochem Cytochem 1982;30:1165-70.
45. Darras V, Thienpon M, Stump DC, Collen D. Measurement of urokinase type plasminogen activator with an enzyme-linked immunosorbent assay (ELISA) based on 3 murine monoclonal antibodies. Thromb Haemost 1986;56:411-4.

46. Ploplis VA, Cummings HS, Castell FJ. Monoclonal antibodies to discrete regions of human glu-1-plasminogen. Biochemistry 1982;21:5891-7.
47. Holvoet P, Lijnen HR, Collen D. A monoclonal antibody specific for lys-plasminogen – application to the study of the activation pathways of plasminogen in vivo. J Biol Chem 1985;260:2106-11.
48. Sim PS, Fayle DRH, Dee WF, Stephens RW. Monoclonal antibodies inhibitory to human plasmin – definitive demonstration of a role for plasmin in activating the proenzyme of urokinase type plasminogen activator. Eur J Biochem 1986; 158:537-42.
49. Elms MJ, Bunce IH, Bundesen PG et al. Measurement of cross-linked fibrin degradation products – an immunoassay using monoclonal antibodies. Thromb Haemost 1983;50:591-4.
50. McCable RP, Lamm DL, Haspel MV et al. A diagnostic prognostic test for bladder cancer using a monoclonal antibody based enzyme-linked immunoassay for detection of urinary fibrin(ogen) degradation products. Cancer Res 1984;44: 5886-93.
51. Haverkate F, Koopman J, Koppert P, Nieuwenhuizen W. Determination of fibrin(ogen) degradation products (FDP) in plasma, using a monoclonal antibody. Scand J Clin Lab Invest 1985;45:153.
52. Alsenz J, Loos M. Simplifed methods for the purification, quantitation and functional estimation of human complement C-1-inhibitor with a monoclonal anti-C-1-inhibitor. J Immunol Methods 1987;96:107-14.
53. Clezardin P, McGregor JL, Manach M, Robert F, Dechavanne M, Clemetson KJ. Isolation of thrombospondin released from thrombin stimulated platelets by fast protein liquid chromatography on an anion exchange mono Q column. J Chromatogr 1984;296:249-56.
54. Lawler J, Derick LH, Conolly JE, Chen JH, Chao FC. The structure of human platelet thrombospondin. J Biol Chem 1985;260:3762-72.
55. Ciaglowski RE, Martinez J, Ryan TJ et al. Monoclonal antibodies to bovine platelet factor 4 – species interaction to platelets and megakaryocytes using indirect immunocytofluorescence. Thromb Res 1986;41:855-65.
56. Johnston GI, Heptinstall S, Robins RA, Price MR. The expression of glycoproteins on single blood platelets from healthy individuals and from patients with congenital bleeding disorders. Biochem Biophys Res Commun 1984;123:1091-8.
57. Montgomery RR, Kunicki T, Taves C, Pidard D, Corcoran M. The diagnosis of Bernard-Soulier syndrome and Glanzmann's thrombasthenia with a monoclonal assay on whole blood. J Clin Invest 1983;71:385-9.
58. Varnon D, Karpatkin S. A monoclonal anti-platelet antibody with decreased reactivity for autoimmune thrombocytopenic platelets. Proc Natl Acad Sci (USA) 1983;80:6992-5.
59. Taylor MA, Anstee DJ. The use of functional and quantitative assays to study glycoprotein Ib in platelets stored under various in vitro conditions. Thromb Haemost 1984;52:271-5.
60. Bloom JW, Mitra G. Monoclonal antibody binding to factor VIII:C. Thromb Res 1986;44:207-16.
61. Thompson AR. Monoclonal antibody to an epitope on the heavy chain of factor IX missing in 3 haemophilia B patients. Blood 1983;62:1027-34.
62. Veerman ECI, Stel HV, Huisman JG, van Mourik JA. Application of sepharose-linked monoclonal antibodies for the immunoradiometric measurement of factor VIII procoagulant antigen. Thromb Res 1984;33:89-93.
63. Battle J, Lopez-Fernandez MF, Lopez-Borrasce A et al. Proteolytic degradation of von Willebrand factor after DDAVP administration in normal individuals. Blood 1987;70:173-6.

64. Rotblat F, Goodall AH, O'Brien DP, Rawlings E, Middleton S, Tuddenham EGD. Monoclonal antibodies to human procoagulant factor VIII. J Lab Clin Med 1983;101:736-46.
65. Bray GL, Thompson AR. Partial factor IX protein in a pedigree with haemophilia B due to partial gene deletion. J Clin Invest 1986;77:1194-200.
66. Smith KJ. Monoclonal antibodies to coagulation factor IX define a high frequency polymorphism by immunoassays. Am J Hum Genet 1985;37:668-79.
67. Wallmark A, Ljung R, Nilsson IM et al. Polymorphism of normal factor IX detection by mouse monoclonal antibodies. Proc Natl Acad Sci (USA) 1985;82: 3839-43.
68. Holvoet P, Boes J, Collen D. Measurement of a free, one chain tissue-type plasminogen activator in human plasma with an enzyme-linked immunosorbant assay based on an active-site-specific murine monoclonal antibody. Blood 1987; 69:284-9.
69. Whitaker AN, Elms MJ, Masci PP et al. Measurement of cross-linked fibrin derivatives in plasma – an immunoassay using monoclonal antibodies. J Clin Pathol 1984;37:882-7.
70. Mahmoud M, Gaffney PJ. Bioimmunoassay (BIA) of tissue plasminogen activator and its specific inhibitor. Thromb Haemost 1985;53:356-9.
71. Corti A, Nolli ML, Cassani G. Differential detection of single chain and 2-chain urokinase type plasminogen activator by a new immunoadsorbent-amidolytic assay. Thromb Haemost 1986;56:407-10.
72. Yoshioka A, Nakagawa O, Uehara Y et al. In vitro characterisation of various heat-treated prothrombin complex concentrates. Thromb Res 1987;47:449-58.
73. Goodall AH, Jarvis J, Chand S et al. An immunoradiometric assay for human factor VIII/von Willebrand factor (VIII:vWf) using a monoclonal antibody that defines a functional epitope. Br J Haematol 1985;59:565-77.
74. Enfield DL, Thompson AR. Factor IX (IX) activation: cleavage of IX and detection of factor IXa by a novel active site directed, immunospecific assay. Circulation 1982;66(suppl 11, ab 694):173.
75. Wotja J, Turcu L, Wagner OF, Korninger C, Binder BR. Evaluation of fibrinolytic capacity by a combined assay system for tissue type plasminogen activator antigen and function using monoclonal anti-tissue plasminogen activator antibodies. J Lab Clin Med 1987;109:665-71.
76. Enayat MS, Hill FGH, Robinson W, Prowse CV, Hornsey VS. Evaluation of monoclonal antibodies to vWf antigen for use in autoradiography vWf multimer analysis. Thromb Haemost 1987;57:217-21.
77. Warhol MJ, Sweet JM. The ultrastructural localisation of von Willebrand factor in endothelial cells. Am J Pathol 1984;117:310-5.
78. Stel HV, van der Kwast TH, Veerman ECI. Detection of factor VIII coagulation antigen in human liver tissue. Nature 1983;303:530-2.
79. Furlong RA, Welch AN, Peake IR. Monoclonal antibodies to factor VIII: Their application in immunoblotting for the visualisation of factor VIII in therapeutic concentrates and plasma. Br J Haematol 1987;66:341-8.
80. Fulcher CA, Roberts JR, Zimmerman TS. Thrombin proteolysis of purified factor VIII procoagulant protein: Correlation of activation with generation of specific polypeptide. Blood 1983;61:807-11.
81. Fulcher CA, Roberts JR, Holland LZ, Zimmerman TS. Human factor VIII procoagulant protein-monoclonal antibodies define precursor product relationships and functional epitopes. J Clin Invest 1985;76:117-24.
82. Foster WB, Tucker M, Katzmann JA, Miller RS, Nesheim ME, Mann KG. Monocolonal antibodies to human coagulation factor V and factor Va. Blood 1983;61:1060-7.

83. Jenny R, Church W, Odegaard B, Litwiller R, Mann KG. Purification of six human vitamin K-dependent proteins in a single chromatographic step using immunoaffinity columns. Prep Biochem 1986;16:227-45.
84. Rotblat F, O'Brien DP, O'Brien FJ, Goodhall AH, Tuddenham EGD. Purification of human factor VIII:C and its characterization by western blotting using monoclonal antibodies. Biochemistry 1985;24:4294-300.
85. Croissant MP, Vandepol H, Lee HH, Allain JP. Characterisation of four monoclonal antibodies to factor VIII coagulant protein and their use in immunopurification of factor VIII. Thromb Haemost 1986;56:271-6.
86. Bourgois A, Delzay M, Fert V. Process for obtaining complex factor VIII/vWf of therapeutical use and resulting products. US Patent 1987;4:670,543.
87. Hornsey VS, Griffin BD, Pepper DS, Micklem LP, Prowse CV. Immunoaffinity purification of factor VIII complex. Thromb Haemost 1987;57:102-5.
88. Bessos H, Prowse CV. Immunopurification of human coagulation factor IX using monoclonal antibodies. Thromb Haemost 1986;56:86-9.
89. Cerkus AL, Ofosu FA, Birchall KJ et al. The immunodepletion of factor VII from human plasma using a monoclonal antibody. Br J Haematol 1985;61: 467-75.
90. Yan SB, Grinnell BW. Characterisation of fully functional recombinant human protein C (rHPC) expressed from the human kidney 293 cells. Fed Proc 1986; 46:2243.
91. Litwiller RP, Jenny RJ, Katzmann JA, Miller RS, Mann KG. Monoclonal antibodies to human vitamin-K dependent protein S. Blood 1986;67:1583-90.
92. Moore KL, Andreoli SP, Esmon NL, Esmon CT, Bang NU. Endotoxin enhances tissue factor and suppresses thrombomodulin expression of human vascular endothelium in vitro. J Clin Invest 1987;79:124-30.
93. Neilsen LS, Hansen JG, Andreasen PA, Skriver L, Dano K, Zeuthen J. Monoclonal antibody to human 66 000 molecular plasminogen activator from melanoma cells – specific inhibition and one-step affinity purification. Embo J 1983;2:115-9.
94. Grondahl-Hanson J, Nielsen LS, Andreasen PA et al. Monoclonal antibodies against human urokinase-type and tissue-type plasminogen activators & their use in indentification of mature proenzyme forms. Haemostasis 1984;14:42(ab).
95. Schleef RR, Sinha M, Loskutoff DJ. Characterisation of two monoclonal antibodies against human tissue-type plasminogen activator. Thromb Haemost 1985;53:170-5.
96. Einarsson M, Brandt J, Kaplan L. Large scale purification of human tissue-type plasminogen activator using monoclonal antibodies. Biochim Biophys Acta 1985;830:1-10.
97. Wang H, Steiner J, Battey F, Strickland D. An immunoaffinity method for the purification of human factor IX. Fed Proc 1986;46:2119.
98. Nielsen LS, Andreasen PA, Grondahl J, Huang JY, Kristensen P, Dano K. Monoclonal antibodies to human 54 000 molecular weight plasminogen activator inhibitor from fibrosarcoma cells – inhibitor neutralisation and one-step affinity purification. Thromb Haemost 1986;55:206-12.
99. Philips M, Juul AG, Thorsen S, Selmer J, Zeuthen J. Immunological relationship between the fast-acting plasminogen activator inhibitors from plasma, blood platelets and endothelial cells demonstrated with a monoclonal antibody against an inhibitor from placenta. Thromb Haemost 1986;55:213-7.
100. Smith KJ. Infusion of monoclonal antibody immunoaffinity purified factor IX in rabbits: Comparison with commercial concentrates. Thromb Haemost 1987;58:349-.

101. Yoshioka A, Ohkubo Y, Nishimura T et al. Heterogeneity of factor IX BM – difference of cleavage sites by factor XIa and calcium in factor IX Kashihara, factor IX Nagoya and factor IX Niigata. Thromb Res 1986;42:595-605.
102. D'Angelo SV, Comp PC, Esmon CT, D'Angelo A. Relationship between protein C antigen and anticoagulant activity during oral anticoagulation and in selected disease states. J Clin Invest 1986;77:416-25.
103. Takase T, Rotblat F, Goodall AH et al. Production of factor VIII-deficient plasma by immunodepletion using three monoclonal antibodies. Br J Haematol 1987;66:497-502.
104. Mazurier C, Samor B, Deromeeuf C, Goudemand M. The role of fibronectin in factor VIII/von Willebrand factor cryoprecipitation. Thromb Res 1985;37:651-8.
105. Suzuki K, Moriguchi A, Nagayoshi A, Mutoh S, Katsuki S, Hashimoto A. Enzyme immunoassay of human protein C by using monoclonal antibodies. Thromb Res 1985;38:611-21.
106. Levine PH, Brettler DB, Sullivan JL, Forsberg AD, Pettilo J, Lamon K. Initial human studies with factor VIII:C purified from plasma by the use of monoclonal antibodies. Thromb Res 1987;(suppl 7):61.
107. Dawson NJ, Kemball-Cook G, Barrowcliffe TW. Assay problems with highly purified factor VIII concentrates. Br Soc Haemost Thromb AGM 1987;(ab 18):107.
108. MacGregor IR, Prowse CV, Micklem LR, James K. A monoclonal antibody which prevents reductions in assayed fibrinogen and $\alpha_2$-antitrypsin in plasma samples containing therapeutic concentrations of tissue plasminogen activator. Thromb Res 1986;44:241-5.
109. Johnston GI, Pickett EB, McEver RP, George JN. Heterogeneity of platelet secretion in response to thrombin demonstrated by fluorescence flow cytometry. Blood 1987;69:1401-3.
110. Dechavanne M, French M, Pages J et al. Significant reduction in the binding of monoclonal antibody (lyp 18) directed against the IIB/IIIA glycoprotein complex to platelets of patients having undergone extracorporeal circulation. Thromb Haemost 1987;57:106-9.
111. Musial J, Niewiarowski S, Hershock D, Morinelli TA, Colman RW, Edmunds LH. Loss of fibrinogen receptors from the platelet surface during simulated extraporeal circulation. J Lab Clin Med 1985;105:514-22.
112. Runge MS, Bode C, Matsueda GR, Haber E. Tissue type plasminogen activator conjugated to an anti-fibrin monoclonal antibody is a 10-fold more efficient fibrinolytic agent than tissue type plasminogen activator alone. Clin Res 1986;34:A469.
113. Bode C, Runge MS, Newell JB, Matsueda GR, Haber E. Characterization of an antibody – urokinase conjugate – a plasminogen activator targeted to fibrin. J Biol Chem 1987;262:10819-23.
114. Liau CS, Haber E, Matsueda GR. Evaluation of monoclonal antifibrin antibodies by their binding to human blood clots. Thromb Haemost 1987;57:49-54.
115. Coller BS, Folts JD, Scudder IE, Smith SR. Antithrombotic effect of a monoclonal antibody to the platelet glycoprotein IIb/IIIa receptor in an experimental animal model. Blood 1986;68:783-6.
116. Pechet L, Tiarks CY, Ghalili K, Humphrey RE. Idiotypes of murine monoclonal antibodies to clotting factor VIII:C. Fed Proc 1986;(ab 45):962.
117. McGraw R, Frazier D, de Serres M, Reisner H, Stafford D. Antigenic determinant in human coagulation factor IX: Immunological screening and DNA sequence analysis of recombinant phage map a monoclonal antibody to residues 111 through 132 of the zymogen. Blood 1986;67:1344-8.

118. Vanzonneveld AJ, Veerman H, Brakenhoff JP, Aarden LA, Cajot JF, Pannekoek H. Mapping of epitopes on human tissue-type plasminogen activator with recombinant deletion mutant proteins. Thromb Haemost 1987;57:82-6.
119. Prowse CV. Monoclonal antibodies and the haemostasis laboratory: Current position. Vox Sang 1986;50:65-70.
120. Griffin BD, Micklem LR, McCann MC, James K, Pepper DS. The production and characterisation of a panel of 10 murine monoclonal antibodies to human procoagulant factor VIII. Thromb Haemost 1986;55:40-6.
121. Nieuwenhuis HK, van Oosterhout JJG, Rozemuller E, van Iwaarden F, Sixma JJ. Studies with a monoclonal against activated platelets: Evidence that a secreted 53 000 molecular weight lysosome – like granule protein is exposed on the surface of activated platelets in the circulation. Blood 1987;70:838-45.

# DISCUSSION

B. Habibi, C.Th. Smit Sibinga

*T.J Hamblin (Bournemouth):* Dr Ploegh, these transgenic mice were specifically unable to produce antibodies against human proteins, because you used an HLA gene. No other gene would have done that. So it had to be an HLA gene that you transfected to the mouse. Is that right?

*H.J. Ploeg (Amsterdam):* The aim is to render these mice tolerant to most of the epitopes commonly seen when you immunize a mouse with a human histocompatibility antigen. So, although we have not been able to produce monoclonal antibodies yet from such transgenic mice, I think the results we have got at the cellular level show that these mice indeed are tolerant to the product of these transgenes. So that sets the stage for using these mice to produce allospecific typing reagents.

*T.J. Hamblin:* Is that simply because they are expressing the human antigen or is it because the human antigen is functional on the mouse lymphocyte?

*H.J. Ploegh:* In order to be able to make reagents that would resemble typing reagents as used in HLA typing, our premise is that these antigens have to be present in the mouse, in the germline and expressed at the appropriate stages of development in the tissues where you normally find them. This is something that we are currently investigating and it would seem as if the regulation of expression of these genes in these mice resembles very much what you find for the endogenous histocompatibility antigens of the mouse and what you find for human antigens in man.

*T.J. Hamblin:* Supposing you wanted to make a mouse tolerant of an antigen present on human liver, could you just stick that gene in and expect the same thing to happen or is it something that is particular significant about HLA?

*H.J. Ploegh:* No, my prediction would be that that would work for any antigen or any molecule that you introduce into the germline of mice through this technique, provided that the site of expression and the mode of expression roughly resembles that which you would expect in the mouse proteins. So, if you would make a mouse transgenic for human albumin and you would introduce this gene with the appropriate elements that control its expression then you could predict that a mouse would result producing human albumin in addition to mouse albumin. This mouse should thus no longer be able to alloimmune respond against that protein.

*C.Th. Smit Sibinga (Groningen):* The presentation of Dr Messeter gave us an idea of how the structure of the different monoclonal antibodies differ. The specificity in the binding therefore discloses different phenotypes of bloodgroups. How does that relate to the presentation of Dr Voak, wherehe illustrated that the use of monoclonal antibodies for the typing of ABO groups showed a variety of antigens specifically in the A group. Could we define this a little further?

*L. Messeter (Lund):* I think it relates very well to what Dr Voak said in his presentation, and also to what has been evident particularly after the recent workshop on monoclonal antibodies in Paris that was referred to.* In this workshop were investigated large numbers of anti-A's and anti-B's. It could be demonstrated by immunochemical means by Dr Oriol and his group that these antibodies see very specific epitopes, which are or are not represented on different types of red cells. I think that this will really lead to a much better understanding of particularly the weak phenotypes of the red blood cells.

*C.Th. Smit Sibinga:* Dr Voak could you comment on that?

*D. Voak (Cambridge):* We are on the limits of what is known and the work is very difficult. Dr Oriol was the only one who had the opportunity of studying the substances prepared. This was rather a pity for the workshop, because nobody was able to compare opinions of different laboratories on data. Ofcourse there are limitations in interpretations made with isolated substances compared to red cell serology, became you have the distributions of epitopes and the limitations of the red cell structure making cross-reference I think rather tentative.

*L. Messeter:* To some degree there was a possibility to make comparison. Dr Oriol's substances were synthetic structures. We had used a couple of natural structures isolated from red blood cells or tissues in the form of sugars or glycolipids. In many instances the reactions were the same, as those obtained by Dr Oriol, but in other instances there was a difference indicating that an antibody might easier recognize a glycolipid than a glycoprotein or anisolated sugar, and that, of course, is important to bloodgrouping.

*C.Th. Smit Sibinga:* That would indeed improve the sensitivity of the tests.

*L. Messeter:* Not only sensitivity, but our understanding. The clarification of what these antigens actually are would help us in typing of the weak groups.

*D. Voak:* Can I make a practical point? The academic research is just getting underway, but if we talk about things like the B(A) phenomena, we have to put it into perspective. What we here demonstrated is that all these group B cells have just a trace of A and because the antibodies that see it are those that see $A_x$, we can not automatically say that it has the same A epitope structure as $A_x$. That may not be true. I think it is probable to say that the non specific activity of B transferase enzymes cause a little A to be on the

---

* Proceedings 1st ISBT International Workshop on Monoclonal Antibodies. Roger P, Salmon Ch (eds), Paris, 1987 (in press).

group B red cells. The B(A) agglutination is fragile, and the antigen sites not clustered, hence a very feeble reaction. I am very cautious in drawing any interpretations from Oriol's data when it comes down to weak red cell epitopes. It is too early.

*B. Habibi (Paris):* Dr Voak, have you not got the feeling that some people are overemphasizing the requirements of those monoclonal antibodies; there is a tendency to tailor monoclonals capable of detecting all such exceptional phenotypes as A$_x$, D VI or D IV, whereas, considering for instance the D VI phenotype, even some potent polyclonals are by definition unable to detect them. So, do you really think that those particular requirements should be included in the criteria for the quality control of those monoclonal antibodies?

*D. Voak:* Selected IgG polyclonal anti-D antibodies detect Rh D category VI by antiglobulin tests. The fundamental difference between monoclonals and polyclonals is that with a polyclonal you only have a small volume. When you obtain a monoclonal especially in a 1,000 liter unit, it is worth your trouble to fully characterize it. It is cheap to do so. However, you can not do that with polyclonals. If we are patient typing we do not care about the detection of weak D (D$^u$) or of the various Rh D categories. We can safely call them Rh D negative. However, if we are donor typing we have two anti-D test procedures which must detect weak D. Where we use automated equipment there is no problem. We use IgG and manual systems adjusted to detect weak D (D$^u$) of significance that we want to see so that we can label a donor as Rh D positive irrespective of the weak D or category type. It is the manual typing where people use the one IgM monoclonal and polyclonal anti-D antibody blend by two-phase saline and anti-globulin test, where we need to know what the reagent will do. We want to be able to detect high grade D$^u$, we care about that in a donor. We do not want anybody to be immunized. I do not think we care about low grade, but the classification is difficult. Paddy Moore in an ISBT meeting said we want to detect D$^u$ if it is detected by a papain anti-D.* And of course, this is a variable into different reagents. It is convenient to select on the basis of Rh D category VI as well as weak D (D$^u$), as category VI is the weakest D variant type that we like to detect in donor blood typing.

*C.Th. Smit Sibinga:* Before we move to the virology, may I come back to part of the discussion from session I regarding the presentation of Dr Holbeck in which we speculated that probably a further typing by sequencing of the DR antigens might predict even better the outcome of an organ transplant. I read from the presentation of Dr Ploegh that he believes more that it is the alertness of the T-cell of the recipient to the antigen being presented, which might determine ultimately the outcome of the transplant. Is that true?

* Moore BPL. Vox Sang 1984;46:95-7.

*H.L. Ploegh:* That is not true. I think that obviously a further molecular characterisation of class II molecules by sequencing will help to refine the sort of associations that have been observed between class II molecules and disease or enable to predict the outcome of transplants, be they bone marrow transplants or simple organ transplants. I think one should not forget that in a situation where MHC molecules are involved, there are probably at least two more polymorphic partners involved, one of which is the T-cell receptor gene family. In these considerations one has to take into account the variation that exists at the level of T-cell receptor genes and you have variability at the B-cell receptor level as well. So, one also has to include the immunoglobulins into the arguments. In most of these cases I will predict that it will be multifactorial. You can not simply point at a particular sequence in a particular class II $\beta$gene and predict whether or not the graft will take. It is more complex than that.

*J.R Aluoch (Nairobi):* My question is more of an epidemiological than of a technological nature. Dr Rouzioux, you showed us that the HIV-2 positivity in the French group that you studied was 6-9% and you were also showing that of the 12 HIV-2 positive cases all of them had a link with West Africa. I did not get quite clearly what the link was. Where these autochthonous French people, who had worked in West Africa or had visited West Africa or were you dealing with West Africans, who are in France?

*C. Rouzioux (Paris):* Two of them were black men from Ivory Coast. One was a white man who lived in Uganda for more than 4 years, is a drug user and now is living in France. But he had numerous sexual contacts in Uganda with women. The others were women who were married with black men from Ivory Coast. In all cases it is very easy to show a link with sexual transmission of HIV to those population irrespective whether they are black or white. So, I think that the epidemiology of HIV-2 is different by time, but not different by the transmission. In Africa the transmission is the same model for HIV-1 and HIV-2 and the problem is heterosexual transmission.

*L.R. Overby (Emmeryville):* Dr Rouzioux, I understand that there is a considerable cross-reaction between the gag proteins and the polymerase proteins of HIV-1 and HIV-2. Then one would expect that the commercial test based on HIV-1 would identify both HIV-1 and HIV-2 seroconversions. But is it not true also that there is a cross-reaction with the gag proteins that are not related to HIV, the P24 only antibodies. So, how would one distinguish then between a positive result on an ELISA. One would not know whether it is true HIV-1, true HIV-2, seroconversion or across-reaction.

*C. Rouzioux:* Concerning the antibodies against P24 only, not related to HIV infection. It is reasonable to think that is cross-reactivity with cellular antigen. It is necessary to follow up these patients. Usually these reactions are stable. The problem of seroconversion is easier to solve now because Western blot tests are better overall for GP160 and GP110. So, true seroconversions are detected by the presence of antibodies directed against P25 associated to those directed to GP160. Another question of this is: Is this really cross-reactivity between HIV-1 and HIV-2 or is it double infection among double positive sera. I think that the cross-reactivity on P25 and P34 are very important for asymptomatic patients, because they have all the antibodies against the virus. The specificity and the sensitivity of the kits is good for all these asymptomatic and, I hope, positive ELISA sera. But the problem I think is very different for AIDS, LAS and ARC cases, because the level of antibody against the P25 and P34 is getting down during the development of the disease. So, it is not possible to see cross-reactivity in these patients between HIV-1 and HIV-2 and AIDS cases. The HIV-1 is not recognized by HIV-2 ELISA kits. That is how we discovered two patients who were totally negative for HIV-1 in ELISA, in Western blot and in radioimmunoprecipitation. We decided out of these real AIDS cases to culture survivors and discovered HIV-2. So, it is possible not to have cross-reactivity during the deadlock month of the disease. It is different if we speak about asymptomatic patients. I think the cross-reactivity may be for the second generation test about 8% of the HIV-2 sera to be detected by an HIV-1 ELISA kit. Sofar, I know only one HIV-2 ELISA kit. Of course, I do not know if the opposite situation is possible to recognize all the HIV-1 by the HIV-2. I think that it is less than 80% at the moment.

*C.Th. Smit Sibinga:* The HIV antigen test was discussed briefly by Dr Rouzioux. We have a new tool for further increasing the safety of specifically the blood supply by trying to eliminate those donations which come from donors in the stage where infectivity is already present but not the classic show up with antibodies. Are the specificity and the sensitivity of the present HIV antigen tests under development such, that we really pick up the mutant expressions of the different viruses within the HIV group which are now known?

*C. Rouzioux:* We have tried different HIV-1 viruses isolated in our laboratory. There was no problem to pick up all the different viruses from supernatant of the culture. Even the Abbott antigen test is able to detect HIV-2 in culture supernatant. In the first development of the antigen test monoclonal antibodies were used and now it is polyclonal.

*C.V. Prowse (Edinburgh):* Dr Highfield, did I get it right you are producing a recombinant e antigen. Is that just c treated in some way?

*P.E. Highfield (Beckenham):* Basically yes. Strictly speaking it is a slightly different construction. We have a number of different core antigens that vary slightly and produce one that is stable and is used to provide the core antigen for our various kits. We produce another which is initially produced as core, but is disaggregated into e. We use that as a source of material for e antigen.

*C.V. Prowse:* Does that tell you anything about quite what the difference between c and e is?

*P.E. Highfield:* No it does not, because we do not have a sufficient range of variations to make any real conclusions. It was a consequence of the way the experiment was done, that I generated two classes of recombinant which differ in this property.

*C.Th. Smit Sibinga:* There are under way test systems in which within one test in a combination both HIV antibodies and hepatitis B surface antigen can be picked up. Applying such a combination does not that affect the sensitivity of the test to both of these markers, Dr Highfield or Dr Rouzioux?

*P.E Highfield:* In our experience it does not. In the combined test formats that we run in house at the moment, both aspects of the test actually are more sensitive. Although to be fair that is not some sort of consequence of just mixing the two sets of reagents. It is because, in trying to devise an assay for two markers at once, the test format has to be changed from that of either marker individually. These changes have meant that the incubation period is longer than it would be for a surface antigen test alone. Therefore the sensitivity for surface antigen has gone up, but that is really just equivalent to running a normal test for a longer period of time. For the HIV antibody aspects of the test; to make that combine with the surface antigen test, we had to change the format and that new format is more sensitive than our currently existing antibody test.

*C.Th. Smidt Sibinga:* Thank you. Would you like to comment, Dr Rouzioux?

*C Rouzioux:* I am not involved in the Blood Bank like some virologists. For a virologist it is impossible to combine two viruses in the same test without losing sensitivity. Moreover, we read two different answers. So, I do not like this sort of test, but I think the problem is different for Blood Banks. For me the problem is the sensitivity. Recently we have discovered in our laboratory new positive sera, but with very, very low HIV antibody titre. I think we need to develop more sensitivity with a second generation test, because it is very difficult to pick up those sera and it is very important for all of us. So, we have to emphasize this part more than to mix viruses at the present time.

*C.Th. Smit Sibinga:* I feel a hesitation in your remarks. Dr Prowse, what I found intriguing is the striking difference in assay results between a monoclonal antibody depleted plasma and a plasma coming from a more natural resource. I am specifically referring to Factor VIII.

*C.V Prowse:* As I said that is only one study and obviously needs confirmation. But if you just take it at face value at the moment, it would appear to relate to the amount of von Willebrand factor that is around in the substrate plasma, when you are trying to assay a product that does not have that in it. Most of the concentrates you buy of the shelf for therapy at the moment have it in, and the assays on these show no discrepancy.

*C.Th. Smit Sibinga:* You mentioned the reagent for an antigen assay developed in the Central Laboratory of the Dutch Red Cross. Maybe we could ask one of the representatives, Dr Over for instance, to give a brief comment?

*J. Over (Amsterdam):* Well, I can hardly comment on that. Dr Prowse has described that perfectly well. We use a combination of I think three mono-clonal antibodies. It is not done in my specific department, so I am not very familiar with it, but I think the procedure is published* and therefore easily available.

*C.V. Prowse:* Can I make two comments? One is that just very recently there has come on the market a second monoclonal hemostasis kit. I have no idea how it performs. That one is for plasminogen activator inhibitor. The second comment is that I think we are going to hear quite a bit about monoclonal antibody purified therapeutic products. There is nothing inherently good about the monoclonal purified product. What is important is what you start with, what the yield is and how easy and safe it is to perform the purification process. It is what is in the bottle at the end of the day that counts. It is not really how you got there.

*D. Voak:* The two factors are the economics and the clearance of viral load. The most important thing is to eliminate the viral load, thereby using the most economic procedure.

---

* Stel HV et al. Thromb Haemost 1983;50:860-3.

# III. Biotechnology and blood components

# MONOCLONAL ANTIBODIES IN THE PRODUCTION OF PURIFIED PROTEINS FROM HUMAN PLASMA

A.B. Schreiber

## Immunoaffinity chromatography applied to human therapeutics

Monoclonal antibodies represent standardized reagents of high specificity and selectivity, that in principle are available in unlimited amounts. Monoclonal antibody technology is by now commonplace to basic research and clinical diagnostic laboratories. *In vivo* and various *in vitro* protocols have been established to allow the economically feasible generation or multi-kilogram amounts of monoclonal antibody preparations, acceptable as raw materials of parenteral quality. The chemistry to couple antibodies to solid supports has been scaled-up to process large volumes of starting material, without appreciable performance loss. With these elements in hand, the application of monoclonal antibody mediated purification is entering the arena of human pharmaceuticals. Therapeutics originating from biological fluids such as plasma or conditioned medium from recombinant DNA engineered cells are usually present in extremely low concentrations in the starting material. Monoclonal antibody purification is particularly well suited to provide the specificity to obtain homogeneous preparations, while removing the majority of unnecessary and undesirable contaminants. In the case of plasma proteins as active ingredients, safety concerns related to viral transmission, add another dimension of paramount importance to use exclusively high purity preparations.

## A. The monoclonal antibody, choise and scale-up

Many practical considerations strongly favor the choice of a monoclonal antibody of the IgG isotype. Antibodies of the IgM isotype are usually of a relative lower affinity and feature poor stability, especially upon freezing and thawing. While it may seem logical to screen for antibodies of the highest affinity for the desired antigen, to ascertain the highest possible degree of selectivity, too strong an interaction between antibody and antigen may necessitate the use of harsh elution conditions in subsequent affinity chromatography procedures. A moderate to high affinity (around $10^8$ $M^{-1}$) is therefore often to be preferred. Of particular interest are screening procedures that identify the appropriate hybridoma cell line, based on the ability of inocuous buffers to mediate antigen-antibody dissociation. An element example is provided by monoclonal antibodies recognizing calcium-dependent conformational epitopes of vitamin K-dependent plasma proteins [1]. In this case, the use of calcium chelating reagents will disrupt in a reversible fashion the antibody binding to the recognized antigen, without altering the antibody viability for repeated use, nor the bioactivity of the vitamin K-dependent protein.

Points to consider and guidelines for the scale-up and manufacturing of monoclonal antibodies used for the preparation of human therapeutics have been issued and recently revised in the US, Japan and Europe. As for any other biological, a great amount of care needs to be addressed to a full characterization of the parent hybridoma cell line and the master cell bank established thereof. Frequent subcloning may be necessary, due to the inherent stability of hybridomas. Generation of large amounts of antibody is feasible by harvesting ascites fluid from the parenteral cavity of histocompatible mice, previously primed with pristane or incomplete Freund's adjuvant. As an example, our laboratories have generated more than a thousand liter of ascites over a period of twelve months, without major operational facilities or manpower involvement. With the identification of a high producer cell line (more than 10 mg/ml ascites), this endeavor can easily yield 5-10 kg of antibody at reasonable cost. The absence of a series of eighteen adventitious viruses is required for the release of ascitic fluids for further purification of the antibody. Only two of these viruses, Reo-3 and lymphochoriomeningitis, are human pathogens and their presence is ensued by the rejection of a batch. Positive titers for any of the sixteen other viruses necessitate retesting at the stage of obtention of purified antibody. In our experience, we did not have to reject a single batch of antibody over the several hundreds of batches produced, amounting to several kg of antibody derived from ascites.

Both for reasons of cost-effectiveness and degree of scale-up, the elegant *in vitro* fermentation techniques for mammalian cells may prevail over ascites. Several formats of bioreactors have established a successful track record to date. The Damon Encapcel® system makes use of alginate microspheres to encapsulate hybridoma cells, with secretion of antibody that can easily be purified away from the microspheres. Other fermentation systems such as that from the Invitron, Celltech and Amicon companies make use of the entrapment of hybridoma cells at high density in microporous or gelatinous beads, upon which continuous perfusion is applied with simultaneous concentration and harvesting of antibody. For all systems, it is advisable to adapt the hybridoma cell culture conditions to serum-free medium. One thousand liter fermentors will produce under optimized conditions about 100 grams of monoclonal antibody in a couple of months at a total cost similar to that obtained from ascites. An obvious and important advantage of the *in vitro* approach is the exclusive presence of the antibody of desired specificity, whereas in ascites the antibody is contaminated with a heterogeneous mixture of naturally occurring antibodies. As some of the latter are necessarily of the same isotype than the desired monoclonal antibody, it may not be straightforward to purify these away. Monoclonal antibodies can usually be purified to near homogeneity from both *in vitro* and *in vivo* sources, by simple salt precipitation followed by ion exchange chromatography. In those instances where antigen is readily available in large amounts, more specific purification approaches can be utilized.

The overall approach for conditions of purifications and quality control release of the monoclonal antibody intended for use in affinity chromatography has to be approached as if the antibody were itself an injectable human therapeutic, despite it really being a raw material. Indeed, as expanded in some detail below, there is an inevitable 'bleed' of the antibody from solid surfaces into the final product, that may raise safety concerns. Antibody preparations must therefore be free of pathogens and have a minimal level of DNA and pyrogen contamination.

## B. The affinity resin, chemistry and performance

Both agarose and acrylamide supports lend themselves for large scale coupling of monoclonal antibodies. The highly reactive cyanogen bromide activation can be controlled in a consistent fashion [2], but generates waste management problems in the manufacturing plant. The formation of aldehyde bonds by reduction chemistry is far more easy to handle and should be preferred as it generates more stable bonds between the antibody molecules and spacer linkers covalently attached to the resins. Less practical experience has been accumulated with inert materials such as silica and perhydrofluorocarbons, but these are anticipated to present the advantage of resistance to pressure allowing high flows, ease of handling and extremely low non-specific binding.

Only a small fraction of the antibody molecules coupled to the resins appears to be functional in terms of their binding capacity. Some extent of denaturation inevitably occurs, but the random coupling of Fc and Fab portions of the antibody molecules has to be invoked with the above mentioned chemistries. An elegant approach to circumvent the latter problem is to oxidate the carbohydrates on the Fc portion of the antibody with periodate, followed by reduction coupling to free amino groups built into a resin.

The quality of an affinity resin is ultimately determined by three criteria, namely:
1. binding capacity and recovery upon elution which will determine yield;
2. the life cycle of a column (the number of useful binding and elution cycles); and
3. the extent of antibody leakage in the eluted product ('bleed').

The optimization for scale-up with the choice of a particular coupling chemistry and elution conditions, becomes a careful evaluation of trade-offs between these three criteria. In our experience, yield considerations have been the primary guide for the selection of the affinity resin, as these impact most on cost-effectiveness and feasibility for product development. The life cycle of the affinity resin appears mostly to be dependent upon careful sterile handling and engineering considerations. Moreover, the net usefulness of a column can be extended by its use in series as a 'scavenger' column. Flow-throughs of a first column can indeed be pooled and re-applied several times to another column (the 'scavenger' column) with incremental improvements in overall recovery. Within the limitations of the first two criteria, bleeds of antibody of murine origin into the final product, becomes a key element for moving forward with product development. Murine monoclonal antibodies have by now been intentionally infused in a large number of cancer patients undergoing immunotherapy [See for example 3]. Surprisingly, despite the observed strong immune reaction to the mouse antigens, these agents have appeared to be well tolerated [4]. In these cases amounts varying from 1 mg to as high as 500 mg per infusion have been used. With proper coupling chemistry, amounts <100 ng/dose of products will appear in a monoclonal antibody purified product. While these amounts are presumably too low to be immunogenic, safety concerns for sensitization and allergic reactions are probably legitimate. Careful and sensitive determination for the presence of mouse Ig during the process and in the final products are therefore required, as well as chronic treatment clinical safety studies.

## Therapeutic preparations

### A. Factor VIII – Monoclate®

Treatment with Factor VIII concentrate isolated from human plasma has played a profound role in the maintenance of hemophilia A patients. Most commercial products presently available for substitution therapy are generally produced by processing of the cryoprecipitate fraction of plasma. Related to the Factor VIII procoagulant content, a typical administered concentrate with a specific activity of about 1 IU of procoagulant per mg of protein is, at best, 0.2% pure. Administration of cryoprecipitate preparations carry the risk for transmission of human pathogenic viruses adventitiously present in the source plasma. While initially the main safety concern surrounded the presence of hepatitis viruses B and NANB, the spreading AIDS epidemic and the possibility of transmission of HIV has become of paramount importance over the last few years.

Fulcher and Zimmerman have described a two-stage chromatographic purification of Factor VIII:C using a solid phase murine monoclonal antibody technique to achieve procoagulant activities greater than 1000 IU per mg of protein [5]. Our laboratories have developed a Factor VIII therapeutic preparation (Monoclate®) employing modifications and improvements of their basic technique so as to make it suitable for large-scale drug manufacture. For the first time, it has been possible to consider and test a therapeutic preparation in which the Factor VIII:C is purified free of the von Willebrand protein. Monoclate® was approved for therapeutic use in the US in October of 1987 and has since been filed with regulatory authorities of most European countries. Clinical studies described in an accompanying report of these proceedings and post-marketing experience have shown that Monoclate® compares favourably with other existing therapeutic factor preparations when safety, in vivo recovery, half-life and efficacy were evaluated.

The basic steps in the processing of Monoclate® are shown in Table 1. In plasma, the Factor VIII procoagulant activity is found in association with von Willebrand factor. Briefly, after conducting human plasma cryoprecipitation, dissolution and absorption with aluminium hydroxide, the purification is accomplished by a two-stage chromatographic process using as the first stage, a solid phase murine monoclonal antibody specific for the von Willebrand factor antigen. Exposure of source material to the solid phase affinity resin results in capture of the Factor VIII complex. The resin is washed free of impurities, after which the Factor VIII complex is dissociated by calcium

*Table 1.* Basic steps: Monoclonal purification
of Factor VIII.

Plasma

Cryoprecipitation

Dissolution & absorption

Affinity purification
Albumin addition

U.F. concentration & re-dilution

Amino-hexyl sepharose chromatography
Albumin addition

Dialysis – final formulation

Sterile filtration & freeze-drying

Heating

Final product

(Monoclate®)

ions. Factor VIII:C is hereby eluted and available for subsequent processing steps, while the von Willebrand factor remains bound to the solid phase. A second step brings about the dissociation of the antibody-antigen complex, thereby regenerating the affinity resin for repeated use. The Factor VIII is eluted from the solid phase as a solution too dilute for therapeutic use. This intermediate is therefore concentrated and the ionic strength is adjusted so as to be appropriate for a secondary chromatography on amino-hexyl agarose.

This second stage serves to further concentrate the activity and to improve purity approximately threefold. The final product is the formulated, filtered, lyophilized and heated. A number of process steps are carried out in the presence of purified pasteurized human serum albumin in order to stabilize and preserve the biologic activity of Factor VIII:C.

The properties of Monoclate® are summarized in Table 2. While the use of albumin improves product stability and allows better recovery of biologic activity during processing, it does not allow for accurate estimates of product purity. Such measurements, therefore, can only be made in concurrent laboratory runs carried out in the absence of albumin. In such albumin-free preparations, the specific activity was established by a combination of bioactivity measurements and protein assays. Mean specific activity of 3500 units per mg of protein were observed. This represents about a 250,000 fold purification from plasma. Other investigators have reported specific activity values in excess of 4500 units per mg [6]. In these instances, protease inhibitors were included throughout the processing in order to prevent proteolytic degradation. The use of these substances is not suitable for therapeutic preparations intended for intravenous administration and Monoclate® was, of

*Table 2.* Properties of Monoclate® .

| Configuration: | 10 ml or 20 ml glass vial, lyophilized diluent – water for injection | Purity (carrier-free lab tests): (in formulation): | >2500 IU/mg 5 IU/mg |
|---|---|---|---|
| Potency: | 250 IU- 2.5 ml 500 IU- 5.0 ml 1000 IU-10.0 ml | Other characteristics: | 99% removal of vWF alloagglutinins almost undetectable |
| Formula components: | Human albumin Mannitol NaCl Histidine CaCl$_2$ | Virus challenge tests: | >6.8-10 logs removal model viruses >7.08-9.1 logs removal LAV/HTLV III |

necessity, purified without additives and formulated with inocuous components. Thanks to the high purity, reconstitution with diluent is practically instantaneous and reconstitution volumes are very small.

The potential contamination of Monoclate® by murine Ig leaking from the affinity resin is assayed both in-process and at the stage of the final product by both *in vitro* specific radioimmunoassay and *in vivo* guinea pig delayed type hypersensitivity assays. Release specifications call for less than 50 ng of mouse Ig/100 IU Factor VIII activity. The sensitivity of the assays is around 10 ng of mouse Ig/ml. In most batches prepared for clinical use amounts of mouse Ig are undetectable by these techniques.

The purity of Factor VIII in Monoclate® is reflected in a number of ways. Firstly, 99% or more of the von Willebrand factor antigen is removed compared to plasma concentrations. Also, the product is virtually devoid of alloagglutinins. Secondly, analysis of Monoclate® by Western blotting techniques with a battery of monoclonal antibodies to various epitopes of Factor VIII:C [7] reveals a thrombin-generated chain composition identical to that of Factor VIII:C in either plasma, cryoprecipitate and Factor VIII:C obtained from conditioned medium of C127 cells engineered with a cDNA plasmid using a bovine papilloma virus vector. Thridly, we conducted studies to demonstrate the reduction in viral titer concommitent with the removal of impurities thanks to the affinity chromatography step in the processing of Monoclate®. Source materials were intentionally inoculated with infectious agents at very high titers. The model viruses were selected according to their resemblance to blood borne human pathogens of interest. Included in the tests were Sindbis virus, pseudorabies and vesicular stomatitis, as well as HIV (LAV strain). Virus titers were assayed by plaque formation and/or production of cytopathology in cell cultures. In each experiment the inoculum titer spiked in cryoprecipitate ranged from 7.6 to >10.9 logs of virus. We obtained more than 6.8-10 logs removal of model viruses and more than 7.1-9.1 logs removal of HIV due to Monoclate® processing. Importantly, about five logs of virus titer removal was achieved by the chromatography steps, irrespective of the virus type studied. Purification of active ingredients from plasma may therefore represent a generic approach to viral safety. Moreover, the combination of monoclonal antibody purification and physical heat inactivation were found to be synergistic in terms of overall virus titer reduction.

## B. Factor IX

Bleeding episodes of hemophilia B patients are currently treated with Factor IX concentrates containing intermediate purity Factor IX of a specific activity of about 1 unit/mg protein, at best containing 0.8% active ingredient. These agents contain all vitamin K dependent proteins and are typically associated with complications, including disseminated intravascular coagulation, thrombotic disorders and viral infectivity [8,9].

Based on our successful experience with Factor VIII, our laboratories set out to devise an immunoaffinity chromatography procedure for purified Factor IX. Clinical supplies are currently manufactured at large scale and we anticipate to conduct safety and efficacy trials in 1988. The obtained Factor IX preparation is nearly homogeneous. The specific activity of the preparation is about 300 IU/mg protein, nearing the theoretical specific activity of HPLC purified Factor IX. Electrophoretic techniques reveal a single band protein with no contaminants. Importantly, bioassays have demonstrated the absence of activated Factor IX, prothrombin and any other vitamin K dependent protein. The integrity of the Factor IX molecule in our preparation was confirmed by N amino-terminal sequencing and tryptic peptide maps. Pharmacology experiments have confirmed the general hemodynamic safety of the preparation and lack of thrombogenicity in the rabbit Wessler model. Viral spiking experiments applied to this process have reproduced the 5 logs of virus titer reduction contributed by the immunoaffinity procedure. Several other virucidal steps have been included in the further processing of this product for an overall viral titer reduction higher than 10 logs.

## C. Protein C

Protein C is a vitamin K dependent, serine protease prozymogen [10]. The activated form of protein C has been demonstrated to prossess both anticoagulant and profibrinolytic activities in animal pharmacology models [11]. Our laboratories have set out to develop processes based on immunoaffinity chromatography for a homogeneous protein C preparation intended for therapeutic use. The starting material chosen was the flow through from the anti-Factor IX affinity resin described above. The specific activity of protein C in this non-bound fraction is about 1 IU/mg protein, thereby providing an immediate fifty fold enrichment over plasma. In addition, by utilizing this fraction that otherwise would be a waste product of Factor IX purification, one can envision a sequential processing from the same unit of plasma to yield in a cost-effective fashion several products. To date, we have generated several preclinical batches of purified protein C of specific activity around 70 IU/mg protein. This compares to a theoretical specific activity of pure protein C at 160 IU/mg protein. Sequence and electrophoretic analysis reveals that our preparations are nearly homogeneous. The specific activity achieved at roughly half of the theoretical is therefore probably due to inactivation during processing as opposed to the presence of contaminants. The obtained preparations were shown to fully retain their bioactivity as measured by amidolytic and anticoagulant assays. Further, we have also confirmed the ability of the preparations of activated protein C to amplify and prolong the effects of tissue plasminogen activator.

## Conclusion

Monoclonal antibody technology has evolved to a stage where procedures are established for immunoaffinity chromatography as applied to human therapeutics. The growing concern for viral infectivity of products derived from human plasma and medical and regulatory standards necessitate the exclusive use of highly purified biological agents. Immunoaffinity chromatography, in our experience, provides a powerful tool to achieve these objectives. The selection and manufacturing of monoclonal antibodies intended as raw materials for immunopurification have to comply with standards set for parenteral products. Optimization of the affinity process is eventually a compromize between factors that affect cost-effectiveness, such as yield of the active ingredient and resin life span, and safety concerns related to leakage of murine protein into the final product. Our laboratories have contributed to the development of Monoclate®, a highly purified Factor VIII:C therapeutic preparation. The key purification step involves immunoaffinity chromatography with a murine monoclonal antibody directed to von Willebrand factor. Our laboratories are currently using similar strategies to develop therapeutic preparations of plasma derived Factor IX and protein C. In our experience, the affinity chromatography step efficiently removes most contaminants, does not impact the biological integrity of the active ingredient and provides for a generic method for viral elimination.

## References

1.  Liebman HA, Limentani SA, Furie B. Immunoaffinity purification of Factor IX (Christmas factor) by using conformation-specific antibodies directed against the Factor IX-metal complex. Proc Natl Acad Sci (USA) 1985;82:3879-83.
2.  Kohn J, Wilchek M. A new approach (cyano-transfer) for cyanogen bromide activation of Sepharose at neutral pH which yields activated resins free of interfering nitrogen derivatives. Biochem Biophys Res Comm 1982;107:878-82.
3.  Shawler DL, Bartholomew RH, Smith LM, Dillman RO. Human immune response to multiple injections of murine IgG. J Immunol 1985;135:1530-5.
4.  Dillman RO, Beauregard JC, Halpern SE, Clutter M. Toxicities and side effects associated with intravenous infusions of murine monoclonal antibodies. J Biol Resp Modifiers 1986;5:73-84.
5.  Fulcher CA, Zimmerman TS. Characterization of human Factor VIII procoagulant protein with a heterologous antibody. Proc Natl Acad Sci (USA) 1982;79:1648-53.

6.  Eaton D, Rodriguez H, Vehar GA. Proteolytic processing of human Factor VIII. Correlation of specific cleavages by thrombin, Factor Xa and activated protein C with activation and inactivation of Factor VIII coagulant activity. Biochemistry 1986;25:505-10.

7.  Fulcher CA, Roberts JR, Holland LZ, Zimmerman TS. Human Factor VIII procoagulant protein. J Clin Invest 1985;76:117-23.

8.  Menache D, Behre HE, Orthner CL et al. Coagulation Factor IX concentrate: Method of preparation and assessment of potential *in vivo* thrombogenicity in animal models. Blood 1984;64:1220-6.

9.  Kasper CK. Thromboembolic complications. Thromb Diath Haemorrh 1975; 33:640-62.

10. Esmon CT. The regulation of natural anticoagulant pathways. Science 1987;235: 1348.

11. Comp PC, Esmon CT. Generation of fibrinolytic activity by infusion of activated protein C into dogs. J Clin Invest 1981;68:1221.

# PRODUCTION OF CLOTTING FACTORS THROUGH BIOTECHNOLOGY

L-O. Andersson

## Introduction

Fractionation of plasma is a way to prepare a number of proteins for clinical use, of great value in treatment and prevention of a number of diseases and disease states. Of special importance are the coagulation factor concentrates used for treatment of hemophilia. In treatment of hemophilia A Factor VIII concentrates are used and for treatment of hemophilia B Factor IX concentrates. Before those concentrates were developed there was essentially no treatment for hemophilia patients and life-expectancy was poor. Average lifespan was around 16 years. With the introduction of the Factor VIII and IX concentrates in the 60ties life has completely changed for hemophilia patients. They now can live an almost normal life.

Thus clotting factor concentrates have been and are very important for treatment of hemophilia. However their use is not without problems. The availability is limited as it depends upon supply of plasma for fractionation. Today the volume of plasma fractionated is to a considerable extend determined by the need of Factor VIII. The cost is high as the cost of plasma is high and much active material is lost during purification. Finally, but not least important, the risk for transmitting certain virus infections is still considerable.

Recombinant DNA technology gives new possibilities to solve those limitations and problems. In principle it allows production of unlimited amounts of material. Further it can probably be produced cheaper than its analogs from plasma. The risk for virus transmission is strongly reduced.

This all sounds very attractive. However, in actual practice it is not that easy, at least not with todays technology. There are still some limitations vîand although some problems may have been solved, some new ones are created instead.

In order to clarify this, this presentation will briefly describe what is required and how a recombinant DNA drug is developed.

## Recombinant DNA technology

Basic principle is to isolate the genetic information how a specific protein is made and transfer this to a producing host organism.

To have a reasonable chance to succeed one needs certain data about the protein in question. They are: molecular weight, general composition, part of amino acid sequence, and biosynthesis site(s). Further, it is advantageous to have antibody against the protein and some knowledge of them RNA.

128

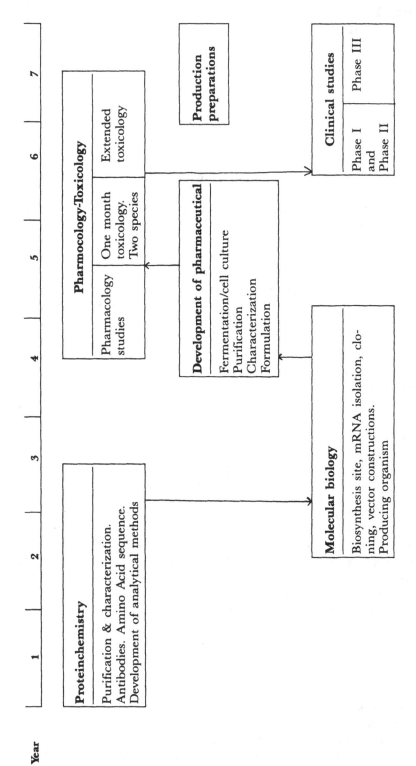

*Figure 1.* Development of recombinant DNA pharmaceutical

In some cases one does not have those data. The protein may not have been purified before. In that case one has to start by purifying and characterizing it. Factor VIII is such an example where a considerable effort had to be put in purifying the plasma Factor VIII, before the molecular biology work really could gain speed.

In the early days of gene technology it was assumed that most proteins could be produced using bacteria as host cells. As bacteria are cheap to feed, grow rapidly and are producing large amounts of protein it was expected that most proteins could be produced cheaply. This also turned out to be the case for the first rather small proteins made: insulin and human growth hormone, that could be produced in Ecoli and give good yields of biologically active protein.

However, this did not work when larger and more complicated proteins were studied. Very little biologically active protein was obtained despite high levels of protein synthesis. What was happening was that those proteins did not fold properly in the bacterial microenvironment They folded incorrectly, were biologically inactive and aggregated to large inclusion bodies in the bacteria.

To solve this problem one has to use mammalian cells as host for the production of recombinant DNA proteins. Mammalian cells do usually have the proper microenvironment. In most cases one has also succeeded to get expression of biologically active protein. In addition to the folding problem for certain proteins there are also other problems with bacteria as expressing systems. Quite a number of proteins contain additonal components such as carbohydrates and other modifications introduced following protein biosynthesis. Bacteria do not have glycosylation systems and thus glycoproteins can not be made in bacteria. At best one obtains a "naked" protein with carbohydrate coverage. Most plasma proteins are glycoproteins so this is a serious problem. Both Factor VIII and Factor IX contain carbohydrate and Factor IX also another post-translational modification, the gammacarboxyglutamic acid residues, which are necessary for biological activity.

## What are the implications?

To use mammalian cell culture for production of proteins is a quite different story than to use fermentation of bacteria. The mammalian cells need more sofisticated food and much more care than bacteria. They grow slowly and produce much less protein.

Consequently it becomes much more expensive to use mammalian cell culture technology than with fermentation of bacteria. It may be a factor between ten and one hundred times more expensive. Depending on specific activity of protein and level of expression obtained, there may be cases where it is very expensive to produce by recombinant DNA technique and that it is not competable with corresponding protein obtained from plasma.

Thus, when there is a producing organism available will every problem be solved? No, far from that. This becomes evident by looking at the entire development scheme as shown in Figure 1.

Purification of recombinant DNA proteins for clinical use is a special problem. The demand on purity is very high because the contaminants are non-human proteins and thus immunogenic. Less then 10 μg of non-human protein per day is allowed to be given. For example with albumin which has to be given in large amounts the demand for purity would be 99.9998% pure, whereas with Factor VIII it would be sufficient with 95% purity.

## What is the situation with coagulation factors?

Actually most of them have been cloned and expressed today: Factor V, VIII, VII, IX and X. Of special interest is of course the Factor IX and Factor VIII as being the clinically used ones. Factor IX was cloned in 1982 by Brownlee and his coworkers [1] and subsequently by Davie and Kurachi [2]. However only trace amounts of Factor IX protein were obtained, biologically inactive as it did not contain the gammacarboxyglytamic acid residues which are essential for activity. Later biologically active protein has been obtained by several groups [3,4]. The key is to choose a host cell that has an active gammacarboxylation system and to give good supply with vitamin K during the cell culture. Expression levels close to that of plasma, that is around 5 μg/ml, have been obtained. So far no major step for making a preparation for clinical use has been taken, however.

Factor VIII is a special story. When Factor IX was cloned there was still large uncertainty about the Factor VIII protein. So the work had to start by purifying plasma Factor VIII. That was accomplished subsequently by several groups: Edvard Tuddenham and coworkers in London [5], Sixma, Hamar and coworkers in Utrecht and our group in Stockholm [6]. Factor VIII is a very large protein, 2331 amino acid residues and presenting just trace quantities in plasma (0.2 μg/ml). To make things worse it is also very sensitive to protease degradation. When more about the protein became known, the molecular biology work could progres and in 1984 the gene was cloned independently by Lawn et al [7] at Genentech and Toole and coworkers [8] at Genetics Institute. The structure of the molecule was unraveled and shown to contain various domains and sequence repeats.

Sequence homology with the copper-containing plasma protein ceruloplasmin was found in two of the domains. Factor VIII contains metalions essential for activity, but it has not been proven yet which metal.

In plasma the Factor VIII is present as a two chain protein with one heavy 200 KD chain and one light 80 KD chain [6]. The two chains are held together by one or several metal ion bridges. In ordinary concentrates for clinical use Factor VIII is presenting various fragmented forms from a heavy 90 KD chain complexed to a light 80 KD chain and upwards to fullsized heavy chain [6]. All forms are active.

Today much is known about the molecule and a model illustrated in Figure 2 can be drawn where the various functional regions are indicated.

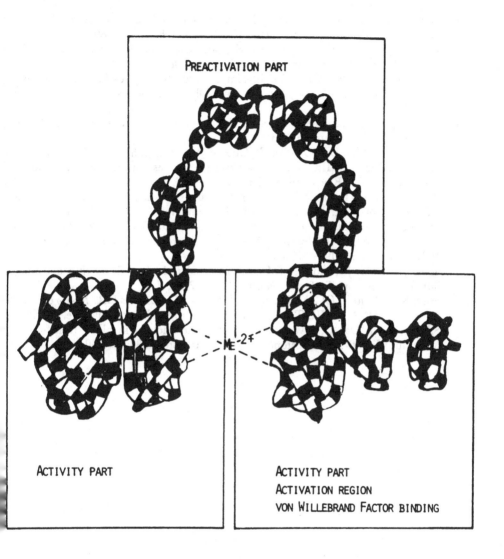

*Figure 2.* Model of Factor VIII molecule.

March 1987 the first injection of recombinant DNA Factor VIII was given to a patient. Response was good and half-life of material was normal [9]. Thus even if there are many problems with this new technology, big achievement can be reached. The Factor VIII story illustrates that clearly. Five years ago we were not sure about what the molecule was and today we know details of structure and structure-function relationships and have given recombinant material to patient.

132

## References

1. Choo KH, Gould KJ, Rees DJG, Brownlee GG. Molecular cloning of the gene for human antihaemophiliac Factor IX. Nature 1982;299:178-80.
2. Kurachi K, Davie EW. Isolation and characterization of a CDNA coding for human Factor IX. Proc Natl Acad Sci (USA) 1982;79:6461-4.
3. De la Salle H, Altenburger W, Elkaim R et al. Activeγ -carboxylated human Factor IX expressed using recombinant DNA techniques. Nature 1985;316: 268-70.
4. Busby S, Kumar A, Joseph M et al. Expression of active human Factor IX in transfected cells. Nature 1985;316:271-3.
5. Rotblat F, O'Brien D.P, O'Brien FJ, Goodall AH, Tuddenham EGD. Purification of human Factor VIII:C and characterization by western blotting using monoclonal antibodies. Biochemistry 1985;24:4294-300.
6. Andersson L-O, Forsman N, Huang K et al. Isolation and characterization of human Factor VIII: Molecular forms in commercial Factor VIII concentrate, cryoprecipitate and plasma. Proc Natl Acad Sci (USA) 1986;83:2979-83.
7. Gitschier J, Wood WI, Goralka TM et al. Characterization of the human Factor VIII gene. Nature 1984;312:326-30.
8. Toole JJ, Knopf JL, Wozney JM et al. Molecular cloning of a CDNA encoding human antihemophilic factor. Nature 1984;312:342-7.
9. High KA, White II GC, McMillan CW, Macik BG, Roberts HR. *In vivo* characteristics of rDNA F VIII: The impact for the future in hemophilia care. In: Smit Sibinga CTh, Das C, Overby LR (eds). Biotechnology in blood transfusion. Martinus Nijhoff Publ: Boston/Dordrecht/Lancaster 1988:223-230.

# MAMMALIAN CELL EXPRESSION AND CHARACTERIZATION OF RECOMBINANT HUMAN ANTITHROMBIN III

G. Zettlmeissl, H. Karges, U. Eberhard

## Introduction

Antithrombin III (AT III) is one of the primary inhibitors of hemostasis [1]. By binding to and inhibiting thrombin, as well as several other activated clotting components (most notably Factors IXa, XIa and XIIa) AT III indirectly influences fibrin clot formation [1]. AT III makes a stochiometric 1:1 complex with thrombin. The complex building rate is increased by the binding of heparin by two orders of magnitude [2]. The physiological importance of AT III in preventing excessive coagulation is demonstrated by studies of individuals whose AT III levels are decreased due to hereditary [3-6] or acquired [7-9] deficiency. Human plasma AT III is a single chain glycoprotein of 432 residues containing three intramolecular disulphide bridges and four N-linked carbohydrate chains [10,11].

To provide the basis for an alternative source for human AT III its cDNA was cloned from human liver cDNA libraries [12-15] and its expression was studied in different systems. Since expression in bacteria and yeast resulted in inactive or only partially biologically active AT III molecules [12,13], we decided to use a mammalian tissue culture system to express a protein with very similar properties as compared to the plasma derived AT III [16].

## Results

### Expression of AT III in mammalian cells

The permanent eukaryotic cell line we used for AT III expression was a Chinese hamster ovary (CHO) cell, which is deficient in the enzyme dihydrofolate reductase (DHFR) [17]. This cell line has already been used successfully to synthesize a variety of human proteins in relatively high amounts [18-20]. After cotransfection of the AT III expression vector pSVATIII [16] with the plasmid pSV2dhfr [21] carrying the mouse DHFR cDNA and subsequent coamplification [22] of the transfected DHFR and ATIII genes cell lines were obatined, which have integrated up to 500 copies of the AT III transcription unit into the chromosome [16]. These cell lines (i.e. CHO AII-A279 resistant to 10 $\mu$M MTX) secreted consitutively 1525 $\mu$g AT III/106 cells/24 hours into the culture medium.

*Table 1.* Purification of AT III from CHO cells.

| | Yield (%) | |
|---|---|---|
| **Step** | **CHO-medium** | **h-plasma** |
| Heparin-sepharose | 50 ± 10 | 50 ± 10 |
| 85% ammonium-sulfate precipiation | >90 | >90 |
| Total | 40 – 50 | 40 – 50 |
| Purity* | >98 | >98 |

* As determined by SDS-polyacrylamid electrophoresis [23] followed by Comassie Blue staining.

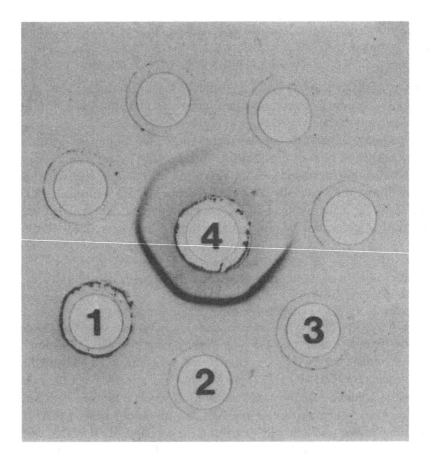

*Figure 1.* Ouchterlony immune diffusion test of recombinant AT III in concentrated serum free CHO culture supernatant (cavity 1), of purified recombinant AT III from CHO cells (cavity 3) and of AT III purified from human plasma (cavity 2), probed with an anti-AT III serum from rabbit (cavity 4).

*Purification of recombinant AT III from CHO supernatants*

A high producing cell line (CHO A11–A279) was grown to mass culture in a fermentation unit (Opticell–bioreactor, KC–biologicals) in the presence of 10% fetal calf serum. Subsequent AT III production was in a serum free medium poor in proteins (Iscove's; Behringwerke AG, Marburg) in order to make the purification process easier. Several hundred milligrams of recombinant AT III were purified by a simple two step purification scheme including adsorption on heparin sepharose, followed by precipitation with ammonium sulfate. During the purification process the recombinant protein behaved identical to AT III from human plasma (Table 1). The total yield of purification was usually 40–50% and the purity of the final product was over 98% as determined by electrophoresis on sodium dodecylsulfate (SDS) polyacrylamid gels according to Laemmli [23; data not shown].

*Characterization of recombinant AT III*

Purified AT III was analyzed by the immunediffusion method of Ouchterlony [24]. The precipitation patterns indicate that recombinant AT III derived from CHO cells is not different from AT III of human plasma origin in this assay (Figure 1).

*Table 2.* Biological activity of purified recombinant AT III..

|  | CHO-medium | h-plasma |
|---|---|---|
| Progressive inhibitor activity (U/mg)* | 5 – 6 | 4,8 – 6,6 |
| Heparin cofactor activity (U/mg)** | 5 – 6 | 4,8 – 6,6 |

U = units
* According to ref. 25, 26.
** According to ref. 27.

*Table 3.* Spectroscopic analysis of purified recombinant AT III.

| Parameter | CHO-medium | h-plasma |
|---|---|---|
| $A_{280\,nm,\,1\,cm}^{1\%}$ [cm²/mg]* | 7,1 | 7,1 |
| $\lambda_{max}^{em}$ [nm]** | 328 | 328 |
| $F_{rel,\,328\,nm}^{em}$ [%]*** | 100 | 100 |
| $\theta_{222\,nm}$ [deg .cm².dmole$^{-1}$]**** | 7600 ± 200 | 7600 ± 200 |

* Absorption coefficient at 280 nm.
** Wavelength of fluorescence emission maximum (excitation at 280 nm).
*** Relative intensity of fluorescence emission at 328 nm (excitation at 280 nm).
**** Far ultraviolet circular dichroism at 222 nm.

At III secreted by CHO cells has the same specific progressive inhibitor [25,26] and heparin cofactor activities [27] as human plasma AT III (Table 2). This means that both the binding to thrombin and the activation by heparin are completely intact in the AT III molecule synthesized by mammalian cells. Besides there is no difference in biophysical properties – like absorption coefficient, fluorescence intensity, fluorescence emission maxima and far UV-circular dichroism – between recombinant and authentic AT III, indicating identical secondary and tertiary structures (Table 3).

Currently we are investigating the biochemical, biophysical and immunologic properties of recombinant AT III in more detail [28] and are performing preclinical studies in order to check the purity, half-life and antigenicity *in vivo*.

## Conclusions

Human AT III can be expressed in mammalian cells and can be purified from culture medium with a yield of 40-50% to a purity greater than 98%. Recombinant AT III from CHO cells is identical to AT III from human plasma concerning biological activity and the immunological, biochemical and biophysical parameters checked up to now. The described expression system can be used to study structure-function relationships of AT III by systematic directed mutagenesis of the molecule.

## Acknowledgments

We would like to thank Prof R. Jaenicke (Regensburg) for help in performing the spectroscopic analyses and M. Cieplik, H. Naumann and E. Veit for excellent technical assistance.

## References

1. Rosenberg RD. Antithrombin III, biochemistry, function, assay and clinical significance. Ann Univ Sarav Med 1983;3:13-4.
2. Damus PS, Hicks M, Rosenberg RD. Anticoagulant action of heparin. Nature 1973;246:355-7.
3. Egeberg D. Inherited antithrombin deficiency causing thrombophilia. Thromb Diath Haemorrh 1965;13:516-41.
4. Sas G, Blasko G, Banhegyi D, Jako J, Palos LA. Abnormal antithrombin III (antithombin III Budapest) as a cause of familiar thrombophilia. Thromb Diath Haemorrh 1974;32:105-15.
5. Sorensen PJ, Dyerberg J, Stoffersen E, Jensen MK. Familiar functional antithrombin III deficiency. Scand J Haematol 1980;24:105-9.
6. Koide T, Odani S, Takahashi K, Ono T, Sakuragawa N. Antithrombin III Toyama: Replacement of arginine-47 by cysteine in hereditary abnormal antithrombin III that lacks heparin-binding ability. Proc Natl Acad Sci (USA) 1984;81:289-93.

7. Abildgaard U, Fagerhol MK, Egeberg D. Comparison of progressive antithrombin activity and the concentration of three thrombin inhibitors in plasma. Scand J Clin Invest 1970;26:349-54.
8. Thaler E, Balzer E, Kopsa H, Pinggera WF. Acquired antithrombin deficiency in patients with glomerular proteinuria. Haemostasis 1978;7:257-72.
9. Fagerhol MK, Abildgaard U. Immunological studies on human antithrombin III. Scand J Haematol 1970;7:10-7.
10. Nordeman B, Nystroem C, Björk I. The size and shape of human and bovine antithrombin III. Eur J Biochem 1977;78:195-203.
11. Franzen LE, Svenssen S. Structural studies on the carbohydrate portion of human antithrombin III. J Biol Chem 1980;255:5090-3.
12. Bock SC, Wion KL, Vehar GA, Lawn RM. Cloning and expression of the cDNA for human antithrombin III. Nucl Acids Res 1982;10:8113-25.
13. Prochownik EV, Markham AF, Orkin SH. Isolation of a cDNA clone for human antithrombin III. J Biol Chem 1983;258:8389-94.
14. Chandra T, Stackhouse R, Kidd VJ, Woo SLC. Isolation and sequence characterization of a cDNA clone of human antithrombin III. Proc Natl Acad Sci (USA) 1983;80:1845-8.
15. Bröker M, Ragg H, Karges H. Expression of human antithrombin III in Saccharomyces cerevisiae and Schizosacchoromyces pombe. Biochim Biophys Acta 1987;908: 203-13.
16. Zettmeissl G, Ragg H, Karges H. Expression of biologically active human antithrombin III in Chinese hamster ovary cells. Bio/Technology 1987;5:720-5.
17. Urlaub G, Chasin LA. Isolation of Chinese hamster cell mutants deficient in dihydrofolate reductase activity. Proc Natl Acad Sci (USA) 1980;77:4216-20.
18. Kaufman RJ, Wasley LC, Spiliotes et al. Coamplification and coexpression of human tissue-type plasminogen activator and murine dihydrofolate reductase sequences in Chinese hamster ovary cells. Mol Cell Biol 1985;5:1750-9.
19. Kaufman RJ, Wasley LC, Furie BC, Shoemaker CB. Expression, purification and characterization of recombinant-carboxylated Factor IX synthesized in Chinese hamster ovary cells. J Biol Chem 1986;261:9622-8.
20. Mory J, Ben-Barak J, Segev D et al. Effective constitutive production of IFN-γ in Chinese hamster ovary cells. DNA 1986;5:181-93.
21. Lee F, Mulligan R, Berg P, Ringold G. Glucocorticoids regulate expression of dihydrofolate reductase cDNA in mouse mammary tumor virus chimaeric plasmids. Nature 1981;294:228-32.
22. Ringold G, Dieckmann B, Lee F. Co-expression and amplification of dihydrofolate reductase cDNA and Escherichia coli XGPRT gene in Chinese hamster ovary cells. J Mol Appl Genet 1981;1:165-75.
23. Laemmli UK. Cleavage of structural proteins during the assembly of the head of bacteriophage T4. Nature 1970;227:680-5.
24. Ouchterlony O. Progr Allergy 1958;5:1-78.
25. Hensen A, Loeliger EA. Antithrombin III assay. Thromb Diath Haemorrh 1963;9(suppl 1):18-29.
26. Kirkwood TBL, Barrowcliffe TW, Thomas DP. An international collaborative study establishing a reference preparation for antithrombin III. Thromb Haemost 1980;43:10-5.
27. Schrader J, Züchner C, Köstering H, Scheler F. Chromogenic substrates for the determination of antithrombin III. Ärztl Lab 1986;32:111-4.
28. Zettlmeissl G, Karges H, Eberhard U. Characterization of recombinant human antithrombin III from mammalian cells. (Unpublished data.)

# PRODUCTION AND TESTING OF rDNA HEPATITS B VACCINE

Ch.R. Bennett, Jr.

## Introduction

Recombinant DNA technology has been described by Burnett and Marsh as the prime biological tool of the 1980's and perhaps of the 20th century [1]. Within the past ten years, we have witnessed the use of recombinant DNA technology to produce insulin as a competitive commercial product. Concurrently, we saw also the birth of a new industry devoted to the development of gene products for both human and veterinary uses.

More recently, in 1986, the first hepatitis B virus vaccine for human use prepared by rDNA technology was introduced. This vaccine, of course, is of particular value to those persons associated with the handling of human blood and blood products.

Hepatitis B vaccines prepared from human plasma have been commercially available since 1983. Hepatitis B plasma-derived vaccine which meets WHO and government regulatory agency requirements has been shown to be completely safe [2,3]. Unfortunately, highly emotional concerns over the theoretical possibility of an infectious agent being present in the plasma and surviving the purification and inactivation procedures has somewhat impeded general acceptance of the plasma-derived hepatitis B vaccine.

**Essential steps in vaccine development.**

Recognize need for vaccine
Isolate and propagate agent
Develop prototype vaccine
Test vaccine in animals
Evaluate feasibility of commercial production
Produce vaccine consistency lots
Test for safety
Begin closed clinical trials (Phase I)
Evaluate closed trials
Expand clinical trials (Phase II)
Begin large field trials (Efficacy studies)
Evaluate field trials
Apply for vaccine license

Examine field trial data
Perform assays on vaccine samples
Review license application } Responsibility of regulatory agency
Issue license

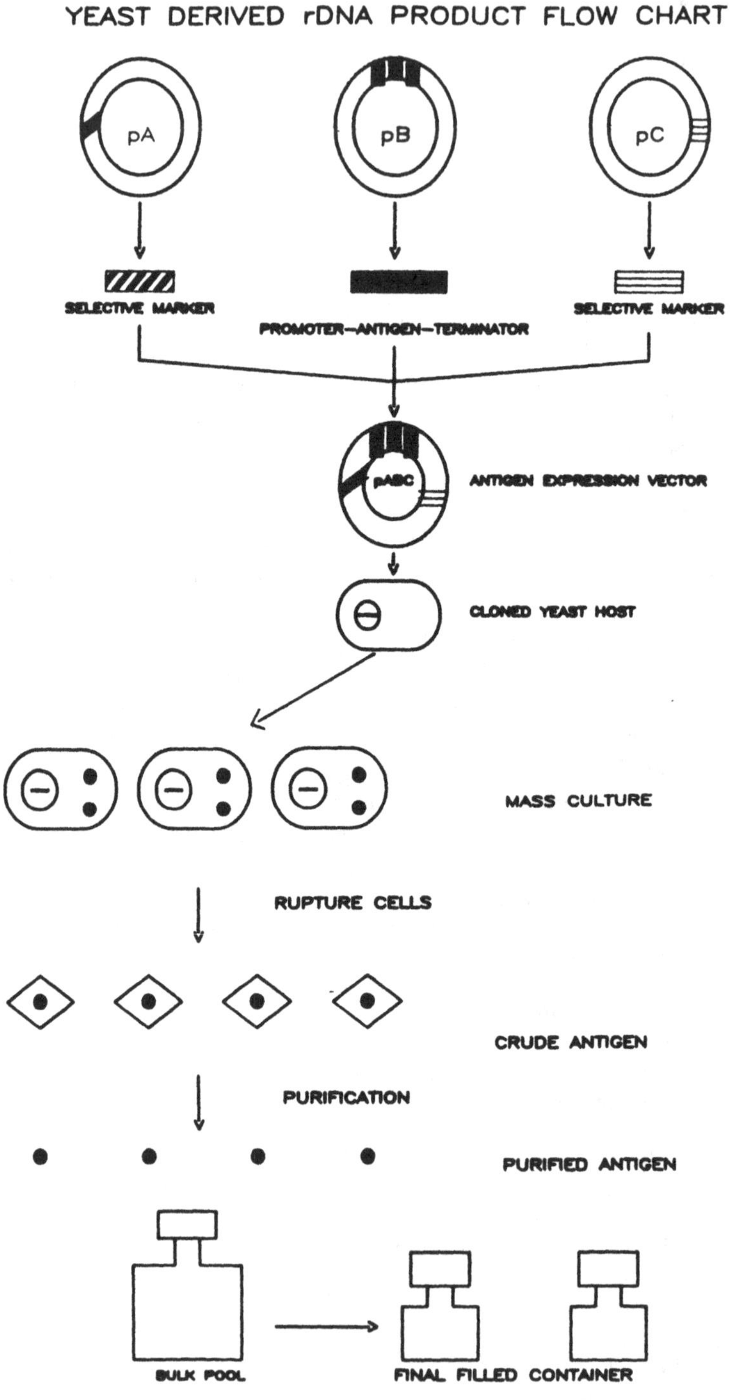

140

*Figure 1.* Flow chart showing basic operational steps in production of rDNA vaccine.

Since the supply of the plasma-derived vaccine is potentially limited to the availability of suitable plasma from carriers of hepatitis B infection, alternative sources of surface antigen (HBsAg) had to be obtained. Research efforts were directed toward rDNA techniques.

As listed, this point of recognizing the need for a vaccine is the initial point in the steps necessary for the development of a vaccine.

However, in the case of recombinant hepatitis B vaccine, additional challenges had to be faced before final licensing could be accomplished. The vaccine prepared by recombinant DNA technology had to meet the challenges of the "Five C's":

Characterization;
Comparison;
Clinical;
Control;
Consistency.

*Characterization* of product through knowledge of its biological, chemical and physical properties.

*Comparison* of the characteristics of the product with the same or similar characteristics of the naturally occurring antigen.

*Clinical* testing to insure safety, efficacy and purity of the product.

*Control* to ensure that the product retains its inherent characteristics.

*Consistency* of production to ensure continued product integrity.

As has been discussed throughout this conference, advances in molecular biology and nucleic acid chemistry have led to the development of laboratory techniques that can identify gene coding for biologically active substances. We can accurately analyze the gene code and we can transfer these genes between organisms to obtain controlled gene expression with the resulting efficient synthesis of products for which they code. We have seen how a gene which codes for a specific product can be isolated and then propagated by extracting the DNA and inserting it into a suitable vector with the aid of enzyme systems which cleave or join the gene insert at precise and specific points to the vector. Then when the vector is introduced into a host organism, clones can be selected which carry the desired gene. The progeny of the clones may then be propagated in mass culture and gene expression obtained.

## Vaccine production using rDNA technology

Let us examine briefly how the use of rDNA applies to a production operation for hepatitis B vaccine. Initially, one must develop an expression vector which codes for the gene producing the hepatitis B surface antigen. In the example expression vector seen in Figure 1, the plasmid pABC is constructed by combining the gene for surface antigen (plasmid B) with other selective marker genes, from plasmids pA, and pC.

Let us assume pA is an auxotropic marker permitting yeast cell growth in a medium deficient in one amino acid in contrast to the requirement of the parent yeast, and pC is a color marker which causes the cells to produce a purple pigmented colony on agar instead of the white colony produced by the parent yeast. Then the final antigen expression vector can be inserted into a yeast cell which can produce the three desired traits. Thus, we have a way in which we can quickly identify the recombinant strain.

Cloning of the progeny from this cell results in a master cell culture or master seed. This concept is most important since the progeny of the master seed will yield quantities of the desired antigen or product in crude form through fermentation processes.

Finally, through intermediate stages of extraction, concentration and purification, the antigen is obtained in a purified form which is held in a bulk pool from which the final filled product is obtained.

*Characterization*

In order for the product to be characterized, let us start with the expression vector. The constructs of the intermediate plasmids and the final expression vector are examined:
1. To confirm presence of correct and complete DNA sequences by nucleotide sequence analysis.
2. To confirm size, location and orientation of inserted sequences by restriction enzyme analysis.
3. To demonstrate that DNA fragments hybridize to specific radiolabelled probes as seen in autoradiograms from the Southern blot technique.

The host system itself must be characterized to show:
a. Passage history;
b. Presence of selective markers.;
c. Description of potential pathogenicity;
d. Phenotype;
e. Presence of any naturally occurring plasmids;
f. Presence of any integrated DNA sequences.

Thus, characterization of the expression vector and the host cell system forms the basis of the master seed concept which provides insurance of continued consistent gene expression.

In the research and development stages, the product also must be characterized:
a. To define chemical structure of the antigen by amino acid analysis and amino acid sequencing.
b. To examine the general structure of the antigen polypeptides by peptide mapping.
c. To determine presence of potential contaminants from host components by chemical and immunological analysis, e.g.,

1. Carbohydrates;
2. Ribosomal DNA;
3. Antigen DNA;
4. Protein.

## Comparison

Equally important to characterization in the overall concept of the 5 C's is the second C – *comparison*. After rigorous identification and characterization of the yeast-derived product by biological and chemical methods, it is necessary to determine the structural, biological or immunological similarities and differences between the recombinant and the naturally occurring HBsAg.

Electron microscopic observation of recombinant vaccine revealed the presence of spherical particles ranging from 17 to 25 nm in diameter (Figure 2).

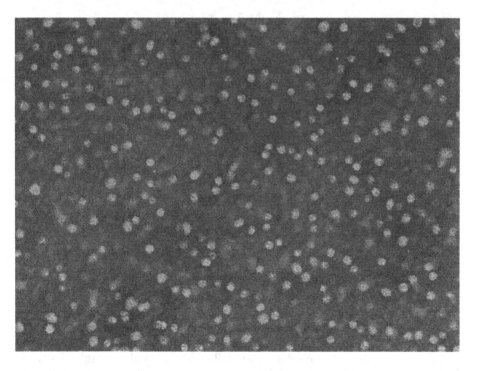

*Figure 2.* Electron microscopic view of HBsAg particles in vaccine prepared from recombinant yeast cells (scale bar = 100 nm).

These particles were found to be similar in size to the naturally occurring particle in the plasma-derived vaccine (Figure 3).

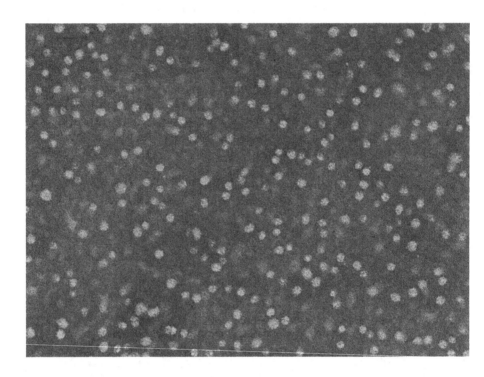

*Figure 3.* Electron microscopic view of naturally occurring HBsAg particles in vaccine prepared from human plasma (scale bar = 100 nm)

Sodium dodecylsulfate polyacrylaminde gel electrophoresis analyses under non-reducing and reducing conditions revealed that the particles are composed entirely of the non-glycosylated 24,000 molecular weight forms of HBsAg and are highly cross-linked with intermolecular disulphide bonds. The particles do not contain the 27,000 molecular weight glycosylated form of HBsAg. This glycosylated form constitutes approximately 25% of the HBsAg found in plasma-derived particles. In addition, the yeast-derived vaccine contains yeast specific proteins. Current production methods, however, yield a product which is greater than 99% HBsAg.

By physical examination, it is evident that some properties of the recombinant vaccine are clearly similar but not identical to those of the plasma-derived product.

It is necessary also to compare the two vaccines by immunological analysis. The plasma-derived vaccine which is composed of the HBsAg of the ad subtype was shown by Hilleman and others to induce protective immunity in chimpanzees against challenge with virus of either ad or ay subtypes [4]. In an identical series of experiments the yeast-derived vaccine, which is of the ad subtype, was shown by Emini and others to induce protective immunity in chimpanzees when challenged by virus of either subtype [5].

In addition, the plasma-derived and yeast-direved vaccine products were used to absorb antibody from serum of persons vaccinated with either of the two vaccines. From these studies Emini showed that the cross-adsorption patterns indicated that the spectra of anti-HBs antibodies elicited by the two products were similar, if not identical.

The results of potency testing of each vaccine in mice are quite similar also. In 33 production lots of plasma-derived vaccines that have been made, a mean potency $ED_{50}$ value of 0.6 $\mu g/ml$ has been seen. Similarly, the mean $ED_{50}$ of the 24 most recent lots of recombinant vaccine has been 0.3 $\mu g/ml$.

*Clinical*

The results of clinical testing to insure safety, efficacy and purity of the product are continuously evolving and even a summary could not be presented in the limited time for this report. A relevant study which can serve to illustrate the clinical "C", however, was that of Zajac in which healthy individuals were vaccinated with 2.5, 5, 10 and 20 $\mu g$ quantities of recombinant DNA vaccine in order to access the degree of seroconversion and the eight of antibody respons [6]. These studies showed that with healthy adults the percentage of vaccines showing seroconversion for anti-HBs (titer greater than 10 IU/l) was similar for all dosages at 3, 6, and 8 months, with 89 to 97% of recipients developing antibody by the 8th month, which was 2 months after the second injection.

The geometric mean titer of vaccine responders at 8 months varied with dosage, with higher GMT's being obtained with 10 and 20 $\mu g$ doses of vaccine than with 2.5 and 5.0 $\mu g$ doses. In the same report, the effect of age of recipient and antibody response was studied also. This portion of the study showed that younger adults in the 20-29 year age group demonstrated more active response to 10 $\mu g$ doses of vaccine than did those older than 50 years of age. The effect of age was evident not only in the seroconversion rates following one or two injections but in the GMT of responders receiving 3 injections of vaccine. Most notable, however, was the fact that three 10 $\mu g$ doses of vaccine produced seroconversion in 91% of adults 50 years of age or older.

*Control*

The time cycle of the first 3 C's extended over a period of several years. Concurrent with the clinical trials, scale-up of the production operation occurred, stability studies were initiated, and assay facilities expanded. Negotiations continued with the personnel of the U.S. Office of Biologics and other regulatory agencies world-wide to establish assay procedures and firm specifications.

Quality control of a biological product is not limited to a series of assays performed on the contents of a few final filled containers, but is based upon overall knowledge and testing of various intermediate steps of processing.

The World Health Organization recommendations issued for hepatitis B vaccines made by recombinant DNA technology state that the novelty of the recombinant DNA derived vaccines and the procedures that are used in their manufacture dictate a need for reasoned caution in their control [7]. This point, however, is tempered by the statement in the WHO recommendations that certain tests should be required on every production batch of vaccine but others will be required only to establish validity, acceptability and consistency of a given manufacturing practice.

Throughout the development of the commercial process and scale-up to final production operations, the concept of in-process control has been emphasized and carried out. This was particularly valuable in defining fermentation parameters which show the structure of the expression vector and characteristics of the host cell prior to full-scale fermentation cycles.

After fermentation, the yeast culture is examined for culture purity and plasmid stability. During intermediate stages of purification, the antigenic content is followed with assays to determine degree of purity. For example, at the final aqueous stage prior to alum adsorption, the following are examples of the tests that are performed on the product.

1.  Sterility.
2.  Antigen and protein content.
3.  Purity
    a.  Gel electrophoresis
        (1) Silver stain to demonstrate presence of P24 antigen;
        (2) Western blot to detect surface antigen and possible yeast impurities.
    b.  HPSEC to determine level of yeast protein.
    c.  Epitope configuration by monoclonal antibody.
4.  LAL for endotoxin.
5.  Reagent analysis.

After alum adsorption, addition tests such as sterility and absence of reagents are repeated and, finally, the contents of the final container are subjected to testing for:
1.  Sterility.
2.  General safety.
3.  Reagent analysis.
4.  Freezing point depression.
5.  Identity.
6.  Endotoxin.
7.  Mouse potency.

*Consistency of process*

In the production of any biological product, the fourth and fifth C's are necessary companions. The consistency of process is the basis of success for any biological product. With the advent of rDNA technology, industry has witnessed the introduction of production and analytical techniques that are capable of producing large quantities of purified proteins and polypeptides that can be precisely analyzed. Nevertheless, although physiochemical characterization can ensure a high degree of purity for a product made by recombinant DNA methods, reliable and sensitive biological tests are needed to detect for trace contamination that may be inherent in biological processes. Recombinant DNA technology is a new tool and relatively little experience has been gained of its use or of the control problems encountered; thus, it is necessary for all manufacturers to show batch-to-batch consistency in identity, purity, and quality of the product.

## Conclusion

This presentation has covered practical considerations involved in the recovery of HBsAg and its application as a vaccine using recombinant DNA technology. Although experience is beginning to show that coding for genes of other virus sub-particles that are capable of eliciting an immune response in man are not making as rapid progress as seen with HBsAg, the concentration of effort that is underway, particularly in the field of AIDS research, promises hope for additional rDNA vaccines in the future.

## References

1.  Burnett JP, Marsh NM. Recombinant DNA technology: Tool of the 1980's. Pharm Tech 1980;Oct 4:42-6.
2.  Hepatitis B vaccine: Evidence confirming lack of AIDS transmission MMWR 1984;33:685-7.
3.  Francis DP, Feorino PM, McDougal S et al. The safety of the hepatitis B vaccine: Inactivation of the AIDS virus during routine vaccine manufacture. JAMA 1986;256:869-72.
4.  Hilleman MR, Bertland AU, Buynak EB et al. Clinical and laboratory studies in HBsAg vaccine. In: Vyas GN, Cohen SN, Schmidt R (eds). Viral hepatitis. Philadelphia: The Franklin Institute Press 1978:525-37.
5.  Emini EA, Ellis RW, Miller WJ, McAleer WJ, Scolnick EM, Gerety RJ. Production and analysis of recombinant hepatitis B vaccine. J Inf 1986;13:3-9.
6.  Zajac BA, West DJ, McAleer WJ, Scolnick EM. Overview of clinical studies with hepatitis B vaccine made by recombinant DNA. J Inf 1986;13:39-45.
7.  World Health Organization. Expert committee on biological standardization: Proposed requirements for the hepatitis B vaccines made by recombinant DNA techniques. (Requirements for Biological Substances No. 39) 1986. WHO/BS/85.1478Rev.3.

# PRODUCTION AND APPLICATION OF MONOCLONAL ANTIBODIES IN T-CELL DEPLETION OF BONE MARROW FOR TRANSPLANTATION

P. Hervé

## Introduction

Recent biotechnological developments have provided an increasingly precise and specific discrimination of cells according to their cell surface marker phenotype [1]. Production and purification techniques of monoclonal antibodies (MoAbs) have become standardized today. Their clinical application (systemic infusion, *ex-vivo* purging) requires purification conditions and control methods which provide the clinician with a perfectly controlled product which is compatible with its therapeutic use. At present, we have a wide panel of MoAbs specific to T-cells at various differentiation levels which provide experimental and clinical investigations so that normal marrow T-cells (GvHD prevention) or leukemia T-cells (minimum residual disease purging) can be removed from the marrow.

In allogeneic bone marrow transplantation, acute and chronic GvH prevention through T-cell depletion is currently the most alluring procedure although its actual future is being widely debated. The ideal procedure would be to remove only those T-cells which cause the GvH reaction while preserving the allo-reactive T-cells involved in graft versus leukemia (GvL) and Host-versus-Graft reactions (HvGR). In autologous marrow transplantation there are multiple purging methods that should kill the residual leukemic cells *in vitro*. It is important to determine that the purging procedure has not adversely affected the hematopoietic potential of the marrow. We must demonstrate that the leukemic cell removal has been achieved with high efficiency. The characteristics of anti T-cell MoAbs at our disposal, and their main applications in the removal of normal and leukemic T-cells in allogeneic and autologous bone marrow will be described here.

## Analysis of T-cell MoAb panel

In spite of its wide application, the essential of the hybridoma technology for making MoAbs has changed little over the years [2]. At the time of the 3rd International workshop on human leukocyte differentiation antigens, 225 antibodies specific to T-lymphocyte antigens were submitted to the analysis [3] The antibodies which showed similar binding patterns were clustered. Clusters of 3 or more antibodies from different laboratories, were given CD designation by the WHO nomenclature committee. Clusters of anti-T cell antibodies CD1 to 8, CD25 and CDW26 were previously defined (Table 1).

*Table 1.* T-cell antigens. Previously and newly defined clusters.

| Antigen designation (from workshop) | Name of antibody | Reactivity |
| --- | --- | --- |
| CD1 | NA1/34,OKT6,D47 | Thymocytes |
| CD2 | OKT11,Leu5,D66,CT2 | Pan-T lymphocyte (sheep eryth. receptor) |
| CD3 | OKT3,UCHT1,Leu4 | Pan-T lymphocyte |
| CD4 | OKT4,Leu3 | T helper/inducer |
| CD5 | T101,A50,OKT1,Leu1 | Pan-T lymphocyte |
| CD6 | MBG6,12.1 | Pan-T; Subpopulation of B |
| CD7 | 3A1,Leu9,WT1,I21 | Pan-T lymphocyte |
| CD8 | OKT8,Leu2,RFT8 | T cytotoxic/suppressor |
| CD25 | 3A3,33B3-1 | Interleukin-2; Receptor |
| CDW26 | 4 Elic 7 | Activated T-cells |
| CD27 | OKT18A,vit14 | Mature T-cell antigen |
| CD28 | 9.3,KOLT-2 | Subpopulation of T-cells |
| CDW29 | K20,4B4 | Subpopulation of CD4-positive cells |

*Table 2.* Applications for marrow purging in allogeneic and autologous marrow transplantation

MoAbs and complement (rabbit, human)
Immunotoxins
– intact ricin (A + B chains)
– ricin A-chain + $NH_4Cl$
Immuno-physical separation
– magnetic immunobeads

Three new clusters were established: CD27, CD28 and CDW29. CD1 was divided into CD1a, CD1b and CD1c recognizing three different glycoproteins [3].

MoAbs identify T-lymphocytes, and have proved to be sensitive and discriminatory. Many of these MoAbs react with immature T-cells; others react with more mature T-cells. Some of these identify antigens found on all T-cells (pan-T MoAbs), whereas others bind only on T cell subsets. MoAbs with important specificities may be difficult to use in the laboratory or clinical situation because they are of classes or subclasses which do not have the required effector functions or which have unfavorable physical or chemical properties (i.e. affinity of the antibody for antigen-bearing cells, association and dissociation rate constants) [4]. MoAbs may be difficult to use for bone marrow purging because they are of an isotype that does not fix complement and cannot mediate C' dependent cytotoxicity (i.e. IgG1). The IgG3 isotype may be relatively insoluble and sometimes precipitate in the cold. IgG2 (a,b) and IgM isotypes appear to be the most effective antibodies in mediating C' lysis of target cells.

The importance of quality control in the production of MoAbs is fully recognized insofar as we intend to use MoAbs both for systemic infusion and for *ex-vivo* marrow purging. De Rie *et al.* have recently described their protocol for the isolation of MoAbs from ascitic fluids [5]. The purification scheme consisted of Ig purification by standard ion exchange column chromatography. Mouse and myeloma cells were tested for the presence of retrovirus. Sterility and pyrogen tests have to be performed to define a suitable antibody for clinical use.

When MoAbs are used in *in vivo* applications, care should be taken to prevent adverse reactions. We need a preparation devoid of aggregates and other foreign proteins. High performance size exclusion chromatography (HP-SEC) seems the most sensitive technique for a biophysical evaluation of purified Ig preparations. For each MoAb used in an assay procedure the methods of production, purification and storage of the antibodies should be documented.

The production of functional chimeric mouse/human antibody consisting of mouse variable regions (idiotype) binding to human constant regions results in a less immunogenic antibody that binds human complement more effectively [6]. That chimeric antibody may have important clinical applications in the future.

## Application of anti-T cell MoAbs to the GvHD prophylaxis

### 1. Graft-versus-Host-Disease (GvDH)

Despite fully matched histocompatibility and the use of immunosuppressive agents after BMT (methotrexate, cyclosporin A, steroids) severe forms of acute GvHD contribute to early mortality. Out of 1,106 patients reported by the EBMTG, the acute GvH rate was as follows: mild (grade I) in 23%, moderate (grade II) in 20% and severe (grade III-IV) in 21%. It was not observed in 36%. Chronic GvH occurred in 24% of the patients (extensive in a third of the cases). Patients who survive severe acute GvHD suffer from the consequences of chronic GvHD, i.e.: immunodeficiency, infectious complications (viral infections), prolonged hospitalization, autoimmune disorders and require immunosuppressive therapy for months if not years [7]. Therefore all efforts have to be made to prevent severe forms of acute and chronic GvHD in most cases, so that allogeneic marrow transplantation becomes a fairly safe procedure.

On the basis of studies in experimental animal models, attempts to prevent GvHD have been made by removing alloreactive T-lymphocytes [8]. It is not yet known today whether all the T-lymphocytes must be removed. Korngold and Sprent [9] found that contamination of the marrow with a low percentage of T-cells (0.3%) was enough to cause a high incidence of lethal GvHD in histoincompatible BMT in mice.

## 2. Removal of GvHD producing T-cells from the allogeneic marrow

A large number of different immunologic methods which have been reported aim to remove >99% of T-cells from the marrow donor (Table 2). Antibody mediated methods have prevailed until now in the pilot clinical studies [10,11].

### a. Complement mediated cytolysis

This method depends on many critical factors reported in Table 3. Based on studies using animal models, pan-T MoAbs ± associated with antibodies that recognize T-cell subsets (CD4, CD8) are highly effective in preventing severe forms of GvHD (magnitude of depletion: 90 to >99%) according to the MoAb cocktail composition and the number of treatments performed. The pioneer work by Prentice *et al.* [12] has recommended T-cell depletion with pan-T MoAbs followed by rabbit C' incubation. This method has provided the investigators with an overall lower incidence and severity of acute GvH. Since the 1st study this technique of T-cell depletion has been widely applied in clinical BMT [13-16].

*Table 3.* Inherent problems associated with *in vitro* puring by means of MoAbs and complement.

---

Antibodies have to bind C'
This technique depends on many variables viz,
- expression of antigen
- cell concentration
- possible anticomplementary activity from bone marrow cells
Multiple MoAbs are more effective than a single one
Rabbit C' is more effective than human C'
Some lots of C' can inhibit normal stem cells
There is a variation in the C' lytic activity from one lot to the other
The cost of baby rabbit C' is high
Following tumor cell lysis there is a possible transfection to normal cells

---

Although the question remains open to discussion, should all T-lymphocytes be removed, or would the removal of a certain subset suffice to prevent GvHD? Most investigators have included one or several pan-T MoAbs in their antibody cocktail [13,15,17,18] To reach a magnitude of >99% T-cell depletion, we need at least 2 cycles of complement. Nevertheless, when using a single treatment, we, with others, reported an effective prevention of severe forms of GvHD [13,17]. Anti-T cell MoAbs, chosen with a view to purging T-cells from the marrow, have been included in the 8 defined cluster groups (CD1 to CD8). All the antibodies fix rabbit C' (IgG2 or IgM isotype). Baby rabbit C' is recommended despite its high cost. It is selected on the basis of the lack of heterohemagglutinins and toxicity on hemopoietic progenitor cells. A constant rate of calcium, magnesium, HU-50 and reproducible cytotoxic activity with MoAbs are needed. Preclinical studies were performed to determine the optimal dosage of each antibody chosen according to the marrow cell concentration ($< 3.10^7$ NC per ml). The identification of residual T-cells was performed either by indirect immunofluorescence (cells were counted by microscope or flow cytometry), PHA culture or by limiting dilution [19]. As a total removal of T-cells is unnecessary in HLA identical BMT, indirect IF proves to be a most suitable method.

Most of the anti-T cell MoAbs were found to be relatively inefficient when human C' was used to obtain lysis, although the ideal method would have consisted of using human C' in the C' mediated lysis system Waldmann *et al.* selected Campath-1 [16], a rat IgM antibody, to remove T-cells from marrow. Campath-1 shows an undefined antigen present on virtually all normal T and B lymphocytes and monocytes.

### b. Ex-vivo immunotoxin (IT) treatment [20]

Preclinical studies have indicated that IT are efficient when compared with the C' mediated lysis method of T-cell depletion [21] It is composed of MoAbs covalently coupled to bacterial or plant toxins. The antibody targets the IT to the cell, while the toxin inhibits protein synthesis and causes cell death following internalization of the IT. Different toxins, including ricin or its A-chain subunit as well as diptheria toxin or Pokeweed Antiviral Protein (PAP), have been used. Ricin is one of the frequently used toxins in the preparation of IT. B-chain in the conjugates facilitates the entry of the toxic A-chain into target cells. The B-chain ricin binds galactose residues to the cell surface and the A-chain inactivates ribosomal subunits enzymatically once it is translocated from the endosomes into the cytosol. Treatment with intact ricin requires the presence of lactose to block the galactose binding site of the B-chain effectively. A-chain ricin IT can be used provided that ammonium chloride is added to the culture medium and pH is alkaline. Whole ricin or the A-chain is linked to MoAbs included in the CD2, CD3, CD5 and/or CD7. It is known to inhibit human T-cell proliferation. Protein synthesis is inhibited both in T-cell lines and normal T-cells. The investigators have used a mixture of either anti T-cell ITs (TA1-IT+CD2-IT+CD5-IT) or a single CD5/T101-IT to pretreat donor marrow. Both approaches were efficient in terms of T-cell inhibition and were suitable for GvHD prevention [22].

### c. Immunomagnetic treatment of bone marrow allografts [23]

In preclinical studies, Vartdal *et al.* have shown that magnetic microspheres coated with MoAbs specific to T-cells may deplete T-cells from the bone marrow without harming the hematopoietic precursor cells [24]. MoAbs of the IgG isotypes were coated indirectly, in a second layer on microspheres precoated with anti-mouse IgG antibodies whereas the MoAbs of the IgM isotype was coated directly on the microspheres. Immunomagnetic T-cell purging was shown to be efficient, leaving less than 0.025% ERFC in the purged marrow. The viability of marrow cells exceeded 99% in all experiments and the recovery of non T-cells, after purging, varied from 43-74%. This technique is a fast and efficient means of T-cell depletion; however a pilot clinical study is needed particularly as stable engraftment was not obtained in the first two patients treated with an immunomagnetic T-cell purged marrow [24].

## GvHD prevention through T-cell depletion – clinical results (Table 4)

An effective prevention of GvHD has been demonstrated in 298 HLA-matched BMT reported by 8 teams throughout the world. Six teams used C'-mediated lysis with a cocktail of 2 to 8 anti-T MoAbs and 2 teams used pan-T MoAbs, linked to ricin (either intact ricin or A-chain only). In 37 patients (12.4%) an acute > grade II GvHD occurred; 56 patients (18.8%) experienced graft rejection and/or autologous marrow recovery. In our institution, compared with our initial experience, i.e. (non graft failure in the first 32 patients) [13], between November '85 and September '86, several patients showed evidence of either non take (2 patients), graft rejection (6 patients) or autologous reconstitution (4 patients). Engraftment failure in most cases was concomitant with viral infection, particularly CMV infection. It was obvious with all but two published clinical studies (especially in 2 randomized studies [14,25]) that leukemia relapse was more frequent in the T-cell depleted group than in the controls [26].

*Table 4.* Incidence of graft failure and actue GvHD

| Methods | Number of patients | Graft failure | Actue GvH > grade II | Reference |
|---|---|---|---|---|
| CD6+8+2C' | 34 | 3 | 3 | Prentice [18] |
| 8 anti MoAbs+1C' | 47 | 13 | 13 | Martin [15] |
| CD2+5+7+1C' | 43 | 8 | 3 | Hervé [13] |
| Campath-A+2C' | 44 | 8 | 0 | Slavin [27] |
| Campath-1+1C' | 39 | 4 | 9 | Apperley [26] |
| CD2+5+7+1C' or CD4+5+8+1C' | 47 | 12 | 3 | GEGMO [25] |
| CD5-Ricin A | 27 | 4 | 2 | GEGMO (unpublished) |
| TA1-CD3+5-whole ricin | 17 | 4 | 4 | Filipovitch [22] |

T-cell depletion remains the best method available in preventing GvHD. Furthermore, we have to point out that the quality of life is excellent. Therefore the main question remains open to discussion: does graft failure and leukemia relapse after T-cell depleted BMT contraindicate this GvHD prevention procedure? We think that additional measures could be taken to overcome complications induced by T-cell depletion; i.e. intensification of conditioning regimen [27], *in vivo* MoAbs to control immune response if one could define and deplete the cells which are responsible for marrow rejection. Therefore, in our current protocol in patients at a standard risk of relapse, those presenting a low GvHD risk (i.e. sex matched, non-reactive mixed epidermal cell lymphocyte culture), and conditioned with fractionated TBI + cytoxan, receive an non-manipulated transplant and GvH prophylaxis with methotrexate. Those presenting high GvHD risk, receive a T-cell depleted transplant (an untreated autologous bone marrow rescue, harvested before the preparative regimen is started) and are conditioned with the TAM proto-col (fractionated TBI+high dose Ara-C+high dose melphalan) in order to overcome the host versus graft reaction and deal with leukemic relapse. In both groups, chimerism is analyzed by restriction fragment lenth polymorphisms (RFLP) to determine the percentage of full chimerism and mixed chimerism respectively. Other investigators are evaluating the effective-ness of *in vivo* MoAbs (pan-T MoAbs, anti human LFA$_1$) to over come the HvGR [29,30]. Preliminary results imply that mismatched BMT (higher than 1 locus disparity) using additional immunosuppression (high dose Ara-C, MoAbs *in vivo*, antithymocyte globulins) and T-cell depleted inoculum could be possible with a low incidence of graft failure or servere GvHD [31,32].

## Autologous bone marrow transplantation (ABMT) in T-cell malignancies. Ex-vivo purging of inoculum with MoAbs

The lymphoid T-cell proliferations show a certain number of differentiating antigens identified by MoAbs. The antibodies have provided a classification, in terms of a differentiation level, of malignant T-cell proliferations. ALL and T-lymphoma in children and adults can be distinguished by their antigenic phenotype. The pan-T MoAbs which belong to the CD2, CD5 and CD7, identify most of the malignant T-cell proliferation [1]. The CD7 reagents alone (WT-1, RFT2, 3A1, Leu 9, I 21) covering the vast majority of T-ALL cases. A panel of anti-T MoAbs provides key reagents for differential diag-nosis (phenotypic analysis of T-lymphoid malignancies) and therapy (*ex-vivo* and *in vivo* purging) [33].

Current ABMT protocol rely on the efficiency of *ex-vivo* techniques which are capable of reducing, to a maximum log, the number of residual conta-minating leukemic cells in the inoculum. Anti-T MoAbs with C' or linked to ricin, may be applied to residual targeting T-ALL cells from the marrow prior to cryopreservation. Campath-1 could also play a part in purging T-ALL bone marrow prior to ABMT [34]. The crucial conditions for purging autologous marrow through C' mediated cytolysis have been defined previously [35]. *Ex-vivo* treatment of the bone marrow should be standardized in terms of cell concentration, choice of MoAbs and precise doses which must be used as well as temperature and incubation time of the C' with the cells. There is no close concordance between the log target having small volumes of cell suspen-sion treated (magnitude of depletion higher than 99.9%) and that obtained

*Table 5.* T-cell depletion from marrow harvested in T-ALL during CR.

| Number T-ALL (harvested marrow) | | T-cells in BM prior to purging | Residual T cells* after purging | Percentage of cytoreduction |
|---|---|---|---|---|
| 8 | mean | 22.7% ± 6.5 | 1.07% ± 0.2 | 98 ± 1.03 |
| | range | (14-35) | (0-1.5) | (96- >99) |

* IF positive, EB negative.

*Table 6.* Quantitative assays in the detection of residual leukemic cells.

| Methods of evaluation | Log killing |
|---|---|
| Indirect IF*/** | 2 |
| Double staining combination*/** (TdT+T-marker) | 4 |
| Flow cytometry*/** | 1.5-2 |
| Hoechst dye technique*/** | 3-4 |
| 51Cr release*/** | 2 |
| Clonogenic*/** | >4 |
| 125 IUDR uptake assay** | 3-4 |
| Rearrangement of the T-cell receptor genes* | 1.5-2 |

* Clinical conditions.
** Preclinical model.

in a clinical situation with large volumes of harvested marrow (Table 5) [36]. A mixture of IT specific to most cases of T-ALL can inhibit > 4 logs of leukemic cells while sparing most hemopoietic progenitor cells [37-39]. Each IT inhibits 1 to 4 logs of clonogenic leukemic cells (i.e. MOLT 3, 4, CEM).

Prior to bone marrow harvesting in acute leukemia we can use more or less sophisticated methods to detect minimal residual disease and to define the quality of the harvested marrow [40]. We need to look at new ways to identify residual leukemic cells to allow us to measure what we are doing. The quantitative assays for detection of residual leukemic cells prior to and after C' mediated lysis are shown on Table 6.

**Commentary**

The availability of a broad panel of T-lymphocytes specific MoAbs has made possible to study T-lineage ontogeny. All maturity steps can now be identified using phenotypic markers of normal T-cells. This knowledge of the pathway of normal T-lymphocyte differentiation has enabled the classification of T-ALL into three groups according to their level of thymic differentiation. MoAb production and purification procedures have been forced to adapt to clinical requirements in order to provide the clinician with a product devoid of pyrogens and bacterial and viral contamination. The MoAb isotype is dictated by the method chosen to treat the marrow graft i.e. for complement dependent lysis IgM or IgG2 isotypes are necessary, while IgG1 isotypes are compatible with immunotoxin use and the magnetic immunobead separation technique.

Whatever the depletion technique employed for either allogeneic (GvH prevention) or autologous (removal of residual leukemic cells) transplantation, the ultimate aim is to deplete the graft of 'unwanted' T cells. However, the two types of BMT are characterized by the choice of MoAb to be employed and the degree of T target cell depletion desired. In autologous BMT total removal of the leukemic T-cell population is desirable. As yet no reliable tests are available to determine the efficiency of this *ex-vivo* depletion. Furthermore the removal of all cells expressing the target T phenotype from the inoculum does not necessarily mean leukemic progenitor cell depletion. It is hoped that with the advent of molecular biology (T-cell receptor genes and DNA sequence amplification) and clonal expansion techniques (spontaneous T-colonies) residual disease detection will become possible. However the depletion efficiency will ultimately be judged by clinical success (disease free survival) and for statistical purposes many more patients are necessary. A different problem rises in allogeneic graft depletion as the identity of GvH T effector cells remains unknown. If these effector cells could be identified, selective depletion would become feasible thus enabling the preservation of GvH and HvG reactions in the allogeneic graft.

The future of T cell-depletion is under constant evaluation: T cell-depletion is undoubtedly the best technique for preventing severe GvH; graft failure or graft rejection (15-20% of cases) and a significant increase in relapse incidence have been reported after T-cell depletion. Despite these latter complications, the survival rate remains identical in both depleted and non-depleted groups. This observation confirms that the acute GvH is one of the major complications responsible for early mortality in non-depleted allogeneic BMT. Thus by employing MoAbs specifically directed against the effector cells of the HvG reaction as well as conditioning reinforcement, specific complications in T-cell depletion might be prevented. The developments in biotechnology will undoubtedly modify marrow graft treatment which up to present has been dominated by complement dependent lysis. The latter serves as a reference model for techniques currently under investigation (anti-T immunotoxins, magnetic immunobeads). Regardless of the technique proposed, the quality control of MoAbs is an essential pre-requisite for their use.

### References

1.  Foon KA, Todd RF. Immunologic classification of leukemia and lymphoma. Blood 1986;68:1-31.
2.  Fazekas de St Groth S, Scheidegger D. Production of monoclonal antibodies: Strategy and tactics. J Immunol Methods 1980;35:1-22.
3.  Mc Michael AJ, Gotch FM. T-cell antigens: New and previously defined clusters in leukocyte typing. III. In: McMichael AJ (ed). White cell differentiation antigens. Oxford University Press 1987:31-68
4.  Underwood PA, Bean PA. The influence of methods of production, purification and storage of monoclonal antibodies upon their observed specificities. J Immunol Methods 1985;80:189-97.
5.  De Rie M, Zeijlemaker WP, von dem Borne AEKr, Out TA. Evaluation of a method of production and purification of monoclonal antibodies for clincial applications. J Immunol Methods 1987;102:187-93.
6.  Boulianne GL, Hozumi N, Shulman MY. Production of functional chimaeric mouse/human antibody. Nature 1984;313:643-46.

7. Santos GW, Hess AD, Vogelsang GB. Graft-versus-host reactions and disease. Immunol Rev 1985;88:169-92.
8. Vallera DA, Soderling CB, Kersey JH. Bone marrow transplantation across major histocompatibility barriers in mice. Treatment of donor grafts with monoclonal antibodies directed against Lyt determinants. J Immunol 1982;128:871-5.
9. Korngold R, Sprent J. Lethal graft-versus-host disease after bone marrow transplantation across minor histocompatibility barriers in mice. J Exp Med 1978; 148:1687-98.
10. Hervé P. Methods for *ex-vivo* purging of bone marrow of residual tumor cells or GvHD-producing T-cells. A review. Plasma Ther Transfus Technol 1985;6: 359-64.
11. Janossy G. Bone marrow purging. Imm Today 1987;8:253-5.
12. Prentice HG, Janossy G, Price-Jones L et al. Depletion of T-lymphocytes in donor marrow prevents significant graft-versus-host disease in matched allogeneic leukaemic marrow transplant recipient. Lancet 1984;i:472-6.
13. Hervé P, Cahn JY, Flesch M et al. Successful graft-versus-host disease prevention without graft failure in 32 HLA-identical allogeneic bone marrow transplantations with marrow depleted of T-cell monoclonal antibodies and complement. Blood 1987;69:388-93.
14. Mitsuyasu R, Champlin R, Gale T et al. Treatment of donor bone marrow with monoclonal anti-T cell antibody and complement for the prevention of graft-versus-host disease. Ann Int Med 1986;105:20-6.
15. Martin PJ, Hansen JA, Buckner CD, Storb R, Thomas ED. Outcomes after transplantation of T-cell depleted HLA-identical allogeneic marrow. XXI Congress of the Intern. Society of Haematol. Sydney 1986:254(abstract).
16. Waldmann H, Hale G, Cividalli G et al. Elimination of graft-versus-host disease by *in vitro* depletion of alloreactive lymphocytes with a monoclonal rat anti-human lymphocyte antibody (Campath-1). Lancet 1984;ii:483-5.
17. Waldmann H, Hale G, Cobbold S. The immunobiology of bone marrow transplantation in leukocyte typing. III. McMichael AJ (ed). White cell differentiation antigens. Oxford University Press 1987:932-7.
18. Prentice HG, Brenner MK, Grob JP et al. HLA-matched T-cell depleted allogeneic BMT in the treatment of acute leukemia in 1st CR. Bone Marrow Transplant 1986;1:91.
19. Martin PJ, Hansen JA. Quantitative assays for detection of residual T-cells of T-depleted human marrow. Blood 1985;65:1134-40.
20. Jansen FK, Blythman H, Carriere D et al. Immunotoxins: Hybrid molecules combining high specificity and potent cytotoxicity. Immunol Rev. 1982;62:185-216.
21. Press OW, Vitetta ES, Farr AG, Hansen JA, Martin PJ. Evaluation of ricin A-chain immunotoxins directed against human T cells. Cellular Immunol 1986; 102:10-20.
22. Filipovich AM, Vallera DA, Youle RJ et al. Graft-versus-host disease prevention in allogeneic bone marrow transplantation from histo-compatible siblings. A pilot study using immunotoxins for T-cell depletion of donor bone marrow. Transplantation 1987;44:62-9.
23. Ugelstad J, Ellingsen T, Berge A. Magnetic polymer particles for cell separation. Bone Marrow Transplant 1987;2(suppl 2):74-7.
24. Vartdal F, Albrechtsen D, Ringden O et al. Immunomagnetic treatment of bone marrow allografts. Bone Marrow Transplant 1987;2(suppl 2):94-8.
25. Maraninchi D, Gluckman E, Blaise D et al. Impact of T-cell depletion on outcome of allogeneic bone marrow transplantation for standard risk leukemias. Lancet 1987;ii:175-8.

26. Apperley J, Jones L, Hale G et al. Bone marrow transplantation for patients with chronic leukemia: T-cell depletion with Campath-1 reduces the incidence of graft-versus-host disease but may increase the risk of leukemic relapse. Bone Marrow Transplant 1986;1:53-66.
27. Slavin S, Or R, Naparstek E et al. Allogeneic bone marrow transplantation for leukemia using T-lymphocyte depletion for prevention of GvHD and total lymphoid irradiation for prevention of allograft rejection. 4th International Symposium on Therapy of Acute Leukemia. Roma 1987:272 (abstr.).
28. Yam PY, Petz LD, Knowlton RG et al. Use of DNA restriction fragment length polymorphisms to document marrow engraftment and mixed hematopoietic chimerism following bone marrow transplantation. Transplantation 1987;43: 399-407.
29. Von Melchner H, Bartlett PE. Mechanisms of early allogeneic marrow graft rejection. Immunol Rev 1983;71:31-56
30. Ferrata J, Mauch P, Murphy G, Burakoff SJ. Bone marrow transplantation: The genetic and cellular basis of resistance to engraftment and acute graft-versus-host disease. Surv Immunol Res 1985;4:253-63.
31. Trigg M, Billing R, Sondel P et al. Clinical trial depleting T lymphocytes from donor marrow for matched and mismatched allogeneic bone marrow transplants. Cancer Treatment Report 1985;69:377-86.
32. Hervé P, Cahn JY, Flesch M, Plouvier E, Racadot E, Noir A. Hematological reconstitution and acute GvH prevention with T-lymphocyte depleted mismatched bone marrow in 13 leukemic transplant recipients. A pilot study. Bone Marrow Transplant 1987;2(suppl 2):143.
33. Macintyre EA. The use of monoclonal antibodies for purging autologous bone marrow in the lymphoid malignancies. Clin Haematol 1986;15:249-62.
34. Hale G, Swirsky D, Waldmann H, Chan LC. Reactivity of rat monoclonal antibody Campath-1 with human leukemia cells and its possible application for autologous bone marrow transplantation. Brit J Haematol 1985;60:41-8.
35. Campana D, Bekassy A, Janossy G. Elimination of leukemic cells with monoclonal antibodies and complement in autologous bone marrow transplantation and complement in autologous bone marrow transplantation. Plasma Ther Transfus Technol 1986;7:83-91.
36. Hervé P, Racadot E, Plouvier E, Flesch M, Cahn JY, Noir A. Autologous bone marrow transplantation for acute lymphoblastic leukemia in remission. In vitro purging of inoculum with monoclonal antibodies and complement in leukocyte culture. Proceedings of the 18th International Conference. La Grande Motte, France. Mani, Dornand, Walter de Gruyter and Co (eds). (In press)
37. Cabellas P, Canat X, Fauser A, Gros O, Laurent G, Poncelet P, Jansen FK. Optimal elimination of leukemic T-cells from human bone marrow with T 101-ricin A-chain immunotoxin. Blood 1985;55:289-97.
38. Strong RC, Uckun F, Youle RJ, Kersey JH, Vallera DA. Use of multiple T-cell-directed intact ricin immunotoxins for autologous bone marrow transplantation. Blood 1985;66:627-35.
39. Rahmakrishnan S, Uckun FM, Houston LL. Anti-T cell immunotoxins containing pokeweed anti-viral protein: Potential purging agents for human autologous bone marrow transplantation. J Immunol 1985;135:3616-22.
40 Favrot MC, Hervé P. Detection of minimal malignant cell infiltration in the bone marrow of patients with solid tumours, non-Hodgkin lymphoma and leukemias. Bone Marrow Transplant 1987;2:117-22.
41. Gale R, Reisner Y. Graft rejection and graft-versus-host disease mirror images. Lancet 1986;i:1468-70.

42. Hervé P. Prévention de la réaction du greffon contre l'hôte par la déplétion lymphocytaire T des greffons de moelle osseuse allogénique. La Presse Médicale. (In press).
43. Cobbold S, Martin G, Oin S, Waldmann H. Monoclonal antibodies to promote marrow engraftment and tissue graft tolerance. Nature 1986;323:164-6.
44. Rigden O, Deeg HJ, Beschorner W, Slavin S. Effector cells of graft-versus-host disease, host resistance and the graft-versus-leukemia effect: Summary of a workshop on bone marrow transplantation. Transpl Proc 1987;19:2758-61.

# LAK CELL PRODUCTION: APPLICATION OF rDNA AND CELL CULTURE TECHNOLOGY

L.F.M.H. de Leij*, M. Elias**, A.G. ter Haar*, C.Th. Smit Sibinga**, T. The*

## Introduction: The concept of immunological surveillance

The immunological surveillance theory, put forward by Ehrlich, Thomas and Burnet [1] in the late fifties and sixties , starts from the idea that transformation of a normal cell into a tumour cell is not a rare event, but occurs quite often during a normal life-time. To counteract the continuous development of tumour foci, the theory predicts that the immune system executes active anti-tumour surveillance. In the normal situation, this results in the immune-mediated destruction of newly formed neoplastic cells. However, if the immune system functions inappropriately or if a tumour cell has a very low immunogenicity, outgrowth of a cancer may occur. Based on this theory, early anti-cancer immunotherapy aimed to restore the apparently diminished immune capacity of cancer patients in order to adjust the imbalance between tumour cell growth and anti-cancer immunity. In most cases, however, this kind of immunotherapy was not very successful as a cancer therapy.

The main presuppositions of the immune surveillance theory, i.e. the continuous generation of tumour cells as well as the ready recognition and destruction of spontaneously formed tumour cells by the immune system, have been challenged by a lot of data since then, and, in effect, the theory as such has been abandoned.

Nevertheless a number of aspects of immunological surveillance are worth while and may be used to construct a new theoretical basis for tumour immunology. A large number of data, obtained both in fundamental and clinical studies, shows that, under the right circumstances, immune cells can recognize and destroy tumour cells. This immune reactivity comprises both 'specific' and 'non-specific' elements of the immune system. Immunotherapy based on 'specific' reactivity has been shown to be effective in experimental animals [2] and even bulky disease can be cured in this way [3]. Although 'specific' anti-tumour immune reactivity appears to be present also in humans [4], the generally poor immunogenicity of human-derived tumour cells has thwarted efforts to induce specific anti-tumour responses in patients. More fundamental studies of the complex events underlying the 'specific' recognition of tumour-associated antigens in humans are clearly needed, before such a problem may be overcome. It has been known for years that the 'non-specific' elements of the immune system can recognize and kill a number of established tumour cell-lines. This natural killing is mainly exe-

* Dept. Clin. Immunology, Univ. Hospital Groningen.
** Red Cross Blood Bank Groningen-Drenthe.

cuted by a specific subset of lymphocytes dubbed according to their function as Natural Killer (NK) cells [5]. NK cells have been shown to belong to a lymphocytic lineage separate from T and B lymphocytes, and to account for about 5-15% of the peripheral blood lymphocytes. they are phenotypically characterized by the expression of the cell markers CD-16 (an Fc Receptor detectable by the monoclonal antibody LEU-11) and NKH-1 (detectable by LEU-19), whereas the T-cell marker CD-3 lacks. More recently it was shown that the 'natural killing' activity of NK cells is markedly enhanced by interferon [6] and interleukin-2 [7,8]. Interleukin-2 can activate also T cells to execute both 'specific' and 'non-specific' killing of tumour cells [9,10]. Since activated NK cells, in turn, can release a number of lymphokines in the same way as T cells do [11], it is clear that complex interrelationships between 'non-specific' and 'specific' elements of the immune system exist in the *in vivo* situation.

The need for an understanding of these interactions is urged by recent biotechnological break-throughs, like the production of monoclonal antibodies and the application of recombinant DNA technology for the production of lymphokines. These new biotechnological tools have greatly enhanced the possibilities to manipulate the *in vivo* immune system.

In the following, current knowledge of the different effector cells operative in immune-mediated cell destruction is given. In addition, the possible use of recombinant interleukin-2 to activate these cells for tumour destruction is indicated.

## Immunological effector cells and the induction of LAK cells

The cellular immune-reactivity against tumours comprises both innate ('non-specific') and acquired ('specific') immune functions. The innate immune functions are executed mainly by NK cells, whereas the acquired immunity is mediated by antigen-specific cytotoxic T lymphocytes (CTL). Although other factors and cells [12] may also play a role, only the NK cells and CTL are dealt with here, since these are thought to be the most important ones in host resistance towards tumour growth.

CTL and NK cells differ concerning their recognition of target molecules on a tumour cell. NK cells recognize a still unknown, *common* target structure present on an array of different tumour cells. CTL interact with a *unique* target molecule that, in addition, is only recognized if specifically presented on an autologous target cell. Recently a new type of CTL has been shown to be present in peripheral blood [13]. This newly discovered type of CTL appears to have a specificity of target recognition that is intermediate to the common tumour cell identification of NK cells and the unique specificity of the above mentioned 'classic' type of CTL.

The effector functions of both CTL and NK cells are under regulatory control. This control is mediated by specific regulator proteins, the lymphokines [14]. Lymphokines are released by specific lymphocytes, but can be produced also by non-lymphocytic cells. Therefore a more correct name would be 'cytokines'. Here the current designation 'lymphokines' is retained, since only their role in the communication between different cells of the immune system will be dealt with. A large number of different lymphokines has been isolated and characterized until now. For instance: the different interleukins, the interferons and tumour necrosis factor (TNF).

Normally, during the local induction of an immune response, lymphokines are released by macrophages and helper T cells. The amount of produced lymphokines is not very high under these circumstances and, because of their short biological half-life, the activity of most of these lymphokines will remain local.

A number of lymphokines can be obtained now in a pure form and in large quantities by means of the recombinant DNA technique. A well-known example of such a lymphokine is interleukin-2, which is a 15,000 dalton glycoprotein normally released by specific helper T cells and which can trigger and amplificate the function of both NK and CTL.

An interesting observation, originally made with crude interleukin-2 preparations was, that lymphocytes incubated in tissue culture medium containing Il-2, developed the ability to lyse freshly obtained human tumour cells [7]. These interleukin-2 activated lymphocytes were much more potent killer cells than the (unstimulated) NK cells mentioned above. This finding, called the lymphokine activated killer (LAK) cell phenomenom, could be extended to the *in vivo* situation, since it was subsequently shown that administration of high doses of rIl-2 mediated the regression of tumour metastases in an experimental animal system [15]. The doses required for tumour regression were very high, however, i.e. just below those causing major toxicity [15].

The first clinical studies with the application of rIl-2 show a similar picture. For instance, a Phase I study at the National Cancer Institute [16] using both natural and recombinant Il-2 indicated dose-limiting toxicity, as manifested by marked malaise and weight gain, at doses of rIl-2 of $10^6$ U/kg as a single bolus or 2000 U/kg/hr. In 2/25 patients (with melanoma metastatic to the lung) partial tumour regression was observed [16], suggesting that Il-2 indeed might stimulate lymphocytes to become LAK cells. However, the doses therapeutically needed are too high.

A combined *in vivo/in vitro* stimulation protocol was subsequently developed by Rosenberg and coworkers [17] to overcome the problem of *in vivo* interleukin-2 toxicity. In this protocol (called the LAK cell protocol), treatment is given in different cycles. One cycle (Figure 1) is started by administration of subtoxic doses of rIl-2 ($10^5$ U/kg tid) to a patient during a relatively short period of time (5 days). Then, after an additional three days, peripheral blood lymphocytes are isolated on a number of consecutive days and these are further stimulated *in vitro* with high doses of rIl-2 (1000 U/ml) during 3–5 days (LAK cell culture). Subsequently these LAK cells are reinfused in the patients, again in combination with rIl-2 ($10^5$ U/kg). The first clinical results with the LAK cell protocol (Phase I study) indicated that the therapy, although still quite toxic, was tolerable for the majority of patients [17]. In addition, objective tumour responses in about 30% of treated patients could be observed. Later studies [a.o. 18] showed tumour responses in 10–20% of treated patients. The fact that relatively long-lasting, complete remissions were seen in a number of these patients justifies a conclusion that LAK cell

# National Cancer Center
# LAK Cell Protocol

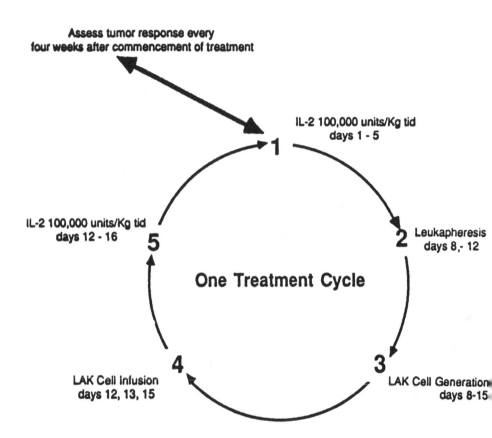

*Figure 1:* National Cancer Center LAK cell protocol.
Treatment is given in a number of cycles.

therapy is a promising treatment option for cancer. It should be kept in mind, however, that the LAK cell protocol is propably not in its final form of development, and that modifications will be brought forward in due time. It can be anticipated that, if this or other forms of anti-cancer immunotherapy can be further improved, just as what happened with the earliest efforts to apply surgery, radiotherapy and chemotherapy to the treatment of cancer, these new treatment options could have major impact for the future therapy of cancer patients.

In the following, some modifications of the LAK cell protocol are indicated and discussed.

# Isolation of peripheral blood lymphocytes by lymphosurge

A problem hampering the routine application of the LAK cell protocol is the difficulty to generate sufficient numbers of LAK cells. These must be handled and cultured aseptically before they can be subsequently used for safe systemic therapy. The elutriation technique used for leukocyte-poor platelet collection (Haemonetics V50-1) can be modified in such a way that sufficient numbers of lymphocytes can be isolated with minimal cross-cellular contamination. In addition, this procedure enables a wash stage and subsequent cell culture in CLX containers.

The lymphosurge elutriation technique is based on differences in sedimentation speed between the different blood cell components (platelets, leukocytes and erythrocytes). Sedimentation of these blood cells during centrifugation is opposed in the technique by applying an adjustable plasma stream (surge) in the reverse direction. This results in concentration and subsequent elutriation of the individual blood cell components. This technique takes into account different donor parameters (like plasma viscosity and cell shape), which are generally not known before the start of the procedure. Figure 2 depicts the sequence of events during a lymphosurge procedure. Three phases are important.

Phase 1: the buffy coat formation phase;
Phase 2: the buffy coat collection phase; and
Phase 3: end of collection.

The quality of cell separation and the width of the buffy coat are determined by the centrifugation speed and time, which, in turn, depend on the draw speed. During the procedure, the plasma optical density is taken as a reference value. When the bowl optics start to detect the buffy coat, the surge pump begins to recirculate the collected plasma with a speed of 80 ml/min. This pump speed is gradually accelerated with 5 ml/min every second, until it reaches the speed necessary to float off the platelets and lymphocytes (surge incremental limit: 'SIL'). The surge pump speed is kept at the SIL value, until the platelet peak (which has the greatest optical density) is detected. In the next phase of the surge, the plasma surge speed is increased according to the platelet/white cell factor (P/WC), which is determined as a proportional increment of SIL (note: in the elutriation technique for leukocyte-poor platelets collection, the pump speed is decreased at this point of the procedure). Once the platelets have left the bowl, the increased speed will also result in the subsequent floating out of the lymphocytes, and then these can be specifically collected. The end of collection is marked by the arrival of the erythrocytes as detected by the bowl optics. The volume of the lymphocyte product is determined by the lymphocyte collection volume (LCV). This volume can be varied. For instance, LCV increases/decreases by starting the collection earlier/later, which will result in a higher/lower yield, but with more/less (platelet) contamination.

## SURGE ELUTRIATION

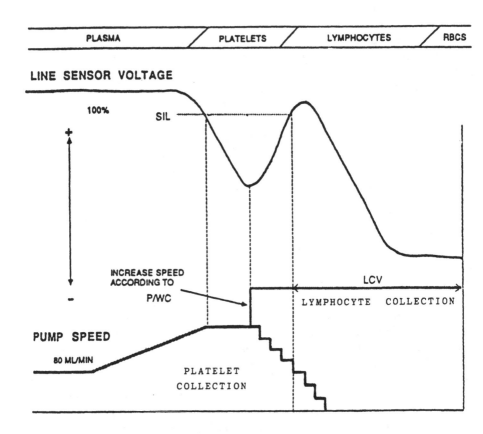

*Figure 2:* Dynamics of the elutriation technique for leukocyte poor platelets collection and its modification for lymphocyte collection.

Our preliminary results with the lymphosurge elutriation technique are summarized in Table 1. In these experiments, the effect of variations in the draw speed and the LCV were investigated. The two other parameters (SIL and P/WC) were kept at a preset value. It is concluded that a draw speed of 60 – 65 ml/min with a LCV of 50 ml is optimal with regard to the final lymphocyte yield ($\bar{x} = 2.5 \times 10^9$) as compared to low contamination with platelets or red cells (as determined with the HCT in Table 1). Attempts to apply a second soft spin to reduce the volume in order to concentrate the product were not very satisfactory in our hands, since this resulted in a considerable loss of lymphocytes (28% loss) and an increase of erythrocytes (as detected by a 13% increase of HCT). Therefore this concentration step is not recommendable.

*Table 1.* Preliminary results of the lymphosurge technique. 4 runs (n = 10).

| Variables | | | | | Lymphocyte product | | | | |
|---|---|---|---|---|---|---|---|---|---|
| draw speed | LCV | SIL | P/WC | Volume | WC $10^9$ | lympho-cyte % | plat $10^9$ | HCT % | Volume processed |
| 65 | 60 | 5 | 2 | 216 | 10.6 | 88 | 60 | 5 | 2214 |
| 60 | 50 | 5 | 2 | 172 | 15.8 | 89 | 30 | 4.5 | 2132 |
| 65 | 50 | 5 | 2 | 167 | 16.8 | 93 | 50 | 4.3 | 2150 |
| | | | | 185 | 14.4 | 90 | 45 | 4.6 | 2165 |

In conclusion, the lymphosurge technique is an elegant procedure for the isolation of large amounts of lymphocytes, since both the yield and the cellular cross-contamination is optimal. The patient as well as the lympho-cytes endure only minimal isolation stress during the procedure.

## Cellular composition of a LAK cell culture

Lymphocytes isolated both by lymphosurge (see above) and by standard isopaque-ficoll density separation can be activated to become LAK cells by incubation with rIl-2 (200 U/ml) containing tissue culture media for 1 to 5 days. We found no clear differences between the two lymphocyte preparations when their cellular composition or rIl-2 induced proliferation capacity was analyzed. In addition, the functional properties of both preparations were similar as tested by determining their lytic activity against the NK sensitive target cell line K562. It can be concluded therefore that the lymphosurge pre-pared lymphocytes are well suited for further 'bulk' LAK cell preparation.

*Table 2.* Phenotype of cells in a LAK cell culture stimulated with 200 U interleukin-2/ml for 5 days.

| Antibody preparation | Percentage at day 0 | Percentage at day 5 |
|---|---|---|
| LEU 4 | 80 | 81 |
| LEU 3 | 38 | 42 |
| Anti-CD8 | 42 | 40 |
| LEU 14 | 11 | 8 |
| LEU 7 | 3 | 4 |
| LEU 11B | 4 | 36 |
| LEU 19 | 6 | 5 |
| A-Il-2Rec | 0 | 21 |

168

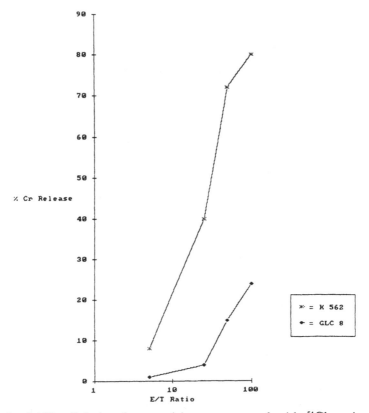

*Figure 3.* LAK cell induced cytotoxicity as measured with [51]Chromium release assay. Target cells (K562 and GLC-8) were labeled with [51]Chromium and incubated with effector cells (LAK cells stimulated for 5 days with 100 U/ml interleukin-2) for 4 hour. Lysis is measured as the amount of [51]Chromium released, expressed as a percentage of the total incorporated [51]Chromium. The assay is done at different effector to target (E/T) ratios.

After 5 days of LAK cell culture about 15% of the cells proved to be in the S-phase of the cell cycle as determined by a 5BrdU incorporation technique. Since this means that about half of the cells are growing and dividing, it was of interest to determine if changes in cellular composition had occurred during culture. No clear differences were observed as compared to the cellular composition at the start of culture (Table 2). This was detected by the mono-clonal antibodies LEU-4 (anti CD-3: pan T), LEU-3 (anti CD-4: T-help), T8 (anti CD-8: T-cytotox/suppr), LEU-7 (HNK-1: a subset of NK cells), LEU-19 (NK cells), and LEU-14 (anti CD-22: pan B). These results indicate that rIl-2 probably induces proliferation in all types of lymphocytes present in the cul-ture and that no clear changes in cellular composition had occurred after 5 days culture yet. With longer culture times (two to three weeks) T cells appear to overgrow the culture (not shown), indicating that T cells grow faster under these conditions than the other cell types.

The only cell markers that were significantly changed at day 5 of culture were the CD-16 molecule (Fc receptor as detected by LEU-11b) and the

IL-2-receptor molecule (Table 2). The induction of these markers was both time- and rIl-2 concentration-dependent: higher rIl-2 concentrations induced more cells in less time to become positive. The fact that 36% of the cells were positive for LEU-11b at day 5 of culture (stimulation with 200 U/ml rIl-2) indicates that the Fc receptor is present not only on (activated) NK cells, but also on the subset of activated T cells.

## LAK cell activity against SCLC derived cell lines: Application of monoclonal antibodies

Until now, most success with LAK cell therapy has been obtained with patients suffering from either melanoma or renal carcinoma [17,18]. In order to determine whether LAK cells may be used to treat also patients with for instance small cell lung cancer (SCLC), we assessed the *in vitro* susceptibility of SCLC cells towards LAK cell culture in medium supplemented with 100 U/ml rIl-2. Figure 3 shows that the 'classic' SCLC derived cell line GvHD-8 is much more resistant to LAK cell induced kill than the control cell line K562. The same result was obatined with the 'variant' SCLC derived cell line GLC-1 (data not shown), indicating that SCLC cells are quite refractory to LAK cell induced kill. 'Variant' SCLC derived cell lines represent a more dedifferentiated form of *in vitro* SCLC as compared to 'classic' SCLC derived cell lines [19].

The reason for the above refractoriness, which is propably a property of more tumour types, is a matter of speculation. LAK cells recognize on tumour cells (a) 'common' target structure(s), which nature is still elusive. Since it is conceivable, however, that on some tumour cells these structures are expressed to a low extent, or, alternatively, shielded off, this could cause a bad recognition of such tumour cells by LAK cells. Thus, in this reasoning, if the regular tumour cell recognition by LAK cells could be bypassed, then also LAK-resistant tumour targets would be sensitive to the lytic action of these LAK cells.

For such a purpose the following strategy may be adopted. During the past years (mouse-derived) monoclonal antibodies have been generated, which, although not really tumour-specific, are directed against highly tumour-restricted antigens. These monoclonal antibodies can be used to retarget LAK cells. The simplest approach to such a procedure would be to make use of the fact that LAK cells have a receptor for the Fc portion of antibodies (i.e. the CD-16 molecule). However, although LAK cells may indeed recognize the Fc portion of a monoclonal antibody via this receptor, this is generally not the case since only a subset of mouse immunoglobulins is recognized by human Fc receptors. Therefore a better approach is to include such an antibody in a 'retargeting device'. Such a device should contain both a site with specificity for a target molecule on the tumour cell (the anti-tumour monoclonal antibody) and a site to which the killer cell can adhere (an anti-killer cell monoclonal antibody). It is necessary that the killer cell adheres via a receptor molecule, which directly or indirectly triggers its lytic machinery. Examples of such receptor molecules are the CD-16 molecule (present in a LAK cell cul-

170

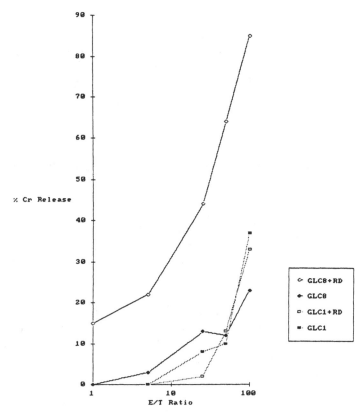

*Figure 4.* The effect of a MOC-31/CD3 retargeting device (RD) on LAK cell induced lysis. The 'classic' GLC-8 (MOC-31 positive) and the 'variant' GLC-1 (MOC-31 negative) SCLC derived cell lines were used as targets. LAK cells were generated in a one day culture (stimulation with 100 U interleukin-2/ml) and pre-incubated with the RD before adding to the targets. Cytotoxicity was measured as indicated in Figure 3.

ture on NK and a subset of T cells), the CD-2 molecule (present on a subset of NK and T cells), and the CD-3 molecule (present on T cells).

We have constructed a retargeting device specific for activated T cells by chemically cross-linking a monoclonal antibody directed against a SCLC-associated molecule (MOC-31: directed against a membrane determinant present on 'classic' but not on 'variant' SCLC derived cell lines) to an anti-CD-3 monoclonal antibody. MOC-31 is not really tumour-specific, since it also reacts with a subset of normal epithelia [20]. Figure 4 shows that LAK cells generated in a one day culture supplemented with 100 U/ml rIl-2 can kill the 'classic' SCLC cell line GLC-8, provided that the MOC-31/anti-CD-3 retargeting device is present in the assay. This killing is specifically directed against the MOC-31+ GLC-8 cells, since the MOC-31⁻ 'variant' GLC-1 cells are not affected. This preliminary result, which is in agreement with recent findings reported by others [21-23], indicates that it is possible to specifically direct the lytic capacity of killer cells towards an otherwise LAK-resistant tumour cell target.

## Discussion

Recombinant DNA technology offers the possibility to obtain various lymphokines in large quantities and in a pure form. Application of rIl-2 has shown that this lymphokine can activate resting lymphocytes to become LAK cells. *In vitro*, LAK cells can induce the lysis of a large array of tumour target cells as well as virus transformed cells. *In vivo*, the application of rIl-2 is limited by its toxicity.

The LAK cell protocol, originally developed by Rosenberg and coworkers, partly overcomes this problem by combining an *in vivo* induction with a further *in vitro* amplification of LAK cell function.

Reinfusion of these LAK cells has resulted in tumour regression in some cases. These results reanimate an old hope, originally inspired by the immune surveillance theory of Burnet, that immunotherapy of cancer may be an achievable goal. However, as Dr. Rosenberg already pointed out in a reply to a letter to the Editor written by Dr. Schulof [24]: "This (LAK cell) treatment has not been proposed as definite or in the final form of its development, but rather as a new treatment approach that one hopes is in its infancy" [25]. One possible improvement could be the use of retargeted LAK cells as discussed in this article. Different retargeting devices all with the same specificity for tumour cells on site, but with different specificities for different, in the LAK cell culture activated, immune cells (e.g. NK cells, CTL, but also T helper cells) on the other site may be used to direct all different kinds of immune cells into a tumour.

In such a concept it is conceivable that different types of tumour-targeted immune cells are usable for different types of tumour therapy [25]. For instance, a tumour largely restricted to the blood circulation, like leukemia, would be best treated with activated NK cells, since these killer cells are not likely to leave the circulation. However, in the case of solid tumours, specific types of CTL appear more suitable, since these cells can leave the capillary bed.

Fundamental as well as clinical studies have to be performed to further develop and establish the value of this new approach to cancer immunotherapy.

## Acknowledgements

The authors thank Gert-Jan Wolbink and Dick-Johan van Spronsen for their help in determining the phenotype of the cells present in LAK cell cultures and Martinus de Jonge for critically reading the manuscript.

172

# References

1. Burnet FM. The concept of immunological surveillance. Progress in Experimental Tumor Research 1970;13:1-27.
2. Herberman RB. Counterpoint: animal tumor models and their relevance to human tumor immunology. J Biol Response Modif 1983;2:39-46.
3. Berendt MJ, North RJ. T cell-mediated suppression of antitumor immunity. An explanation for the progressive growth of an immunogenic tumor. J Exp Med 1980;151:69-80.
4. The TH, de Leij L. Search for tumorantigens. In: Veldman EJ (ed). Immunobiology, histophysiology and tumorimmunology in otolaryngology. Proceedings 2nd International Academic Conference. Utrecht, The Netherlands. Kugler Publications, Amsterdam/Berkeley, 1987:387-92.
5. Trinchieri G, Perussia B. Human natural killer cells: biologic and pathologic aspects. Lab Invest 1984;50:489-513.
6. Krown SE. Cytokines. Interferons and interferon inducers in cancer treatment. Seminars in Oncology 1986;13:207-17.
7. Grimm EA, Mazumder A, Zhang HZ, Strausser JL, Rosenberg SA. Lymphokine activated killer cell phenomenon: Lysis of natural killer resistant fresh solid tumor cells by interleukin-2 activated autologous human peripheral blood lymphocytes. J Exp Med 1982;155:1823-41.
8. Herberman RB, Hiserodt J, Vujanovic N et al. Lymphokine-activated killer cell activity. Characteristics of effector cells and their progenitors in blood and spleen. Imm Today 1987;8:178-81.
9. Ochoa AC, Gromo G, Alter BJ, Sondel PM, Bach FH. Long-term growth of lymphokine-activated killer (LAK) cells: role of anti-CD3, beta-Il-1, interferon-gamma and -beta. J Immunol 1987;138:2728-33.
10. Reynolds CW, Ortaldo JR. Natural killer activity: The definition of a function rather than a cell type. Imm Today 1987;8:172-4.
11. Scala G, Djeu JY, Kasahara T et al. Cytokine secretion and noncytotoxic functions of human large granular lymphocytes. In: Lotzova E, Herberman RB (eds). Immunobiology of natural killer cells. CRC Press, Boca Raton, Florida 1986:133-44.
12. Levy MH, Wheelock EF. The role of macrophages in defense against neoplastic disease. Adv Cancer Res 1974;20:131-63.
13. Borst J, van de Griend RJ, van Oostveen JW et al. A T-cell receptor gamma/CD3 complex found on cloned functional lymphocytes. Nature 1987;325:683-8.
14. Dinarello CA, Mier JW. Current concepts: Lymphokines. N Engl J Med 1987;317:940-5.
15. Rosenberg SA, Mule JJ, Shu S, Spiess P, Schwartz S. Systemic administration of recombinant interleukin-2 leads to the regression of established tumor in mice. J Exp Med 1985;161:1169-88.
16. Lotze MT, Matory YL, Rayner AA et al. Clinical effects and toxicity of interleukin-2 in patients with cancer. Cancer 1986;58:2764-72.
17. Rosenberg SA, Lotze MT, Muul LM et al. Observations on the systemic administration of autologous lymphokine-activated killer cells and recombinant interleukin-2 to patients with metastatic cancer. N Engl J Med 1985;313:1485-92.
18. Rosenberg SA, Lotze MT, Muul LM et al. A progress report on the treatment of 157 patients with advanced cancer using lymphokine-activated killer cells and interleukin-2 or high-dose interleukin-2 alone. N Engl J Med 1987;316:889-97.
19. Gazdar AF, Carney DN, Guccion JG et al. Small cell carcinoma of the lung: Cellular origin and relationship to other pulmonary tumors. In: Greco FA,

Oldham RK, Bunn PA (eds). Small cell carcinoma of the lung. Grune and Stratton, New York 1981:145-75.

20. De Leij L, Postmus PE, Poppema S, Elema JD, The Th. The use of monoclonal antibodies for the pathological diagnosis of lung cancer. In: Hansen H (ed). Lung cancer: Basic and clinical aspects. Martinus Nijhoff Publishers, Boston 1986:31-48.

21. Perez P, Hoffman RW, Titus JA, Segal DM. Specific targeting of human peripheral blood T cells by heteroaggregates containing anti-T3 crosslinked to anti-target cell antibodies. J Exp Med 1986;163:166-78.

22. Titus JA, Garrido MA, Hecht TT, Winkler DF, Wunderlich RT, Segal DM. Human T cells targeted with anti-T3 cross-linked to antitumor antibody prevent tumor growth in nude mice. J Immunol 1987;138:4018-22.

23. Titus JA, Perez P, Kaubish A, Garrido MA, Segal DM. Human K/Natural killer cells targeted with hetero-cross-linked antibodies specifically lyse tumor cells in vitro and prevent tumor growth in vivo. J Immunol 1987;139:3153-8.

24. Schulof RS. Treatment of cancer with lymphokine-activated killer cells and interleukin-2. N Engl J Med 1987;317:961-2.

25. Rosenberg SA. Reply to the letter of Dr Schulof. N Engl J Med 1987;317:662-3.

26. Hersey P, Bolhuis R. "Nonspecific" MHC-unrestricted killer cells and their receptors. Imm Today 1987;8:233-9.

# BIOTECHNOLOGY OF HEMOPOIETIC CELLS IN CULTURE

J.D. Lutton, R.D. Levere, N.G. Abraham

## Background

In the past few years, advances in biotechnology and gene cloning have contributed much to the culture and identification of specific hemopoietic cells and to the therapeutic application of blood cells or cell products in clinical medicine. Recent insights on the regulation of hematopoiesis and the applications of new technologies now permit growth of significant quantities of blood cells. Furthermore, these advances have permitted a more precise kinetic analysis of hemopoietic growth induced by natural and synthetic growth factors. Growth factors are new powerful tools which can be used clinically for the manipulation of the hemopoietic milieu during disturbed hemopoietic states. Clonal culture is useful in that it can be used to examine the viability of stem cells from specimens that have been stored for various time periods such as is commonly done in blood banks. Evaluation of stem cell viability by such clonogenic assays and the separation of specific cell populations may be of particular significance to the area of bone marrow transplantation. In particular, recognition and quantitation of immediate progenitor cell compartments within a specimen is possible and the response of specific cell populations within the specimen to various biological response modifiers can be evaluated. Additionally, clonal culture is a useful tool for examining stem cell kinetics and growth patterns by bone marrow cells from disturbed hematological states.

Stem cells are considered to be ancestral cells that persist in post-natal life which have extensive self-renewal capacity and provide the organism with specialized end cells [1,2]. Hemopoietic stem cells are thought to arise from embryonic blood islands after which they populate the liver, spleen, blood and bone marrow tissues during embryonic and neonatal life. The bone marrow becomes the major source of stem cells in the normal human adult organism. However, reduced numbers of precursor cells are also found circulating in peripheral blood.

Kinetic studies suggest that stem cells do not have to be in a continuous cell cycle, but instead may be in a $G_0$ phase and are able to shift into an active $G_1$ phase under certain conditions. Such a shift into a $G_1$ phase and active cycle is thus vital for the eventual differentiation into a specialized committed cell series. Pluripotential stem cells are those that possess the capacity to become specialized along several routes or compartments, whereas unipotential stem cells are those that form a series of committed cells within a compartment terminating in end cells of one kind. End cells may be perma-

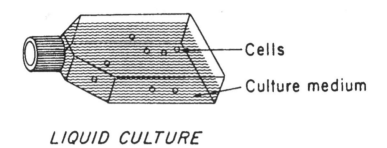

*LIQUID CULTURE*

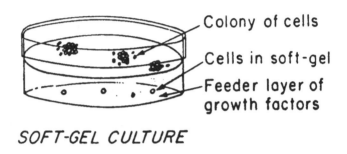

*SOFT-GEL CULTURE*

*Figure 1.* Commonly used culture systems.

nent end cells (static) or nonpermanent end cells that can cycle or expand under specific conditions.

The *in vitro* growth of hemopoietic stem cell compartments into progeny of differentiated cells requires specialized culture conditions and the presence of specific growth factors or hemopoietins such as erythropoietin (Epo) and colony stimulating factor(s) (CSF). When appropriate *in vitro* conditions are obtained, colonies of cells may be obtained which represent cell lineages of hemopoietic compartments including erythroid, myeloid, lymphoid and megakaryocytic lineages [1,2].

Two types of tissue culture systems have been commonly used for analyzing growth and differentiation of hemopoietic cells and their regulator molecules [3-6]. They are the classical liquid culture and the so-called soft-gel culture method. The liquid culture allows for mass growth of cells in a suspension or as adherence to a culture flask. The soft-gel procedure allows for clonal growth of immobilized cells in a semi-solid matrix, such as agar or methyl-cellulose which has a soft-gel texture (Figure 1).

In the mid-sixties, Pluznik and Sachs in Israel [7] and Bradley and Metcalf in Australia [8] reported the use of soft-gel method for the growth of individual mouse bone marrow cells into colonies. These procedures employed a double layer or semi-solid agar with the bone marrow cells seeded on the top layer while the lower layer consisted of feeder leukocytes as the source of stimulants or growth factors for bone marrow cells. After a period of incubation, colonies or clusters of cells were found on the upper layer which subsequently were identified to be composed of granulocytes and macrophages. The colonies were derived from the bone marrow precursor cells with the colony forming activity produced from the cells in the lower layer. *In vitro* generation of such colonies has been shown to be derived from precursor cells called colony-forming cells which are found in the bone marrow. These colony forming cells are actually recognized as cells at a particular stage of differentiation and not the true stem cells. Both the liquid suspension culture and the soft-gel method has been used as assay tools for the cells as well as the regulators. The liquid culture provides an advantage of assaying cells at any given time while the other technique is advantageous for observing clonal development of cells.

Blood cell types of normal or leukemic origin have been used as *in vitro* model systems that include human and various species of mammals. To investigate the controls of cell proliferation and differentiation, various cell lines have been established [9]. These lines have specific characteristics at different stages of development and in some cases may be arrested at specific stages of the developmental process. Their growth characteristics and their development toward maturer stages can be monitored and the regulator molecules involved in this process can be studied. For example, the mouse Friend erythroleukemia cell line (FELC) and the human HL-60 promyelocytic leukemia line have been employed extensively for the respective investigations relating to red blood cell and myeloid cell growth and differentiation.

As indicated, growth of stem cell compartments into progeny of differentiated cells requires specific growth factors or regulator molecules such as CSF [10]. These molecules initiate a series of events such as limited proliferation of a specific cell type followed by the induction of differentiation and a depression of proliferation. Changes in myeloid colony forming cells undergoing differentiation include: a cell cycle shift from S-phase to $G_1$ phase and proliferation cessation; loss of immature cell antigens and acquisition of new membrane antigens and phenotypes; IgG and complement (C3) receptor development and alterations in cell shape and adherence; changes in enzymes such as myeloperoxidase, esterases, lysozymes and the development of functional enzymes for heme, respiratory cytochromes and the cytochrome P-450 systems; acquisition of specific functions such as phagocytosis, drug metabolism and immunological cooperation.

## Maturation and autocrine factors

Specific lymphokines or other factors distinct from Epo or CSFs have also been decribed which specifically induce differentiation, whereas other factors induce replication of autologous cells without initiating differentiation. Thus, autocrine and paracrine factors may regulate cell proliferation [11].

Chiao et al [12-14] have characterized, isolated, and purified a human myeloid maturation inducer or D-factor which is produced by T-lymphocytes and will induce terminal differentiation in normal and leukemic cells. Autostimulatory growth factors (ASF or ASA) have also been described which are distinct from D-factors in that they are produced by a specific cell type and are capable of stimulating replication of the same cell type. Heil et al [15]

178

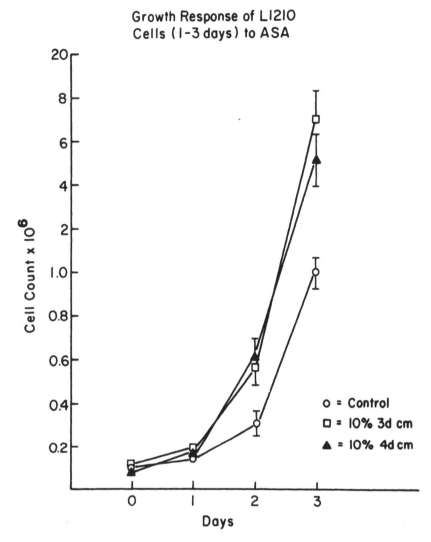

*Figure 2.*    Growth curves for L1210 cells grown in suspension cultures in the absence or presence of 3-4-day conditoned media (CM) containing ASA. All cultures were innoculated with $1 \times 10^5$ cells/ml at day 0 and then incubated at 37°C with 5% $CO_2$ + 95% air. Results represent M ± SE, n=6.

have characterized ASA for human HL-60 myeloid leukemia cells and we have described an ASA for murine L1210 leukemia cells [16]. The effect of L1210 conditioned media (CM) containing ASA on L1210 replication is shown on Table 1 and Figure 2 where it can be seen that ASA significantly enhanced cell growth and $^3$H-TdR uptake over controls. Furthermore, on Table 2 it can be seen that L1210 CM also contains CSF activity which is specific for myeloid colony growth (CFU-GM). Note on this table that L1210 CM has no effect on erythroid colony growth (CFU-E), whereas 10% L1210 CM stimulated 115±10 CFU-GM. ASA appears to be distinct from other CSFs since addition of various CSFs to L1210 cultures had no enhancing effect on L1210

*Table 1.* Autostimulatory activity determined by $^3$H-Thymidine ($^3$H-TdR) uptake into L1210 cells exposed to conditioned media (CM) containing ASA*.

| Culture Period (days) | CPM of $^3$H-TdR | |
|---|---|---|
| | Control | CM |
| 1 | 19,651 ± 808** | 39,129 ± 3832 |
| 2 | 49,678 ± 1583 | 61,697 ± 1870 |
| 3 | 63,024 ± 1458 | 114,718 ± 912 |

* L1210 cells were plated into microtiter wells ($1 \times 10^4$ cells/well) without (control) or with 10% L1210 CM and incubated for 1-3 days. Cultures were labeled with 0.4 μC: $^3$H-TdR.
** M ± SE.

*Table 2.* The effect of L1210 conditioned media (CM) on murine erythroid and myeloid bone marrow colony growth.

| Additions | No. bone marrow colonies/$10^5$ cells* | |
|---|---|---|
| | CFU-E** | CFU-GM*** |
| Epo | 342 ± 39 | ND**** |
| Epo + 10% CM | 345 ± 22 | ND |
| Epo + 20% CM | 320 ± 28 | ND |
| — | 0 | 2 |
| 10% CM | 0 | 115 ± 10 |

* M ± SE.
** CFU-E were cultured in plasma clots with 0.4 U/ml erythropoietin (Epo).
*** CFU-GM were cultured in metylcellulose for 7 days.
**** Not determined.

*Table 3.* Effects of different sources of colony stimulating factor (CSF) on 2-day L1210 growth.*

| Source of CSF | Cell counts $\times 10^5$ after 2-day growth |
|---|---|
| Controls | 3.5 ± 0.2** |
| 10% ASA | 6.4 ± 0.3 |
| 10% GCT | 3.1 ± 0.2 |
| 10% Mo-T | 2.0 ± 0.3 |
| 10% L-cell | 3.7 ± 0.1 |
| 10% WEHI | 3.6 ± 0.2 |

* Cultures were plated with $1 \times 10^5$ L1210 cells/ml ± CSF, and incubated for 2 days at 37°C.
** M ± SE, n=4.

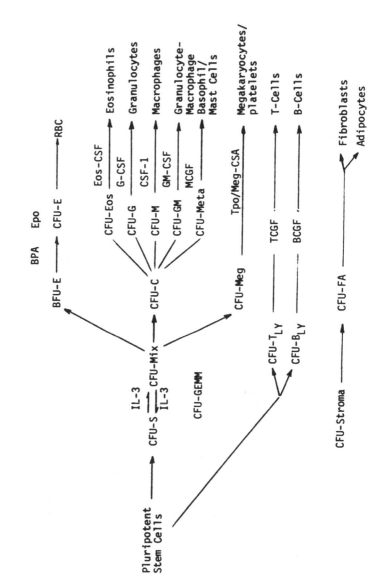

Figure 8. Hierarchical Stem Cell Model

growth (Table 3). Note on Table 3 that 2-day cell culture counts for controls was $3.5 \times 10^5$, and cultures with GCT, Mo-T, L-cell or WEHI CSF contained 3.1, 2.0, 3.7 and $3.6 \times 10^5$ cells/ml. In contrast, cultures with ASA had $6.4 \times 10^5$ cells after 2 days of growth. Therefore, L1210 cells appear to elaborate factors such as ASA and CSF, and CSFs may be distinct from ASA in that they have no growth enhancing effect on L1210 tumour cells.

## Stem cell hierarchy

Enrichment of specific cell populations and identification of specific regulator molecules such as CSFs along with morphological and kinetic studies have provided data which help to clarify the hemopoietic stem cell hierarchy [1,2]. Such a scheme represents stages of stem cell differentiation into specific steps which portray cells with increasing commitment and decreasing self-renewal capacity. Figure 3 represents a stem cell hierarchy and illustrates the colony forming units (CFU) within the various compartments, along with the presumed growth factors. Pluripotent multilineage progenitor colonies are designated as CFU-GEMM, and are grown in the presence of IL-3 or PHA conditioned media, plus Epo [2]. The erythroid compartment is represented by the primitive erythroid colony forming cell (BFU-E) and the more differentiated Epo dependent erythroid colony or CFU-E [17]. A substance generated by other cell populations enhances BFU-E growth and is called burst promoting activity (BPA). BPA is found in preparations of IL-3 and GM-CSF, however, its exact nature is not clear [18]. Megakaryocytic colonies are designated as CFU-Meg, and their growth is thought to be regulated by undefined substance(s) called thrombopoietin (Tpo) and/or Meg-CSA [19]. Meg-CSA is found in thrombocytopenic and aplastic anemia sera whereas Tpo has been obtained from human embryonic-kidney cell conditioned medium.

The myeloid compartment (CFU-C) includes multiple CFUs such as granulocyte (G), macrophage (M), GM-colonies (CFU-G, CFU-M, CFU-GM) which are under the regulation of recently defined growth factors (G-CSF, CSF-1, GM-CSF) [3,10]. Basophil/mast cell colonies have also been described [20,21], however, their regulators are not yet clearly defined. The lymphoid (CFU-Ly) and stromal cell compartments (CFU-stroma) are also represented on this figure. It is important to note that long term hemopoietic growth requires the interaction of the various unipotent compartments with the stromal cell compartment, whereas short term hemopoiesis of the unipotent compartments ensues in the absence of the stromal compartment [5,22,23]. Various examples of hemopoietic colonies grown *in vitro* are represented in Figure 4.

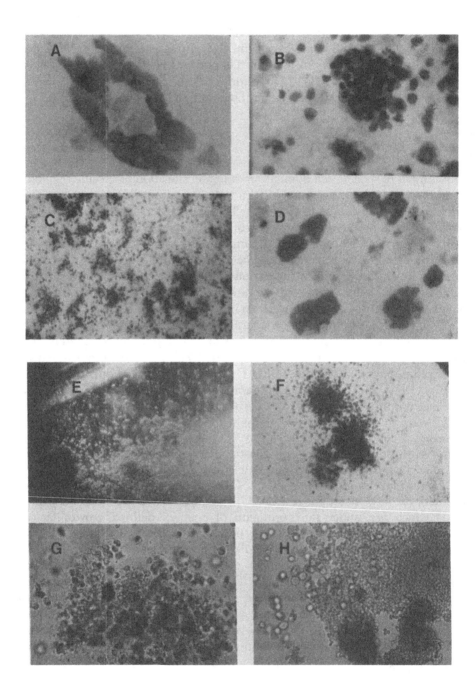

*Figure 4.* Representative bone marrow hemopoietic colonies grown *in vitro.*
(A) Human bone marrow erythroid colony (CFU-E). (B) Cord blood CFU-E. (C)
Human fetal liver CFU-E. (D) Mouse CFU-E. (E) Human burst colonies (BFU-E).
(F,G) Granulocyte-macrophage colonies (CFU-GM). (H) Human multilineage colony
(CFU-GEMM).

# General methodology for hemopoietic colony cultures

In order to obtain an enrichment of colony-forming cells, nonadherent bone marrow cells are used in most cultures. When murine cells are to be used, bone marrow cells are flushed from the femurs of mice and then incubated at 37°C in Iscove's Modified Modified Dulbecos Medium (IMDM) containing 20% FCS in Falcon plastic petri dishes (100 mm). Usually $20\text{-}30 \times 10^6$ cells are incubated in 10 ml of media. After 60 minutes the plates are swirled, the nonadherent cells removed, washed, resuspended in IMDM + 20% FCS and incubated in petri dishes in a similar manner. After two hours of incubation the cells are removed, washed and resuspended to the desired concentration in IMDM + 2% FCS. These cells are then used in culture experiments.

When human cells are to be employed, bone marrow or peripheral blood are collected in heparinized syringes after informed consent, diluted (1:1) with IMDM and layered over a Ficoll-Hypaque gradient (density=1.077); centrifuged at $400 \times G$ for 30 minutes. The cells are then washed twice, counted and concentration adjusted to $5 \times 10^6$ cells/ml in IMDM with 20% FCS. The cells are applied to FCS coated dishes and incubated for 60 minutes, 30°C, 5% $CO_2$. Nonadherent cells are removed, washed twice and counted. Less than 3% monocytes (nonspecific esterase positive cells) should be present in the nonadherent population. In some cases T-cell depleted fractions can be obtained from the monocyte depleted population by the use of the AET-treated sheep red blood cells (AET-SRBC) rosetting method. Cell viability can be routinely determined by the Trypan Blue exclusion technique. Cell counts are done using a hemocytometer, and all results are expressed as percentage viable cells.

*Hemopoietic stem collony assays (CFU-E, CFU-GM, GFU-GEMM)*

Bone marrow cells (human or mouse) or peripheral blood mononuclear cells can easily be simultaneously cultured in both plasma clot and methylcellulose culture systems in the absence or presence of an appropriate cytokine such as Epo or CSF. Both culture systems have been described in detail previously [3,17,24-27]. Plasma clot cultures are advantageous since the cultures can be removed, fixed onto slides and stained for permanent record. Methylcellulose cultures are useful for enzyme assays since the cultures can be collected and cell material prepared as a pellet for assays. For erythroid plasma clot cultures, the cells $(0.5\text{-}8 \times 10^5/\text{ml})$ are incubated in 0.1 ml clots at 37°C in an atmosphere of 5% $CO_2$ + 95% air in a fully humidified incubator. Briefly, 0.1 ml of the desired cell concentration is added to 1.0 ml of culture medium which contains 0.3 ml of heat-inactivated fetal calf serum; 0.1 ml of 10% deionized bovine serum albumin in phosphate buffered saline; 0.1 ml beef embryo extract; 0.1 ml $\alpha$-thioglycerol; (1:10,000 in NCTC-109) 0.1 ml asparagine (2 mg/ml in NCTC-109) 0.1 ml NCTC-109; 0.1 ml citrated bovine plasma; 0.1 ml erythropoietin (Epo) (Toyobo) in NCTC-109 (0.25-2.0 units/ml), and a source of burst promoting activity for BFU-E cultures (Mo conditional medium). Erythroid colonies (CFU-E, BFU-E) are detected after

2-14 days of incubation by benzidine staining of gluteraldehyde fixed clots. Clusters of greater than eight cells are scored as colonies. Murine and human CFU-E are detected after 2½ and 7 days, and BFU-E on 9 and 14 days respectively. Myeloid colonies (CFU-GM) can also be grown in this sytem by substituting 5-10% CSF for Epo. CFU-GM are then scored after 7-14 days of growth.

Methylcellulose culture technique has been described by Iscove et al [28]. The medium contains 30% FCS, methylcellulose (0.8%), cells and various growth factors in IMDM. Cultures are plated as multiple 1 ml cultures in 35 mm Falcon culture dishes. Erythroid colonies are scored at various times of growth as described previously [17], and meyloid colonies (CFU-GM) are scored after 7-14 days of growth. When myeloid colonies (CFU-GM) are to be grown, the methylcellulose culture system is essentially the same as that for erythroid colonies except that $1-2 \times 10^5$ cells/ml are employed with 5-10% CSF. Agar may also be employed and is usually used as 0.3% (Difco) in place of methylcellulose.

Culture of pluripotent hemopoietic progenitors (CFU-GEMM) has been described in detail by Messner [2] and essentially utilizes modifications of techniques described above. Briefly, $1 \times 10^5$ light density bone marrow cells are cultured in 1 ml cultures of IMDM containing 30% human plasma, 5% PHA-LCM (lymphocyte conditioned media prepared with PHA), 1.0 U/ml Epo, $5 \times 10^5 M$ 2-mercaptoethanol and 0.9% (w/v) methylcellulose (or 0.3% agar). Il-3 may be substituted for PHA-LCM. After incubation for 14 days at 37°C with 5% $CO_2$ + 95% air, mixed colonies (CFU-GEMM) are iden-tified by their morphology and staining of smears.

Megakaryocyte colony culture (CFU-Meg) can also be done using modifi-cations of the previously described plasma clot and methylcellulose culture systems [19]. For culture of human bone marrow, separated mononuclear cells ($5 \times 10^5$ cells/ml) are cultured in 35 mm petri dishes. The plasma clot culture is modified to contain heat-inactivated human AB serum, $\alpha$-medium, nonessen-tial amino acids (0.02 mM/ml), L-glutamine (0.4 mM/ml) and sodium pyru-vate (0.2 mM/ml). Also, a source of Meg-CSF (CSA) and/or thrombopoietin (Tpo) must be added and in some cases 2 U/ml Epo may also be included. These factors have been obtained from thrombocytopenic plasma (Meg-CSA) and human embryonic kidney cell conditioned media (Tpo) [29,30]. Cultures are incubated for 12-14 days after which the clots are harvested and fixed onto glass slides. CFU-Meg can be identified with immunofluorescence by using antiserum to purified human platelet glycoproteins (PGP). The PGP prepar-ation is incubated with the fixed plasma clot cultures for 60 min, washed with PBS and then reincubated with fluorescein-conjugated goat anti-rabbit IgG for 60 min (0.36 mg protein/ml). The slides are then washed and counter stained with Evan's Blue (7 min), dried and CFU-Meg scored using a fluor-escence microscope . CFU-Meg are scored as clusters of 3-4 fluorescent cells.

*Serum free cultures*

In some experiments, methylcellulose cultures of bone marrow cells can be maintained in serum free media similar to the methods of Breitman et al [31] with some modifications. Basically, the medium consists of a 1:1 mixture of

Ham's F-12 and RPMI 1640 (GIBCO, Grand Island, NY) supplemented with $3 \times 10^{-8}$ M selenium, 5 $\mu$g/ml transferrin and 5 $\mu$g/ml insulin (Collaborative Research, Inc., Lexington, MA). Purified or recombinant growth factors (Epo, CSF) are also employed and the cultures incubated as described above.

*Evaluation of morphology, differentiation and proliferation*
Myeloid colonies consisting of at least 40-50 cells are usually detected as tight (granulocytic, CFU-G), mixed (granulocyte-macrophage, CFU-GM) and loose (macrophage, CFU-M). In some cases, myeloid colony morphology can be determined *in situ* by staining with chloracetate and nonspecific esterases. A staining kit (No. 90) from Sigma Chemical Co., (St. Louis, MO) provides the appropriate reagents to detect monocytes ($\alpha$-naphtyl acetate esterase), neutrophils (naphthol AS-D-chloroacetate esterase) and eosinophils (Luxol Fast blue). Staining of hemoglobin in erythroid colonies is accomplished by utilizing a 1% benzidine in ethanol preparation which is allowed to react in 3% $H_2O_2$. Plasma clot slides are also counter stained with hematoxylin for myeloid and nuclear morphology. Erythroid colonies (CFU-E) are scored as colonies containing at least 8 benzidine positive cells, and BFU-E may consist of several hundred cells of erythroid and multiple cell types.

Morphological criteria of the cells and differential count analysis can be used to assess maturation and to determine the proportion and absolute number of each cell type. Smears of cells are made with a cytocentrifuge and stained with May-Grünwald Giemsa. The morphology of granulocytes and macrophages is characteristic and useful in determining the presence of such cells. One of the early indications of monocytic cell differentiation is the development of cells adhering firmly to the surface substrate of the culture containers. Macrophage-like cells are the predominant cell type among the adherent cells. Cells firmly attached to a surface substrate of culture containers after rigorous pipetting can be detected with an inverted microscope.

The frequency of colony growth by normal human specimens shows considerable variation from sample to sample and the growth patterns may be markedly different when samples are from various hematological disorders [25,32-35]. For example, the frequency of normal human bone marrow CFU-GEMM ranges from $3-30/2 \times 10^5$ cells; CFU-GM ranges from $20-110/10^5$ cells and CFU-E ranges from $150-230/10^5$ cells. CFU-Meg counts range from $2-32/5 \times 10^5$ cells. In contrast, CFU-E and CFU-GM frequencies from a patient with CML in erythroblastic transformation may be as high as 800-1000 CFU-E/$10^5$ cells and 200-400 CFU-GM/$10^5$ cells [34]. CFU-E numbers generated by specimens from patients with polycythemia vera may even be greater than 1000 CFU-E/$10^5$ cells [32].

*Long term hemopoietic cultures*

Early observation by Allen, Dexter and others [22,23] revealed that when murine marrow preparations were seeded into culture dishes under specific conditions, adherent cells became established that included many fat-containing cells and other fibroblast-like endothelial cells and macrophages. Closely associated with these adherent cells were nonadherent hemopoietic cells in various stages of differentiation. Cultures could then be recharged by adding fresh medium and marrow suspension cells after 3-4 weeks. Nonadherent cells removed during feeding could then be tested for colony growth (CFU-E, CFU-GM, etc.) or for their ability to form mouse spleen colonies (CFU-S). Early studies indicated that by using long term culture, human CFU-GM colony forming ability could persist for 20 weeks, whereas BFU-E, CFU-E and CFU-Meg persisted for shorter time periods [22,23].

The basic medium for the original Dexter system consists of Fisher's medium (GIBCO) + 25% horse serum (HS). Adipocytes are usually seen by week 4 in this culture. After recharging the cultures with a second marrow innoculum, a weekly removal of 50% volume of cells and medium change can be done so that $10^5$-$10^6$ nonadherent cells can be removed per week. Greenberger et al [5] has modified the Dexter system so that CFU-GM are obtained after more than 65 weeks in culture. The medium consists of Fisher's medium, 25% HS or FCS and $10^{-7}$ M hydrocortisone. The presence of FCS + HS and hydrocortisone markedly improves the long term viability of the system.

The basic methodology for culture of human monocytes (MO) and marrow fibroblastoid stromal cells in long term culture has been described by Broudy et al [36] and is outlined below.

Monocytes are isolated from peripheral blood of healthy volunteers and the low-density cells are obtained by Ficoll-Hypaque (Pharmacia Fine Chemicals, Piscataway, NJ) centrifugation. Low-density cells (less than 1.077 g/ml) are incubated with sheep red blood cells and E rosettes removed by density centrifugation. Monocytes are isolated from the E rosette-negative population by adherence to serum coated dishes. Monocytes thus isolated are usually 90% nonspecific esterase positive and 95% viable by Trypan Blue exclusion. The monocytes are cultured at a concentration of $1 \times 10^5$ cells per ml in RPMI 1640 (GIBCO, Grand Island, NY) supplemented with 2 mmol/L L-glutamine and 15% lactoferrin-depleted FCS. After three days of incubation at 37°C in an atmosphere of 7.5% $CO_2$ in air, the conditioned media is harvested and centrifuged to remove cell debris.

Marrow fibroblastoid stromal cells (MFSCs) can be cultured according to the procedures of Broudy et al [36] using bone marrow from healthy adults. Low-density marrow cells are obtained from single-cell suspensions of heparinized marrow aspirates using Ficoll-Hypaque. These cells are incubated in Medium 199 (GIBCO) supplemented with 20% FCS and 2 mmol/L L-glutamine. Cells are seeded at $5 \times 10^6$/ml in T flasks and are incubated at 37°C in a humidified atmosphere of 5% $CO_2$ in air. The medium is changed twice weekly and usually reaches confluence by 3 to 4 weeks. The cells are maintained for up to 6 months in culture. Primary outgrowths of cells at confluence are detached from the culture flasks with 0.02% EDTA-trypsin, washed, diluted 3:1, and replated.

The cells are characterized by cytochemical staining with acid phosphatase, $\alpha$-naphthylacetate esterase, alkaline phosphatase, periodicacid Schiff (PAS), and myeloperoxidase by standard techniques [36]. Surface antigenic characteristics of the cells are determined with the monocyte-specific monoclonal antibodies M1 and M120, followed by a fluorescein-labeled second antibody, and are then examined by fluorescence microscopy.

# Regulators of hemopoiesis

Little was known about the physiological regulation of growth of bone marrow cells until the development of clonal culture techniques in the 1960's. In such cultures, individual progenitor cells of a particular lineage are able to proliferate and generate a clone of mature cells provided the proper conditions and growth substances are present. Clonal culture permitted the growth of bone marrow myeloid, erythroid and lymphoid cells and the colony of cells is referred to as the colony forming unit (CFU). Since cell proliferation and colony formation are dependent upon specific regulatory molecules, these molecules have been referred to as colony stimulating factors (CSF) or colony stimulating activity (CSA). Regulatory molecules that are mediated by cells have also been referred to as 'cytokines', and those of lymphocyte origin have been termed 'lymphokines'. Colony stimulating factors can be found circulating in many biological fluids, however, the number of cells in man that produce and release CSF is rather limited. Basically the CSFs are named so as to designate the hemopoietic cell lineage they stimulate in an *in vitro* clonogenic assay. Thus, granulocytic colonies are stimulated by granulocyte CSF (G-CSF), macrophage clonal growth by macrophage CSF (M-CSF) and mixed colonies of granulocytes and macrophages by GM-CSF. In some instances, different nomenclature has been ascribed such as CSF $\alpha$, $\beta$, 1, 2, etc.

## Role of stromal cells

Experiments by Cronkite et al [37], Gordon et al [38,39] and others revealed that murine bone marrow fibroblastoid stromal cells have marked modulatory effects on hematopoiesis by nonadherent cells. The influence of different stromal cell populations on *in vitro* hemopoietic colony growth is summarized

*Table 4.* Effects of stromal cell types on *in vitro* hematopoiesis.

| NABM plus additions | Relative bone marrow colony growth | |
| --- | --- | --- |
| | CFU-GM | BFU-E |
| CSF | + + | |
| Fb | ± | |
| Fb + CSF | + + + + + | |
| St + CSF | + + | |
| MO + CSF | + | |
| Epo | | + + + + |
| Epo + Fb | | – |
| Epo + St | | + + |
| Epo + Mɸ | | + + + + |

NABM = Non adherent bone marrow cells; CSF = Colony stimulating factor; Epo = Erythropoietin; Fb = Fibroblasts; St = Stromal cells (Fb + fat cells); Mɸ = Macrophages.

188

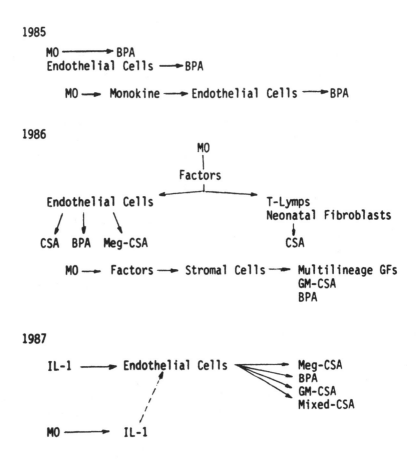

*Figure 5.* Summary of growth factor production by human stromal-endothelial cells.

on Table 4. It is apparent that when fibroblasts are included in the colony cultures, there is an enhancement of CFU-GM growth whereas BFU-E growth is suppressed [37-39].

Experiments with human systems have indicated important roles for stromal cells in the regulation and maintenance of hematopoiesis. In these studies, it was found that specific stromal cell-nonadherent cell interactions are involved in the regulation and/or modulation of hematopoiesis [36]. Results from experiments demonstrated that mononuclear phagocytes actually recruit stromal cells of the marrow to produce multilineage growth factors *in vitro* [36]. It was also found that phagocytes constitutively produce soluble factor(s) that stimulate T-lymphocytes, fibroblasts and endothelial cells to produce colony stimulating activity *in vitro* [40-42]. Additionally, monocytes produce a factor that stimulates the production of burst-promoting activity (BPA) and megakaryocyte colony stimulating activity (Meg-CSA) by endothelial cells [43,44].

A brief summary of some of the experimental findings regarding stromal cell interactions is outlined on Figure 5. In 1985, Zuckerman et al [43] established that human monocytes (MO) produce a monokine that in turn stimulates the production of BPA by umbilical vein endothelial cells. Later (1986) it was found that MO recruit stromal cells (monocyte recruiting activity or MRA) to produce multilineage growth factor *in vitro* [36,45]. The MO derived activity was also able to stimulate T-lymphocytes and neonatal fibroblasts to release CSA or CSFs. By 1987, Bagby and his collaborators established that MRA was actually IL-1 (interleukin-1) and that IL-1 elaborated by MO induced the release of multilineage growth factors [46,47].

It is clear from these studies that the microenvironmental and stromal cell interactions play critical roles in the maintenance and regulation of hematopoiesis *in vitro* and *in vivo*. Activation of specific genes through cellular interactions may result in specific production of a CSF or lymphokine. For example, the gene for human GM-CSF resides on the long arm of chromosome 5 [48]. The locus of the gene is near the position of genes for other growth hormones and hormone receptors. Stimulation of the gene may occur by agents that activate macrophages, and activated macrophages may then induce resting T-lymphocytes to express the GM-CSF gene. Thus, these studies emphasize the importance of complex cell-cell interactions in the regulation of hemopoiesis-lymphopoiesis.

*Colony stimulating factors*

The majority of the CSFs are acidic glycoproteins which may exist as monomeres consisting of a molecular weight (MW) range between 21-28,000, of which approximately 40% is carbohydrate [10]. They also exist as dimers (MW=70,000) of several polypeptide subunits each with a MW of approximately 14,000. Deglycosylation experiments have suggested that the carbohydrate portion is not of major importance for the *in vitro* growth stimulating activity [10]. Several types of CSFs controlling the production of hemopoietic cells in animals and humans have now been isolated, purified and cloned by recombinant DNA technology.

*Granulocyte macrophage colony stimulating factors*
Granulocyte-macrophage-CSF (GM-CSF) has been isolated and also has been referred to a CSF-α or CSF-2 [10]. It is a glycoprotein with a MW of approximately 23,000, and the murine form has been purified from endotoxin treated mouse lung. Elution studies from hydrophobic columns have identified at least two separable forms of human CSF that can stimulate human granulocyte-macrophage colony formation [49,50]. These have been designated as CSF-α (non-binding) and CSF-β (binding). CSF-α has been purified to homogeneity and may represent the natural form of GM-CSF. CSF-β has not been fully purified, but is able to stimulate differentiation of murine WEHI-3 leukemia cells.

Human GM-CSF has been obtained from medium conditioned by the Mo hairy T cell leukemia line [51]. It was purified to homogeneity and found to have a MW of approximately 20-23,000. Clones of cDNA were then isolated by direct expression screening of cDNA libraries from Mo leukemic cell mRNA [52] or a human T-cell line [53]. Transfection of these clones to monkey COS cells produced a GM-CSF that was active on human cells. Sequencing studies indicated that the polypeptide contains 127 amino acids (MW=14,000) with four cysteine residues. The recombinant GM-CSF produced by transfected COS cells had a MW of 19,000 and a specific activity of $4 \times 10^7$ U/gm protein [54].

The cellular receptor for GM-CSF has been isolated and its MW is approximately 52,000 [55]. It has been estimated that resting non-induced HL-60 cells have about 50 high affinity receptors/cell [55], whereas DMSO induced HL-60 cells may have more than 1,000 receptors/cell. All normal granulocytes and monocytes bear receptors for GM-CSF and the numbers decrease with increasing cellular maturation.

GM-CSF has now been cloned from three species including mouse, gibbon ape and human [55,56]. Both human and ape GM-CSF cDNA clones revealed substantial sequence homology of the amino acid sequence. GM-CSF has also been shown to stimulate eosinophil colony formation and to initiate multipotential erythroid and megakaryocyte colony formation [57].

Production of recombinant human GM-CSF has permitted the evaluation of its *in vivo* effects in primates [58]. Continuous infusion of human recombinant GM-CSF into healthy monkeys elicited a dramatic leukocytosis and substantial reticulocytosis. A similar effect was observed in a pancytopenic immunodeficient monkey. These studies provided the opportunity to test the potential clinical use of GM-CSF in various disorders such as in the treatment of some types of cytopenias. Thus, clinical trials on monkeys demonstrated that GM-CSF is a potent stimulator of primate hematopoiesis *in vivo.*

*Macrophage colony stimulating factor*
Macrophage CSF (M-CSF, CSF-1) is a glycoprotein that stimulates growth and differentiation of cells from the mononuclear phagocyte lineage. CSF-1 has been purified to homogeneity and the molecule is a 65-80,000 MW sialoglycoprotein composed of two similar chains linked by disulfide bonds [10]. Recently a human CSF-1 analogous to murine CSF-1 has been cloned [59]. Sequence studies of the cDNA clone indicates the existence of a pre-pro CSF-1 of 252 residues which is then further processed to a more active form. In other experiments it has been reported that the product of the c-Fms proto-oncogene is identical to the receptor for CSF-1 [60]. It is significant that the c-Fms gene is located on human chromosome 5 and that a deletion in this chromosome (5q) in bone marrow cells is frequently associated with a syndrome that may develop into myeloid leukemia [48] or polycythemia vera [61]. It is known that the CSF-1 receptor is similar to the epidermal growth factor (EGF) receptor and c-Fms proto-oncogene product. These receptors possess tyrosine kinase activities, and antibodies to Fms protein will precipitate the CSF-1 receptor complex [60,62].

*Granulocyte colony stimulating factor*

Murine granulocytic CSF (G-CSF), which has been isolated and purified from mouse lung conditioned media, stimulates the production of granulocytic colonies *in vitro* [63]. Polyacrylamide gel electrophoresis revealed that G-CSF is a distinct molecular species different from GM-CSF and separated as one band with a MW of 25,000. The human analogue of murine G-CSF has also been isolated from human placental conditioned media and was referred to a CSF-$\beta$ [64]. The murine and human G-CSF molecules demonstrated almost complete biological and receptor-binding cross-reactivities to normal and leukemic murine or human cells. Both G-CSFs were able to induce the production of terminally differentiated cells from WEHI-3B and other myeloid leukemia cell lines and to suppress renewal and leukemogenicity of leukemia cells [63,64].

Iodinated forms of murine G-CSF and human CSF-$\beta$ were found to bind specific bone marrow target cells and cells from several forms of human leukemia such as acute myeloblastic leukemia, chronic myeloid leukemia, acute promyelocytic leukemia, preleukemia and the cell line HL-60. Acute myelomonocytic leukemias showed little binding and unlabelled G-CSF could competitively inhibit the binding of the iodinated CSF in a dose-dependent manner, whereas unlabelled M-CSF, GM-CSF or multi-CSF were without effect [64,65].

Recently a human pluripoietin growth factor with G-CSF growth and differentiation-like activities has been isolated from conditioned media produced by a human bladder carcinoma cell line 5637 [66]. In addition, the gene for human pluripoietin CSF was cloned and a recombinant form of the growth factor has been produced [67]. Because of the similarities to murine G-CSF, the factor was referred to as human G-CSF or hG-CSF. The similarities to murine G-CSF include the ability to stimulate growth and development of granulocytic colonies *in vitro* and to induce terminal differentiation of WEHI-3B (D+) cells. However, unlike murine G-CSF, recombinant hG-CSF supported early erythroid and mixed colony formation. The secreted form of the protein produced by the cell line was found to be 0-glycosylated, had an isoelectric point of 5.5 and a molecular weight of 19,600. It is important to note that the G-CSF like molecules described above have a differentiation inducing activity which was consistently found to co-purify or be associated with an activity stimulating growth. In addition, hG-CSF had pluripoietin-like activity on erythroid and multiple lineages. It remains possible that a true biological G-CSF may be specific only for the granulocytic lineage. However, others distinguish that differentiation inducing activity is due to a separate molecule and have subsequently purified it to homogeneity. In fact, two different cDNAs and mRNAs for human G-CSF have recently been isolated and could account for differences in growth and differentiating activities [68,69].

A human squamous cell line, CHU-2, was found to produce large amounts of G-CSF that was very specific for the human and murine granulocytic lineage [68]. Purification of the factor to homogeneity revealed that the factor did not stimulate other types of colony growth nor did it induce differentiation in leukemia cells such as $KG_1$ or HL-60. It was found that the concentration of the factor required to obtain one-half maximum colony formation ($2.37 \times 10^{-11}$ M) was equivalent to the value reported for pluripoietin. The molecule is a hydrophobic glycoprotein, molecular weight 19,000, isoelectric point 6.1, with possible 0-linked glycosides. Amino acid sequence determination of the molecule gave a single $NH_2$ terminal sequence which had no homology to corresponding sequences of other CSFs previously reported. Utilizing oligonucleotides as probes, two clones were isolated containing G-CSF complementary DNA from the cDNA library prepared with mRNA from CHU-2 cells. Complete nucleotide sequences of the cDNAs were determined and hybridization analysis with monkey cells suggested that the human genome contains only one gene for G-CSF. This gene is interrupted by four introns and a comparison of the cDNAs structures indicated that two mRNAs are generated by alternative use of the sequences in the second intron of the gene. The finding of two mRNAs for the G-CSF polypeptide suggests that specific functional differences exist. Therefore, it may be necessary to produce each G-CSF molecule on a large scale by recombinant DNA technology, and study the function of each *in vitro* and *in vivo*.

*Interleukin-3*

Other murine and human growth factors called multi-CSFs or interleukin-3s (IL-3) have been purified and genetically cloned [70,71]. The cDNAs and gene sequences for human and murine forms appear to have significant sequence homology and the factors appear to be functionally related. IL-3 supports the growth of multilineage colonies and in this respect, human GM-CSF does exhibit some multilineage activity that is similar to IL-3. Thus, IL-3 and GM-CSF are two separate molecules with some overlapping biological activities. Both IL-3 and GM-CSF often show coordinate expression which suggests that the gene may be transcriptionally linked in some T-cells and expressed in response to the appropriate stimulus [72].

*Erythropoietin*

Erythropoietin (Epo) is the major regulator for erythropoiesis and there is considerable information on the physiology and biochemistry of this hormone. For a recent review, see Spivak 1986 [73].

Epo is produced primarily by the kidney and has 166 amino acids with a molecular weight of 39,000. The molecule is heavily glycosylated and salic acid accounts for 40% of the carbohydrate. Epo can be inactivated by proteolytic enzymes, alkylation and by iodination. With the application of recombinant DNA technology, human Epo has been molecularly cloned, sequenced and expressed in a biologically active form in mammalian cells. There are now several sources of human recombinant Epo available on the market.

The major effect of Epo is on erythroid progenitor cell growth and differentiation (hemoglobin synthesis) in Epo responsive cells. Clonal assays have demonstrated that early erythroid progenitors, BFU-E may be regulated by Epo, and the mature progenitor or CFU-E requires Epo for terminal differentiation. There is considerable evidence which indicates that Epo is the natural regulator of erythropoiesis *in vivo*.

*Other factors*
Recently a human pluripotent CSF has been prepared and apparently has properties that encompass the activities of IL-3 and GM-CSF [74]. Another area of overlap in growth stimulating activity is seen with IL-3 and GM-CSF so that at least 3 molecules influence CFU-Eos. Bartelmez et al [75] has isolated a small molecular weight peptide (MW 5,000) capable of stimulating eosinophil colony growth *in vitro* (Eos-CSF). Others have described eosinophil differentiating factor(s), however, the relationship of differentiating factor to colony stimulating factor has not yet been clarified. Less information is available regarding thrombopoietin, the presumed regulator of thrombopoiesis [19]).

The primary growth factors for lymphoid growth are B-cell growth factor (BCGF) and T-cell growth factor (TCGF, IL-2) [76]. In brief, it is possible to grow T-cell clones with purified TCGF and B-cell clones using partly purified BCGF. The response of T-lymphocytes to IL-2 depends on both the TCGF concentration, and the number of TCGF receptors. There is no apparent structural relationship between TCGF and BCGF. Continuous B-cell clones have been derived in the presence of BCGF and monoclonal antibodies have been made specific for the clones.

The production of immunoglobulin by B cells is also influenced by factors elaborated by T-cells [77,78]. In particular, B-cell differentiating factors stimulate IgM secretion and the release of another differentiating factor, BCDF. BCDF induces a type of IgG class switching rather than a new clone of cells. Thus, growth, differentiation and functions of lymphocytes themselves depend upon the complex production and interaction of regulatory molecules.

*Clinical applications*
There are many potential clinical applications for the use of recombinant forms of CSF. These molecules may be used in situations where there is a granulocytic deficit. For example, chemotherapy is frequently associated with leukopenia and CSFs could be administered before and after chemotherapy to accelerate leukocyte regeneration. Preliminary studies in Japan and the United States suggest that therapeutic administration of CSF has potential for improving the engraftment of transplanted bone marrow cells. Recently, administration of r-GM-CSF helped hematologic recovery in a Brazilian patient accidently exposed to radioactive cesium. It has also been suggested that CSFs could be useful for differentiation therapy. In this respect, treatment of chronic myeloid leukemia with CSF could induce the leukemia cells to differentiate rather than replicate, and the differentiated macrophages could then possess direct anti-tumour activity [79-81].

Studies are currently underway at several Medical Centers studying the potential usefulness of CSF-therapy in patients with acquired immune deficiencies such as AIDS [80,81]. It is thought that CSFs may increase the host defenses and possible enhancement of antibody-dependent cell mediated cytotoxicity (ADCC) against viral infected cells.

Epo therapy may prove to be useful in improving the anemia of chronic renal failure (CRF). Patients with kidney disease which receive hemodialysis treatment frequently develop anemia along with other hematological problems. In some instances, insufficient Epo production and/or ineffective Epo activity due to inactivation are thought to be involved in the etiology of the anemia. Clinical trials are currently underway at a number of institutions (Seattle, UCLA) utilizing r-Epo to maintain an adequate hematocrit in anemic patients with CRF. Preliminary results appear to be promising and it is possible that similar therapy may be useful in a variety of other anemic states [79-81].

## Cell separation techniques

Improvements in hemopoietic culture have been made possible in part due to the application of refined cell separation procedures. Numerous techniques are available, however, only a limited number are routinely used to prepare cells for hemopoietic culture. Such techniques include depletion of adherent cells, isopycnic centrifugation, velocity sedimentation, elutriation, immuno-logical panning and fluorescent activated cell sorting (FACS). Removal of cells by adherence usually involves the attachment of adherent cells (such as macrophages) to the surface of a petri dish containing medium with 15% FCS, and then rinsing the nonadherent cells away. In isopycnic sedimenta-tion, cells sediement to a point in a density gradient equivalent to their own density. Usually percoll, metrizamide or Ficoll are employed to establish a gradient. Velocity sedimentation or centrifugal elutriation employ a principle whereby sedimentation is influenced mainly be cell size and to some degree by surface area and density.

### Removal by adherence

Removal of adherent cells (monocytes, MO; macrophages, MØ) can be accomplished by the following procedures. Washed bone marrow or peripheral blood mononuclear cells are suspended in IMDM + 15-20% FCS, at a concentration of $2 \times 10^6$ cells/ml. The preparation is then incubated in 35-90 mm petri dishes (Falcon) (2-10 ml/plate) for two hours at 37°C in 5% $CO_2$ + 95% air. After incubation, the nonadherent cells are removed with a Pasteur pipette, washed and then diluted with fresh medium to the desired concentration. Removal of cells in this manner will eliminate most of the MO or MØ from the sample and enrich the number of erythroid colony forming cells per ml of sample [27].

### Ficoll-Hypaque separation

A conventional method to enrich buffey coat cells from blood or bone marrow is to use density gradient centrifugation on Ficoll-Hypaque (Ficoll-Paque, Pharmacia, or Ficoll-Isopaque or Lymphoprep, Nyegaard Co.) [82]. The method is simple, rapid and inexpensive, however the cells are also contamin-ated with platelets. Platelets can be eliminated by isopycnic centrifugation on Percoll. In brief, heparinized blood (or bone marrow) is diluted 50:50 in

HBSS (Mg$^{++}$-Ca$^{++}$ free) and then 6-8 ml is layered onto 3 ml of Ficoll-Hypaque. The tubes are then centrifuged at 450×g for 30 min (room temperature) and the interface cells removed with a sterile Pasteur pipette. The cells are then washed twice (HBSS, Mg$^{++}$-Ca$^{++}$ free) and resuspended to the desired concentration. Total lymphocyte-mononuclear cell recovery by this method is 50-85% (1-3% MO and granulocytes), depending upon the separation medium and specimen source [83,.

An isokinetic-gradient sedimentation employing a linear gradient of Ficoll in medium has been adapted to isolate erythroid progenitor populations from bone marrow. This technique is rapid and efficient and it has been previously shown that erythroid colony progenitors can be separated into three distinct model populations [84]. Furthermore, the gradient can be used to separate megakaryocytes and pluripotent stem cells (CFU-S) from bone marrow.

*Separation of T-cells by rosettes*

T-cell popultions can be removed by the methods described by Levitt et al [85] or the AET-SRBC method of Kaplan and Clark [86]. Suspensions of bone marrow or peripheral blood mononuclear cells (PBMC) (5x10$^6$/ml) are treated with neuraminidase-treated sheep erythrocytes (SRNC) (5% suspension in IMDM) so as to form rosettes. The cell preparations are then layered on Ficoll-Hypaque and the buffey coat separated by standard procedures. The nonrosetting interface is then treated with pan-T lymphocyte McAb with or without complement. The McAb should be an antibody similar to 17F12/Leu (Levitt et al) which is a complement fixing antihuman McAb that recognizes a 67,000 MW glycoprotein antigen on all T-lymphocytes and thymocytes. PBMC are then recovered from the rosetted pellet by treatment with 0.155 mol/L NH$_4$$^+$. The T-cell enriched fractions recovered are usually 96-100% rosette positive and should contain less than 3% monocytes [85,86].

*Panning*

Monoclonal antibodies (McAb) permitted a useful solid-phase immuno-absorption (panning) technique for separation and sorting of specific cell populations. For example, the method is useful for immunologic marrow T-cell depletion similar to that done by gated fluorescence activated cell separation of cytofluorometry. The technique has been described by Levitt et al [85] and can be performed as follows: polystyrene petri dishes are coated with 100 μg of purified goat anti-mouse IgG (or IgM), diluted in buffer, incubated for 40 min at 23°C, after which the overlying buffer is decanted and the dishes washed with PBS. Human marrow cells (20×10$^6$ in AB serum) are then coated with McAb (50-100 μg Leu-1 or TM-1), incubated for 20 min (4°C), washed and then added to the antibody-coated dishes (indirect panning) and incubated for 70 min at 4°C. Bound and nonbound cells are then separately recovered by elution with cold PBS + 1% FCS. In most cases, the majority of bound cells (>95%) will stain positive for the McAb used for panning.

Thus, cell populations can be separated depending upon McAb specificity and therefore offer a unique way of separating specific cell populations. Problems exist regarding the cost of some McAb preparations and the efficiency of cell recovery. In this respect, panning of human bone marrow is not easily applicable to the large volume of marrow that would need to be processed in clinical transplantation, and the extent of T-cell depletion with this procedure may not be optimal.

*Separation by flow cytometry*

A unique sophisticated method for sorting small numbers of cells is by the use of fluorescence-activated cell sorting (FACS). This can be done using a laser (488 nM) with an Ortho 50-H cytofluorograph coupled to a 2150 computer (Ortho Diagnostics, Westwood, MA), or a modified FACS II system (B-D FACS Systems, Becton Dickinson & Co., Sunnyvale, CA). Cells are usually labeled with some fluorescent conjugated material such as an antibody or a lectin like wheat germ agglutinin conjugated to fluorescein isothiocyanate (WGA-FITC). This complex binds bone marrow stem cells (CFU-S) and by using light scatter characteristics it was found that the CFU-S population could be enriched by 100 fold [87,88]. Refinements can be made in order to sort specific cell populations such as H-2K positive cells. This involves the removal of WGA-FITC and the subsequent labeling of cells with antibody (in this specific case, anti H-2K-biotin and fluorochrome). Using such technology, it has been possible to sort individual cells into micro-culture wells (Terasaki trays) so as to perform limiting dilution analysis of small numbers of cells (1,2,4-400/well etc.) and then to grow the cell cultures *in vitro* or examine the preparations by electron microscopy. Sorting and culture of individual or small numbers of cells allowed for the detection and identification of stem cells which give rise to individual myeloid colonies (CFU-GM) [87,99].

Cell cycle distribution profiles can also be determined by quantitating DNA and RNA content in cell samples. The DNA content is usually visualized by staining the cells with fluorescent propidium iodide. Although this methodology is very sophisticated, it has disadvantages in that the equipment is very expensive, and that large scale fractionation of blood or bone marrow is impractical at the present time.

There are other numerous methods that may improve bone marrow separation and concentration and are not discussed here. These methods include the utilization of an IBM cell processor, sepharose cellular immunoabsorption column and ricin-conjugated McAbs [85].

*Unit gravity sedimentation*

This technique is very useful for separation and enrichment of hemopoietic progenitor cells [89,90]. It is reproducible and provides enriched fractions of progenitor cells in culture media which have not been exposed to agents such as Ficoll or agents that may have questionable effects on cells. However, the technique is very time-consuming and the resolution and enrichment is not the best. Cells are separated into a number of fractions on the basis of cell size, by velocity-unit gravity sedimentation in a chamber containing a gradient of FCS (3-30%) in culture medium at 4°C. An upper streaming limit exists in the starting band of cell sample which varies with the type of cell, cell number and type of gradient. In time, cells will sediment in the chamber at specific sedimentation velocities (mm/hr) after which the bands of cells are collected at various intervals as fractions. It has been found that sedimentation velocity (mm/hr) approximately equals $r^2/4$ (r = cell radius in microns) and that specific hemopoietic progenitor cells differ in size and can therefore quantitatively be separated by this technique. The apparatus consists of a glass cylindrical chamber (11.5 cm dia) with a conical cone base. The chamber is loaded with cells ($8 \times 10^7$ total) and a gradient established by introducing a linear gradient of 15-30% FCS in media or PBS ($\sim 500$ ml) under the cell band. After 3-4 hours, the chamber is drained by removing the cone volume and then collecting 10-15 ml fractions. All procedures can be done under sterile conditions.

We have separated adult human bone marrow and fetal liver progenitor cells by velocity sedimentation. Human fetal liver cells (12-20 wks) were obtained through the collaboration of Dr R. Rieder at SUNY Downstate Medical Center [91]. Results on Table 5 show the sedimentation velocities of human hemopoietic colony forming cells for adult bone marrow and fetal liver. It is clear that granulocytic progenitors (CFU-GM) sediment at different velocities than erythroid CFU-E or BFU-E. Human fetal liver erythroid progenitors appeared to sediment as several distinct populations which appeared in culture as 4-,7-,10- and 14-day colonies. Note that progenitors for 4-day colonies sedimented at 4.2 and 8.8 mm/hr, 7-day colonies at 7 and 7.9 mm/hr, whereas 10-day colonies sedimented at 7 and 7.3 mm/hr and 14-day colonies sedimented at 6.5 and 4.0 mm/hr. In contrast, normal human bone marrow 7-day colonies sediment at 6.1 mm/hr and 14-day colonies at 3.8 mm/hr. Thus fetal liver appears to contain a spectrum of erythroid progenitors, some of which may or may not develop or seed hemopoietic tissues such as the bone marrow in later development.

*Table 5.* Unit gravity sedimentation profiles of human hematopoietic cells.

| Tissue | Sedimentation velocity mm/hr | | | |
| | CFU-GM | CFU-E | BFU-E | RBC |
|---|---|---|---|---|
| Bone Marrow | 7.5–8.8 (14d)<br>7.5–8.1 (G)<br>8.0–8.8 (M) | 6.1 (7d) | 3.8 (14d) | 2 |
| Fetal Liver | | 4.2, 8.8 (4d)<br>7, 7.9 (7d) | 7, 7.3 (10d)<br>6.5, 4.0 (14d) | |

Bone marrow cells were obtained by aspiration from the posterior iliac crest from 4 normal donors.

Three fetal liver specimens were obtained at post-mortem examination from 13-20-week prostaglandin induced abortuses. The livers were minced, filtered through gauze and then separated on a Ficoll-Paque gradient.

d = day of culture; G = granulocyte; M = macrophage.

*Table 6.* Characterization of fractionated HL-60 cells by elutriation according to Heil and Chiao [96].

| Cell fraction | Particle diameter – μM (sedimentation Vel – mm/hr) | Percentage of cells in | | | Yield (%) |
|---|---|---|---|---|---|
| | | $G_1$ | S | $G_2M$ | |
| Unfractionated HL-60 | — | 48 | 43 | 9 | 100 |
| $G_1$ fraction | 8.5 (7) | 96 | 4 | 0 | 10 |
| Intermediate fraction | 10.0 (10) | 68 | 30 | 2 | 48 |
| $S/G_2$ fraction | 35.0 (125) | 20 | 61 | 19 | 28 |

**INTRACELLULAR LOCALIZATION OF ENZYMES AND INTERMEDIATES OF THE HEME BIOSYNTHETIC AND DEGRADATIVE PATHWAYS:**

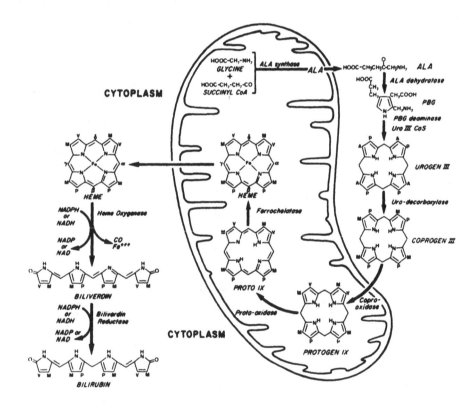

*Figure 6a.* Intracellular localization of heme biosynthetic and degradative enzymes.

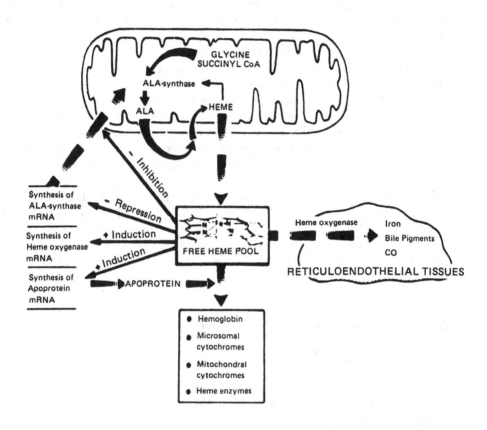

*Figure 6b.* Schematic model for the regulation of heme metabolism and heme proteins.

*Elutriation*

Centrifugal elutriation provides a rapid means of separating large numbers of cells on the basis of their sedimentation properties [92]. Basically, cells are elutriated in culture medium or HBSS supplemented with 5% FCS or gelatin. A special centrifuge 100 rotor is kept cool (4°C), a flow rate adjusted to about 30 ml/min and the cells injected into the rotor over a period of about 2 min. Usually $10^8$-$10^9$ cells are used with the smaller rotors such as the Beckman JE6-B, however a larger rotor is available for larger cell number (Beckman JE-10X). Fractions are then recovered at different counter flow rates of 30-48 ml/min, after which the fractions (usually 3-4) are washed. All procedures are done under sterile conditions and in fact a semi-closed system has been adapted which makes use of disposable transfer packs of blood products.

This technology may have valuable clinical application such as in bone marrow transplantation where elutriation may be used for the rapid preparation of specific enriched bone marrow populations. In this respect, centrifugal elutriation has been used to deplete lymphocytes from bone marrow cells to be used for allogeneic transplantation [93] and also to isolate and purify human pancreatic islet cells for transplantation [94]. Such procedures provide an enrichment of stem cells and reduce the incidenicnce of Graft-versus-Host disease without compromizing engraftment.

Nijhof et al [95] have utilized centrifugal elutriation to obtain a 3-5-fold enrichment of murine spleen CFU-E. When this elutriated preparation was then placed on a Percoll gradient, further enrichment was obtained so that the overall CFU-E recovery was about 70%. Heil & Chiao [96] have utilized elutriation to separate cell populations into specific cell-cycle phases. Results from their studies demonstrate that highly pure populations of cells can be obtained efficiently without any chemical treatment which may affect cellular physiology. A summary of some of their studies depicting the separation of HL-60 cells into specific pure populations is represented on Table 6. These results demonstrate that a highly purified fraction of cells in $G_1$ phase could be recovered (96%) containing a minimal contaminant (4%) and a total recovery of about 86%. Therefore, this technique may be very useful for obtaining large numbers of purified cells that are virtually free of chemical treatment.

## Heme metabolism in hemopoietic colonies

### Heme enzymes in CFU-E, BFU-E

Heme synthesis and degradation play pivotal roles in the regulation of growth and differentiation of hematopoiesis. In this regard, it is well-known that a variety of disturbances in hematopoiesis accompany abnormal heme metabolism [97]. The cellular heme pool directly influences a multitude of cellular processes including hemoglobin formation, microsomal cytochromes (cyto), such as cyto P-450, mitochondrial cytochromes, peroxidases and the enzymatic synthesis and degradation of heme itself. Of major importance are the rate limiting enzymes for heme synthesis (δ-aminolevulinic acid synthase, ALAS) and heme degradation (heme oxygenase, HO). The activity of these two enzymes is critical to regulating the level of heme within the cell. Figure 6a-b is a schematic representation of heme and its interrelationships within the cell. It is important that adequate levels of heme are maintained in order for hematopoiesis to ensue, and in this respect a fall in HO may be a prerequisite for erythroid differentiation. Therefore, the enzymatic events of heme synthesis and degradation must be carefully regulated or maintained in order to obtain adequate growth of hemopoietic cells.

We have characterized the heme biosynthetic and degradative enzymes in bone marrow hemopoietic colonies. Modifications of methodology were made so that enzymes could be measured from erythroid colony (CFU-E, BFU-E) methylcellulose cultures. Methylcellulose cultures are used because the technique allows one to dissolve the semi-solid matrix and prepare a sample of colonies. Special micro-methods were developed for the specific heme enzymes ALAS, ALAD and HO [27,98-100]. Figure 7 summarizes the chronologic changes in heme enzyme activities during human bone marrow CFU-E growth. It can be seen that as growth and differentiation of CFU-E occurs, activity of the degradative enzyme HO ($\triangle$) drops, while the biosynthetic enzymes ALAS ($\bigcirc$) and ALAD ($\square$) increase in activity. These enzyme patterns are accompanied with an increase in heme synthesis ($\blacktriangle$), with maximal activity between 7-8 days. A similar developmental profile is seen with murine CFU-E development, however maximal developmental activity occurs between 48-56 hours (Figure 8, solid lines, ALAS ($\bullet$), ALAD ($\blacktriangle$), HO ($\blacksquare$)). In addition, this figure demonstrates that cycloheximide (dotted lines), which is an inhibitor of cytoplasmic protein synthesis, inhibits the activities (or synthesis) of all three heme enzymes.

The heme biosynthetic enzyme urobilinogen deaminase (URO) has also been measured in human BFU-E colonies. Results from our experiments are represented on Figure 9 and indicates the levels of URO and HO in human BFU-E under different conditions [100]. Note that heme synthesis, represented as URO, favors heme degradation (HO) in control cultures. Addition of hemin or conditioned media from PHA stimulated lymphocytes (PHA-LCM) were found to stimulate URO activity. In contrast, addition of excess iron (Fe) or conditioned media from adherent macrophages (MØ) stimulated heme degradation or HO. Results from these studies clearly indicate the importance of maintaining adequate levels of heme for maximal erythroid colony growth and development.

*Cytochrome P-450 system in CFU-E, CFU-GM*

We have also characterized a cytochrome (cyto) P-450 system in developing hemopoietic colonies [101]. The cyto P-450 system is important for a variety of cellular functions including chemical-drug metabolism and detoxification, and more recently the metabolism of arachidonic acid [102]. In this respect the cyto P-450 system may play important roles in the growth and differentiation of hemopoietic cells. The cyto P-450-dependent aniline hydroxylase (AHH) system has been measured in developing CFU-E and CFU-GM growth in methylcellulose cultures. Figure 10 shows the activity profile of AHH ($^{14}C$ counts in benzopyrine metabolites) in developing bone marrow CFU-E. Table 7 shows the activity of AHH in developing CFU-GM colonies. It can be seen that maximal AHH activity in CFU-E occurred by 64 hrs of culture, whereas activity is significantly elevated in 6-7-day cultures of CFU-GM. Additionally, exposure of cultures to 3-methylcolanthrene (3-MC) resulted in a significant enhancement oᶠ AHH activity (Table 7).

202

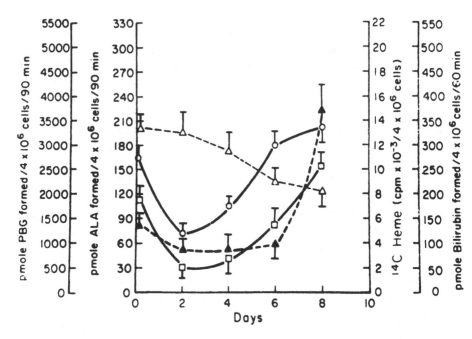

*Figure 7.* Chronologic changes of ALAS (○), ALAD (■), ¹⁴C-ALA incorporation into heme (▲) and heme oxygenase (△) during normal human bone marrow CFU-E growth. Values are from four normal marrows (± SEM).

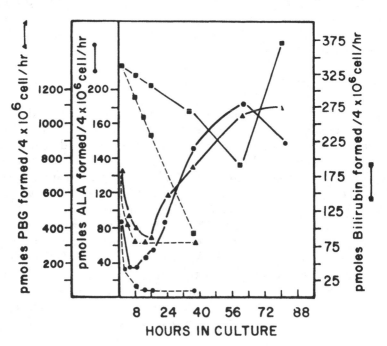

*Figure 8.* Chronologic changes of ALAS (●), ALAD (□) and heme oxygenase (▲) during murine bone marrow CFU-E growth in the absence (——) or presence (---) of cycloheximide.

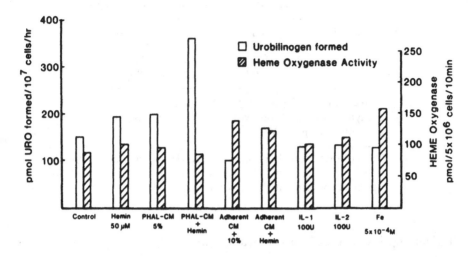

*Figure 9.* Effect of growth factors and other agents on heme oxygenase and uroporphobilinogen deaminase in human BFU-E colonies.

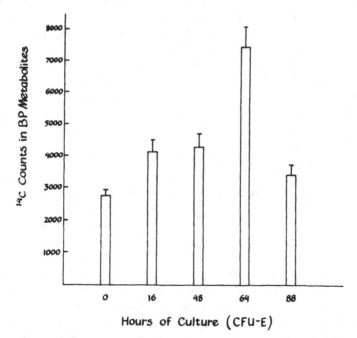

*Figure 10.* Developmental pattern of arylhydrocarbon hydroxylase (AHH) activity in mouse bone marrow CFU-E colony culture. CFU-E were grown in methylcellulose with erythropoietin. The cells harvested from 4-5 plates/assay after the desired incubation period (37°C) and AHH activity determined using 0.5 μCi $^{14}$C-BP.

*Table 7.* Developmental pattern of arylhydrocarbon hydroxylase (AHH) activity in murine bone marrow CFU-Gm culture.*

| | AHH activity $^{14}$C counts in BP metabolites | |
| Days of culture | Control | + 3-MC |
|---|---|---|
| | 6,630 | ND |
| 6-7 | 9,027 | 16,908 (88)** |

\* Mouse bone marrow CFU-GM were grown at 37°C in methylcellulose cultures with colony stimulating factor with or without 40 $\mu$g 3-MC.
() = % increase.
The cultures were harvested and AHH activity determined with $5 \times 10^6$ cells/assay and 0.5 $\mu$Ci $^{14}$C BP.
\*\* Significantly different from control, p < 0.001.

## Clinical significance of hemopoietic culture

Advances in hemopoietic culture technology have contributed to a better understanding of hematological disorders in clinical medicine. The potential clinical applications of CSFs or growth factors have been briefly discussed previously in this report. Insufficient production of any of the growth factors *in vivo* could result in neutropenic and anemic states. A variety of hematological disorders are also associated with disturbances in colony growth and/or heme metabolism. We will not review these findings, but only mention a few examples to illustrate how colony assays may serve as useful tools to further characterize these disorders. Early studies revealed that the frequencies of bone marrow agar colony forming cells were considerably elevated in chronic myelogenous leukemia (CML) whereas they were markedly depressed or absent in AML. Upon remission, normal growth patterns could be achieved [103]. Studies on erythropoiesis revealed that plasma clot cultures of bone marrow from polycythemia vera patients grow endogenous CFU-E in the absence of exogenous Epo [32]. This property appears to be distinct from secondary polycythemia where exogenous Epo is necessary for growth. Bone marrow from patients with nutritional deficiencies (iron, B-12) or maturational blocks, and certain leukemic states (CML in erythroblastic crises) grow large numbers of CFU-E when adequate conditions exist [33,34,99]. Poor or absent CFU-E growth is obtained from aplastic marrows [104] whereas sideroblastic anemia (SA) bone marrows may generate large numbers of CFU-E in methylcellulose, but not plasma clot cultures [33]. Heme metabolism is disturbed in the SA cells in that ALAS activity is reduced and HO activity elevated [98]. Upon culture of the SA bone marrow in methylcellulose for CFU-E, ALAS activity becomes elevated and HO drops. Thus, normal erythropoiesis and heme metabolism may ensue in the proper culture environment. Elevated HO activity has been associated with several disturbances where CFU-E growth and hematopoiesis is impaired. For example, benzene, phenol, heavy metals, iron overload and SA are all associated with elevated levels of HO and depressed colony growth [26,98,106,107]. Attempts to depress HO activity by experimental agents are currently in progress and may have definite clinical application for the therapy of anemia.

In conclusion, hemopoietic culture provides a means of culturing large numbers of blood cell progenitors under defined conditions. Recombinant DNA technology has provided the means for production of specific growth factors necessary for the culture of stem cells and their hemopoietic compartments. Future advances in immunohematology, growth factor biology and large scale culture technology will serve to enhance the establishment of hemopoietic stem cell banks which could then serve as a permanent source of bone marrow or blood cell progenitors.

## Acknowledgements

This work was supported by the National Institute of Arthritis for Diabetes and Digestive Kidney Diseases (N.G.A.) (AM 29742). N.G.A. is a recipient of a Research Career Development Award of the National Institutes of health (AM 00781).

## References

1. Boggs S, Boggs D. Multipotent stem cells *in vivo*. In: Golde D (ed). Hematopoiesis. Churchill Livingstone Pubs, NY 1984:1-72.
2. Messner HA. Multipotent stem cells *in vitro*. In: Golde D (ed). Hematopoiesis. Churchill Livingstone Pubs, NY 1984:73-86.
3. Kurland JI. Granulocyte-monocyte progenitor cells. In: Golde D (ed). Hematopoiesis. Churchill Livingstone Pubs, NY 1984:87-122.
4. Rozenszain LA, Radnay J, Nussenblatt R, Sredni B. Human lymphoid cells and their progenitors: Isolation, identification and colony growth. In: Golde D (ed). Hematopoiesis. Churchill Livingstone Pubs, NY 1984:150-79.
5. Greenberger JS. Long-term hematopoietic cultures. In: Golde D (ed). Hematopoiesis. Churchill Livingstone Pubs, NY 1984:203-42.
6. Preisler H, Kirshner J, Early AP. Leukemia cell cultures. In: Golde D (ed). Hematopoiesis. Churchill Livingstone Pubs, NY 1984:243-68.
7. Pluznik DH, Sachs L. The cloning of normal mast cells in tissue culture. J Cell Comp Physiol 1965;66:319-25.
8. Bradley TR, Metcalf D. The growth of mouse bone marrow cells *in vitro*. Aust J Exp Biol Med Sci 1966;44:287-93.
9. Harris P, Ralph P. Human leukemia models of myelomonocytic development: A review of the HL60 and U937 cell lines. J Leuk Bio 1985;37:407-12.
10. Metcalf D. The molecular biology and functions of the granulocyte macrophage colony stimulating factors. Blood 1986;67:257-67.
11. Sporn MD, Todaro G. Autocrine secretion and malignant transformation of cells. N Engl J Med 1980;303:878-80.

12. Chiao JW, Freitag WF, Steinmetz JC, Andreeff M. Changes of cellular markers during differentiation of HL-60 promyelocytes to macrophages as induced by T lymphocyte conditioned medium. Leuk Res 1981;5:477-83.

13. Chiao JW, Andreeff M, Freitag WB, Arlin Z. Induction of in vitro proliferation and maturation of human aneuploid myelogenous leukemic cells. J Exp Med 1982;155:1357-64.

14. Leung K, Chiao JW. Human leukemia cell maturation induced by a T cell lymphokine isolated from medium conditioned by normal lymphocytes. Proc Natl Acad Sci (USA) 1985;82:1209-13.

15. Heil MF, Chiao JW. Cell cycle effects of an autologous growth promoter from human leukemia cells. Exp Cell Res 1985;157:282-7.

16. Lutton JD, Ascensao JL, Chiao JW, Levere RD. Divergent production of autostimulatory activity and colony stimulating activity by L1210 leukemia. Exp Hemat 1986;14:531.

17. Ogawa M, Leary AG. Erythroid progenitors. In: Golde D (ed). Hematopoiesis. Churchill Livingstone Pubs, NY 1984:123-32.

18. Donahue RE, Emerson SG, Wang EA, Wong GG, Clark SC, Natan DG. Demonstration of burst-promoting activity of recombinant human GM-CSF on circulating erythroid progenitors using an assay involving the delayed addition of erythropoietin. Blood 1985;66:1479-81.

19. Mazur EM, Hoffman R. Human megakaryocyte progenitors. In: Golde D (ed). Hematopoiesis. Churchill Livingstone Pubs, NY 1984:133-49.

20. Leary AG, Ogawa M. Identification of pure and mixed basophil colonies in culture of human peripheral blood and marrow cells. Blood 1984;64:78-83.

21. Denburg JA, Messner H, Lim B, Jamal N, Telizyn S, Bienenstock J. Clonal origin of human basophil/mast cells from circulating multipotent hemopoietic progenitors. Exp Hemat 1985;13:185-8.

22. Allen TD, Dexter TM. Cellular interrelationships during in vitro granulopoiesis. Different 1976;6:191-4.

23. Dexter TM, Allen TD, Lajtha LG. Conditions controlling the proliferation of hematopoietic stem cells in vitro. J Cell Phy 1977;91:335-44.

24. Lutton JD, Osborn DC, Zanjani ED, Wasserman LR. Stimulation inhibition of granulocyte and mononuclear colony formation by conditioned medium from mouse peritoneal cells. JRES 1975;18:186-95.

25. Lutton JD, Schmalzer EA, Rao AN, Rao SP, Levere RD. Erythroid colony studies on sickle cell anemia in hypoproliferative crisis. Am J Hemat 1981;8:15-21.

26. Lutton JD, Abraham NG, Friedland M, Levere RD. The toxic effects of heavy metals on rat bone marrow in vitro erythropoiesis: Protective role of hemin and zinc. Env Res 1984;35:97-103.

27. Abraham NG, Lutton JD, Levere RD. The role of haem biosynthetic and degradative enzymes in erythroid colony development: The effect of haemin. Brit J Haemat 1982;50:17-28.

28. Isocove NN, Sieber F, Winterhalter KH. Erythroid colony formation in cultures of mouse and human bone marrow: Analysis of the requirement for erythropoietin by gel filtration and affinity chromatography on agarose-concanavalin A. J Cell Phy 1974;83:309-20.

29. Mazur EM, Hoffman R, Bruno E. Regulation of human megakaryocytopoiesis. J Clin Invest 1981;68:733-41.

30. Yang HH, Bruno E, Hoffman R. Studies of human megakaryocytopoiesis using an anti-megakaryocyte colony stimulating factor antiserum. J Clin Invest 1986;77:1873-80.

31. Breitman TP, Collins SJ, Keene BR. Replacement of serum by insulin and transferrin supports growth and differentiation of the human promyelocytic cell line HL-60. Exp Cell Res 1980;126:494-8.
32. Lutton JD, Levere RD. Endogenous erythroid colony formation by peripheral blood mononuclear cells from patients with myelofibrosis and polycythemia vera. Acta Haemat 1979;62:94-9.
33. Lutton JD, Abraham NG, Hoffman R, Ritchey AK, Levere RD. Sideroblastic anemia: Differences in bone marrow erythroid colony growth responses to erythropoietin in plasma clot and methylcellulose cultures. Am J Hemat 1984;16: 219-26.
34. Lutton JD, Chiao JW, Ascensao JL, Arlin Z, Atamer M, Levere RD. Humoral dependent hemopoiesis and flow cytometric analysis of chronic myelogenous leukemia in erythroblastic transformation. Acta Haemat 1987;77:120-3.
35. Friedland M, Lutton JD, Spitzer R, Levere RD. Dyskeratosis congenita with hypoplastic anemia: A stem cell defect. Am J Hemat 1985;20:85-7.
36. Broudy VC, Zuckerman KS, Jetmalani S, Fitchen JH, Bagby GC. Monocytes stimulate fibroblastoid bone marrow stromal cells to produce multilineage hematopoietic growth factors. Blood 1986;68:530-4.
37. Cronkite EA, Miller ME, Garnett H, Harigaya K. Regulation of hematopoiesis: Inhibitors and stimulators produced by a murine bone marrow stromal cell line (H-1). In: Killman SV, Cronkite EP, Muller Borat CN (eds). Haemopoietic stem cells. Munksgaard Pub Co, Copenhagen 1982:266-82.
38. Gordon MY. Granulopoietic effects of factors produced by cultured human marrow fibroblasts. Stem Cells 1982;1:180.
39. Gordon MY, Kearney L, Hibbin JA. Effects of human marrow stromal cells on proliferation by human granulocytic (GM-CFC), erythroid (BFU-E) and mixed (MIX-CFC) colony forming cells. Brit J Haemat 1983;53:317.
40. Bagby GC, Rigas VD, Bennet RM, Vanenbark AA, Gared HS. Interaction of lactoferrin, monocytes and T-lymphocyte subsets in the regulation of steady-state granulopoiesis in vitro. J Clin Invest 1981;68:56-63.
41. Bagby GC, McCall E, Bergstrom KA, Burger D. A monokine regulates colony-stimulating activity production by vascular endothelial cells. Blood 1983;62: 663-8.
42. Bagby GC, McCall E, Layman DL. Regulation of colony-stimulating activity production. Interactions of fibroblasts, mononuclear phagocytes and lactoferrin. J Clin Invest 1983;71:340-4.
43. Zuckerman KS, Bagby GC, McCall E et al. A monokine stimulates production of human erythroid burst-promoting activity by endothelial cells in vitro. J Clin Invest 1985;75:722-5.
44. Segal GM, McCall E, Stueve T, Bagby GC. Monokine-stimulated endothelial cells promote human megakaryocyte and mixed-cell colony growth. Blood 1985; 66:464a.
45. McCall E, Rathbun RK, Riscoe M, Wilkinson B, Bagby GC. Human placental conditioned medium contains monocyte derived recruiting activity (MRA). Exp Hemat 1986;14:789-93.
46. Bagby GC, Dinarello CA, Wallace P, Wagner C, Hefeneider S, McCall E. Interleukin-1 stimulates granulocyte macrophage colony stimulating activity release by vascular endothelial cells. J Clin Invest 1986;78:1316-23.
47. Segal GM, McCall E, Stueve T, Bagby GC. Interleukin-1 stimulates endothelial cells to release multilineage human colony stimulating activity. J Immunol 1987; 138:1772-8.

48. Sokal G, Michaux JL, Van den Berghe H et al. A new hematopoietic syndrome with a distinct karyotype: The 5q chromosome. Blood 1975;46:519-33.
49. Begley CG, Metcalf D, Lopez AF, Nicola NA. Fractionated populations of normal human marrow cells respond to both colony-stimulating factors with granulocyte-macrophage activity. Exp Hemat 1985;13:956-62.
50. Nicola NA, Metcalf D, Johnson GR, Burgess AW. Separation of functionally distinct human granulocyte macrophage colony stimulating factors. Blood 1979; 54:614-22.
51. Gasson JC, Weisbart RH, Kaufman SE et al. Purified human granulocyte macrophage colony stimulating factor: Direct action on neutrophils. Science 1984;226:1339-42.
52. Wong GG, Witek J, Temple PA et al. Human GM-CSF: Molecular cloning of the complementary DNA and purification of the natural and recombinant proteins. Science 1985;288:810-5.
53. Lee F, Yokota T, Otsuka T et al. Isolation of cDNA for a human granulocyte-macrophage colony-stimulating factor by functional expression in mammalian cells. Proc Natl Acad Sci (USA) 1985;82:4360-5.
54. Metcalf D, Begley CG, Johnson GR et al. Biologic properties in vitro of recombinant human granulocyte-macrophage colony-stimulating factor. Blood 1986; 67:37-45.
55. Park LS, Friend D, Gillis S, Urdal DL. Characterization of the cell surface receptors for human granulocyte/macrophage colony stimulating factors. J Exp Med 1986;164:251-62.
56. Cantrell MA, Anderson D, Cerretti DP et al. Cloning, sequence and expression of a human granulocyte macrophage colony-stimulating factor. Proc Natl Acad Sci (USA) 1985;82:6250-4.
57. Metcalf D, Johnson GR, Burgess AW. Direct stimulation by purified GM-CSF of the proliferation of multipotential and erythroid precursor cells. Blood 1980; 55:138-47.
58. Sehgal PK, Mather DG, Clark SC. Stimulation of hematopoiesis in primates by continuous infusion of recombinant human GM-CSF. Nature 1986;323:872-5.
59. Kawasaki ES, Ladner MB, Wang AM, van Arsdell J, Warren A. Cloning of a cDNA encoding human macrophage-specific colony stimulating factor (CSF-1). Science 1985;230:291-4.
60. Sacca R, Stanley ER, Sherr CJ, Rettenmier CW. Specific binding of the mononuclear phagocyte colony-stimulating factor CSF-1 to the product of the v-fms oncogene. Proc Natl Acad Sci (USA) 1986;83:3331-6.
61. Wisniewski LP, Hirschhom K. Acquired partial deletions of the long arm of chromosome 5 in hematologic disorders. Am J Hematol 1983;15:295-300.
62. Rettenmier CW, Chen JH, Roussel MF, Sherr CJ. The product of the c-fms proto-oncogene: a glycoprotein with associated tyrosinekinase activity. Science 1985;228:320-3.
63. Nicola A, Metcalf D, Matsumoto M, Johnson GR. Purification of a factor inducing differentiation in murine myelomonocytic leukemia cells: Identification as granulocyte colony-stimulating factor (G-CSF). J Bio Chem 1983;258:9017-23.
64. Nicola NA, Begley CG, Metcalf D. Identification of the human analogue of a regulator that induces differentiation in murine leukemic cells. Nature 1985;314:625-8.
65. Nicola NA, Metcalf D. Binding of the differentiation-inducer, granulocyte-colony stimulating factor, to responsive but not unresponsive leukemic cell lines. Proc Natl Acad Sci (USA) 1984;81:3765-70.

66. Welte K, Platzer E, Lu L. Purification and biochemical characterization of human pluripotent hematopoietic colony-stimulating factor. Proc Natl Acad Sci (USA) 1985;82:1562-31.
67. Souza LM, Boone C, Gabrilove G et la. Recombinant human granulocyte colony-stimulating factor: Effects on normal and leukemic myeloid cells. Science 1986;232:61-9.
68. Nomura H, Imazeki I, Oheda M et al. Purification and characterization of granulocyte colony stimulating factor (G-CSF). EMBO Jour 1986;5:871-6.
69. Nagata S, Tsuchiya M, Asano S et al. Molecular cloning and expression of cDNA for human granulocyte colony stimulating factor. Nature 1986;319:415-8.
70. Yang YC, Ciarletta AB, Temple PA et al. Human IL-3 (Multi-CSF): Identification by expression of cloning of a novel hemopoietic growth factor related to murine IL-3. Cell 1986;47:3-10.
72. Barlow DP, Bucan M, Lehrach H, Hogan LM, Gough NM. Close genetic and physical linkage between the murine haemopoietic growth factor genes GM-CSF and multi-CSF (Il-3). EMBO Jour 1987;6:617-23.
73. Spivak JL. The mechanism of action of erythropoietin. Int J Cell Clon 1986;4:139-66.
74. Platzer E, Welte K, Gabrilove JL et al. Biological activities of a human pluripotent hemopoietic colony stimulating factor on normal and leukemic cells. J Exp Med 1985;162:1788-95.
75. Bartelmez SH, Dodge WH, Mahmound AAF, Bass DA. Stimulation of eosinophil production *in vitro* by eosinophilopoietin and spleen cell derived eosinophil growth stimulating factor. Blood 1980;56:706-13.
76. Rozenszajn LA, Radnay J, Nussenblatt R, Sredni B. Human lymphoid cells and their progenitors: Isolation, identification and colony growth. In: Golde D (ed). Hematopoiesis. Churchill Livingstone Pubs, NY 1984:150-79.
77. Noell RJ, Snow EC, Uhr JW, Vitetta ES. Activation of antigen specific B cells: Role of T cells, cytokines and antigens in induction of growth and differentiation. Proc Natl Acad Sci (USA) 1983;80:6628-33.
78. Howard M, Paul WE. Reguation of B cell growth and differentiation by soluble factors. Ann Rev Immunol 1983;1:307-14.
79. Dexter TM, Moore M. Growth and development in the haemopoietic system: the role of lymphokines and their possible therapeutic potential in disease and malignancy. Carcinogenesis 1986;7:509-16.
80. Golde D. Clinical role, therapeutic promise of CSFs. In: Oncology Times 1986;Oct:3.
81. Lymphokines and monokines in the clinic. Imm Today 1986;7:185-7.
82. Boyum A. Separation of leukocytes from blood and bone marrow. Scand J Clin Lab Invest 1968;21:7-13.
83. Mizobe F, Murtial E, Colby-Germinario S, Livett BG. An improved technique for the isolation of lymphocytes from small volumes of peripheral mouse blood. J Immunol Meth 1982;48:269-79.
84. Misiti J, Spivak JL. Separation of erythroid progenitor cells in mouse bone marrow by isokinetic-gradient sedimentation. Blood 1979;54:105-16.
85. Levitt L, Kipps TJ, Engleman EG, Greenberg PL. Human bone marrow and peripheral blood T-lymphocyte depletion: Efficacy and effects of both T-cells and monocytes on growth of hematopoietic progenitors. Blood 1985;65:663-79.
86. Kaplan ME, Clark C. An improved rosetting assay for detection of human lymphocytes. J Immunol Meth 1974;5:131-5.

87. Visser JWM, Eliason JF. *In vivo* studies on the regeneration kinetics of enriched populations of haemopoietic spleen colony-forming cells from normal bone marrow. Cell Tiss Kinet 1983;16:385-92.

88. Visser JWM, Bauman JGJ, Mulder AH, Eliason JF, DeLeeuw AM. Isolation of murine pluripotent hemopoietic stem cells. J Exp Med 1984;59:1576-90.

89. Miller RD, Phillips Ra. Separation of cells by velocity sedimentation. J Cell Physiol 1969;73:191-202.

90. Heath DS, Axelrad AA, McLeod DL, Shreeve MM. Separation of the erythropoietin-responsive progenitors BFU-E and CFU-E in mouse bone marrow by unit gravity sedimentation. Blood 1976;47:777-92.

91. Hassan MW, Lutton JD, Levere RD, Rieder RF, Cederquist LL. *In vitro* culture of erythroid colonies from human fetal liver and umbilical cord blood. Brit J Haemat 1979;41:477-84.

92. Lindahl PE. Principle of a counter-streaming centrifuge for the separation of particles of different sizes. Nature 1948;161:648-9.

93. DeWitte T, Raymakers R, Plas A, Koekman E, Wessels H, Haanen C. Bone marrow repopulation capacity after transplantation of lymphocyte-depleted allogenic bone marrow using counter flow centrifugation. Transplant 1984;37:151-5.

94. Sharp DW, Lacy P. Human islet isolation and transplantation. Abstract. Am Diabetes Assoc 1985.

95. Nijhof W, Wierenga PK. Isolation and characterization of the erythroid progenitor cell CFU-E. J Cell Biol 1983;96:386-92.

96. Heil MF, Wu JM, Chiao JW. Cell-cycle differences of HL-60 leukemia cells fractionated by centrifugal elutriation. Biochim Biophys Acta 1985;845:17-20.

97. Abraham NG, Friendland ML, Levere RD. Heme metabolism in erythroid and hepatic cells. In: Brown E (ed). Progress in Hematology 1983;XIII:75-130.

98. Abraham NG, Lutton JD, Levere RD. Regulation of heme metabolism in normal and sideroblastic bone marrow cells in culture. J Lab Clin Med 1985;105:593-600.

99. Abraham NG, Lutton JD, Levere RD. Heme metabolism and erythropoiesis in abnormal iron states: Role of $\delta$-aminolevulinic acid synthase and heme oxygenase. Exp Hemat 1985;13:838-43.

100. Brown A, Lutton JD, Nelson J, Abraham NG, Levere RD. Microenvironmental cytokines and expression of erythroid heme metabolic enzymes. Blood Cells 1987;12:123-36.

101. Lutton JD, Solangi K, Ran JY et al. Development of a cytachrome P-450 monooxygenase system in clonogenic hemopoietic cells. Res Comm Chem Path Pharm 1987;56:87-99.

102. Schwartzman ML, Pagano PJ, McGiff JC, Abraham NG. Immunochemical studies on the contribution of NADPH cytochrome P-450 reductase to the cytochrome P-450 dependent metabolism of arachidonic acid. Arch Biochem Biophys 1987;252:635-45.

103. Metcalf D. Hemopoietic Colonies: *In vitro* cloning of normal and leukemic cells. Springer-Verlag, NY. 1977:1-227.

104. Hoffman R, Zanjani ED, Lutton JD, Zalusky R, Wasserman LR. Suppression of erythroid colony formation by lymphocytes from patients with aplastic anemia. N Engl J Med 1977;296:10-3.

105. Abraham NG, Lutton JD, Levere RD. Benzene modulation of bone marrow hemopoietic and drug metabolizing systems. Biochem Arch 1985;1:85-96.

106. Abraham NG, Lutton JD, Freedman ML, Levere RD. Benzene modulation of liver cell structure and heme-cytochrome P-450 metabolism. Am J Med Sci 1986;29:81-6.

# DISCUSSION

G. Jacquin, P.C. Das

*H.V. Beer (München):* Dr Andersson, the topological structure you have shown for Factor VIII, how was it derived.

*L.O. Andersson (Stockholm):* It is based on the sequence data, the domain structure and also the type of fragments you obtain by protein degradation. There is no X-ray data available on Factor VIII and I think that will take still quite a while. Essentially this model is based on amino acid sequence data.

*A.B. Schreiber (King of Prussia):* I enjoyed your talk. I can not let you go before you make a prediction of when I could prescribe a vial of recombinant Factor VIII for hemophilia patients.

*L.O. Andersson:* Clinical studies have started in the United States now and I would guess that it will take some two, three years before they are completed. Then regulatory authorities would take one or two years maybe less because of the risks involved in present concentrates. So, I would guess on the order of five years, but there may be people in the audience knowing better.

*C.Th. Smit Sibinga:* Just another question related to the final production as you described. What was not quite clear to me is, whether the actual rDNA production is now aimed for the totality of the molecule or is still aimed as it was in earlier stages to just one part, the gag part, the low kilodalton part.

*L.O. Andersson:* That is an important question. Actually several groups are working today on the recombinant Factor VIII. Some have chosen to take the full size molecule at the genome level, but then what you actually get out from the producing cells is not the single chain molecule. It is them mixture of all the material that you do find in a normal commercial concentrate. So, even if you have the full size gene you are getting a mixture out, because the host cell is also processing it and you have in the cell culture added the calf serum, which also gives a chance for thrombin formation causing degradation of the molecule. But there are also some groups like ours who are working with the smaller molecule.

*C.Th. Smit Sibinga:* Second question if I may. We learned from Dr Schreiber's presentation that in the highly purifying methods through immuno-adsorption, you need a stabiliser eventually for the Factor VIII. How does that look like in the rDNA. Do we need a similar stabiliser?

*L.O. Andersson:* Yes, because the specific activity of Factor VIII is so high that you probably have to add another protein in order to make it stable, not adsorbing to the walls. Of course normal human albumin is a candidate for that.

*D. Voak (Cambridge):* Dr Schreiber, how many times can you recycle the monoclonal antibody to Factor VIII to get a more economic utilization of the antibody for the biosynthesis or immunopurification of Factor VIII.

*A.B. Schreiber:* That is an excellent question in the sense that any recycling or additional improvement in the number of recyclings of the columns is more important in terms of cost economics than improvements in yield or cost of the antibody can be. The decision to retire a column is also an economical one in terms of defining satisfactory yields. We have experience with more than 50 recyclings of the same resin upon which yields start to drop off and it really pays more to start with a new column than continue to use it. I think this is particular to the Factor VIII and to plasma applications. We have other projects where we use the same column over a hundred times. Presumably proteases in plasma start chewing on the antibody resin. To answer your question it really depends on the resin material; 40 to 50 is a reasonable number, but we are still improving.

*B. Habibi (Paris):* Dr Schreiber could you talk a little more about the yield of that preparation and could you give us, if at all possible, an indication on the price of the product you are preparing I know it should be considered as a premature question, but it is important.

*A.B. Schreiber:* In terms of yield I will give my classical answer, which is that it is higher than some pasteurized preparations where you really take a great loss in yield. It is obviously somewhat lower than current preparations as there are additional processing steps. We have improved our yield over the learning curve to make it quite satisfactory in terms of making it feasible. I can not give you the precise percentage, but it is somewhere in between the low and the high end of the spectrum. For terms of pricing I can refer you to the business people. We do not feel the production price will remain the same as we continue to improve the technology. Our policy as pharmaceutical house is to bring any improvement in technology directly over to the primary prescriber and the hemophiliac community. As this is a costly technique and we can not supply the whole world, we are more than amenable to learn about improvements and technology from other people as the purpose is truly to give the best medically useful products to the hemophiliac community. In terms of local prices, for marketing in the United States, as you know the products have kept the same price for the last 15 years. So the differential will be high. I think that in Europe they will be somewhat higher, but I can not tell you the exact price. I will be more than happy to refer you to our representatives.

*H.V. Beer:* You mentioned very small volumes for Factor VIII Monoclate®. I would estimate at least 10% loss in the infusion devices. If for example you deliver 2.5 ml or 5 ml you would lose considerable activity in the devices.

*A.B. Schreiber:* In fact that was a concern especially at the price that it costs, as you do not want to lose the 10% that usually stays in the butterfly. We are bringing out a new device that would minimize that loss in the tubing. We are also thinking and actually working on some improvements focussed on surgical applications and pediatric applications. We have now data on the stability in dry state as a lyophilized product, at both 4°C and room temperature for more than 3 years. It appears to have a fairly good stability also once it is reconstituted. We are thinking of making different formats more applicable to continuous infusions. In fact I would like to take this time to make a comment. Dr Smit Sibinga asked whether human albumin is a necessary evil in the recombinant product. In our product it is currently used as stabiliser. We have a prototype product that is devoid of any extraneous human proteins, basically an albumin free product. You can replace the human albumin at least at the small scale we are working at, by just playing with ionic strength and using some other formulations. So it is not unfeasible though a bit more difficult.

*J.-C. Faber (Luxemburg):* If I understand correctly your yield is 15% in this method. Do you have an explanation why you lose 85% of the Factor VIII.

*AB. Schreiber:* I am not sure how you arrived at the numbers.

*J.-C. Faber:* Is the yield 15%, is that correct?

*A.B. Schreiber:* No, it is higher.

*J.-C. Faber:* Yes, but do you have an explanation why you can not extract the rest of the Factor VIII.

*A.B.. Schreiber:* Well, there is nothing as frustrating as starting from plasma. When you go from plasma to cryoprecipitate as probably all of you in the fractionation industry know, there seems to be at least 35% of the Factor VIII bioactivity that somewhere disappears. So one could say why start with cryoprecipitate if you lose right at the top 35% of your yields. Considering the volumes that you have to load, the logistics, at least, at the scales that we are working at, make it impossible and unfeasible to start straight from plasma although the technique will work. You can take small volumes of plasma and work at that. The losses are not that high in the affinity chromatography step. It is starting with 35% off the top and then all the other steps that you usually do to make a parenteral; the filtration, lyophilization and so on.

*P.C. Das:* Dr Bennett, the rDNA vaccine, is it going to replace the plasma vaccine completely and how soon.

*C.R. Bennet (West Point):* Eventually it will be replaced. At the present time in our company it is a matter of trying to outguess the market place. As I mentioned in my talk the acceptance of the plasma vaccine was low to begin with and then as time proceeded it increased such that we reached the point where we were nearly out of stock. What we had planned to do was to replace the plasma derived vaccine with the recombinant vaccine as soon as possible. However, with the increase in sales and distribution of the plasma vaccine and the delay in getting the recombinant vaccine accepted, the lines overlapped. Consequently we have been back in production with both the plasma vaccine and the recombinant vaccine to meet the market demands. When the present supply of plasma vaccine is depleted then it will be completely recombinant.

*B. Habibi:* Dr Zettlmeißl, how soon do you expect your rDNA antithrombin III to go through the clinical trials or if possible on the market.

*G. Zettlmeißl (Marburg):* A plasma concentration of 83% represents about 150 mg per litre. In our middle scale fermentation unit, which means about hundred litres, we get now between 30 and 40 mg/l. This means a factor 3 to 5 less than human plasma. What we are trying to do now is try to increase the yield by changing media and fermentation techniques. So, I think personally it will last at least 3 to 5 years until we can start clinical trials with this recombinant material.

*S. Mouslichan (Jakarta Selatan):* Dr Hervé, you mentioned that the monoclonal antibodies used for T-cell depletion in leukemia give a high percentage of relapse. How if we use this for bone marrow transplantation in thalassemia patients.

*P. Hervé (Besançon):* It is not possible to use such GvH prevention for thalassemia, because in these cases we have already a graft failure between 20 to 30%. At the present for aplastic anemia and thalassemia I do not recommend to use T-cell depletion, because of the rather high percentage of graft failure.

*T.J. Hamblin:* I agree with that. Actually, I think you give much less preparation to such patients and there is evidence that cyclosporin is very good for thalassemia and aplastic anemia GvH prevention. Just a comment to Dr The, because the system he was describing with LAK cells directed to monoclonal antibodies is something we have been working on. I was pleased to see that he gets exactly the same results as we do using mouse monoclonals and LAK cells. This is because LAK cells do not have a receptor for mouse Fc. What we have done to try to get around this, is to make chimeric antibodies with human Fc and mouse Fab and I can say that these do in fact enhance the effectiveness of LAK cells against tumour targets. The other thing that we have been doing is making bispecific antibodies just as he is doing, except that we have been using the CD16 (anti-CD16) as the other half of the bispecific antibody. This again enhances the killing. We are going for the NK1 or the LAK1 type of receptor. Have you got any further results on your T3 biospecifics?

*T.H. The (Groningen):* No, not yet.

*T.J. Hamblin:* Dr Hervé, I want to know if you really believe that we can separate the Graft-versus-Host leukemia in different subsets of T-cells.

*P. Hervé:* A crucial question, because at the present we do not know really what kind of T-cells are responsible of GvL effect and GvH reaction. The problem is to identify each population in the bone marrow and to use a specific monoclonal antibody for each specific set.

*W.G. Ho (Los Angeles):* Dr Hervé, how strongly do you feel that purging of autologous marrow should be carried out before the transplant? Somewhat disturbing evidence is accumulating that if one looks at the increasing number of autologous transplants over the past decade, some of which have been purged with antibodies against residual leukemic cells and some of which have not, the overall results of the purged and unpurged marrow transplants are about the same. In those patients who received purged marrow transplants there is perhaps about a 20 to 25% long term survival for ALL while in the unpurged situation the overall disease free survival is around 15 or 20%. In addition, when one does what could be considered the control experiment for an autologous transplant in ALL i.e. a transplant from a genetically identical twin in which it is certain that the marrow being infused does not contain leukemic cells (a situation which can never be certain with the purged marrow), the relapse rate has been reported to be as high as 60%. So, is purging really necessary?

*P. Hervé:* To reach better disease free survival it is necessary to increase both *in vivo* purging as well as adapt conditioning regimens. Concerning the bone marrow purging at the present we do not know. It is necessary first to assess the residual disease, second maybe to combine different purging techniques like chemotherapeutic agents plus monoclonal antibodies. But the problem is to demonstrate by clinical setting that purging is effective or not.

*H. Keable (Paris):* My comments are addressed to the first part of Dr Hervé's talk and essentially concern the indications for T-cell depletion. We have had similar experience with T-cell depletion. The quality of the T-cell depletion varied according to the modalities used. We consistently obtained more than three logs T-cell depletion with immunotoxins and we very rapidly reserved that type of depletion for the miss-match transplant. With a cocktail of antibodies (either CD2, 3 and 7 or 4, 5 and 8) we obtained only two log T-cell depletion and with Campath I, it was extremely variable (between one and three logs depletion). Regarding the status of the patients studied: When the cocktail of different antibodies or T101 were used we had indeed a take of the graft. But with Campath I we had a tremendous increase of bone marrow rejection and failure as late as 9 months after BMT. None of these patients could be rescued, except the one for whom we had cryopreserved marrow. For the patients who survived more than a year (in leukemic setting), we determined the status of the chimera with molecular probes. We observed that they had either autologous or mixed chimera. It was in contrast with our aplastic anemia patients, who had full engraftment. So I like to ask you to specify for what type of patients you now do reserve bone marrow depletion.

*P. Hervé:* We treated only CGL, AML and ALL patients, but if you look at the bone marrow graft we observe a high percentage of mixed chimera's. So, the engraftment seems very good and it is important to carefully look at the full chimera and the mixed chimera's using T-cell depletion. In fact we know that mixed chimerism is compatible with long term disease free survival – the major question concerns its biologic importance of the allo BMT.

*P.C. Das:* Dr Lutton, I think it is quite clear you have opened a new vista particularly in relation to all these growth factors and stroma cells. Could you tell us what do you think the future would be for the cell count and cell culture?

*J.D Lutton (Valhalla):* The future for cell culture with respect to cultivation of all the elements, the stroma and non-adherent cells, I think is quite bright. I think there are various areas such as utilizing foetal tissue like liver cells, where we might be able to in fact expand and grow hematopoietic elements and then utilize these cells. Such has been done for transplant purposes, and I believe it certainly has a bright future. So, that would be one area that certainly has promise.

# IV. Clinical application and future directions

# USE OF GENE PROBES FOR CARRIER DETECTION AND PRENATAL DIAGNOSIS IN HEMOPHILIA A

E. Briët, A.H.J.T. Bröcker-Vriends

## Introduction

For a number of years the estimation of gene product (Factor VIII) concentrations was used for genotype assignment in potential carriers as well as in prenatal diagnosis of hemophilia A. The difficulty with this method for carrier testing is the probabilistic nature of the result. The Factor VIII assay is converted into a likelihood ratio favouring carriership and this ratio is combined with the genetic chance to yield a final probability of carriership [1-3]. In practice, however, it is very difficult for the women to base their decisions on this kind of information.

In prenatal diagnosis the problems of gene product assays are of a different nature. Fetal blood sampling is a difficult procedure that can be carried out only in specialized centers. Moreover, the fetus must be about 19 weeks old before the procedure is applicable and if an abortion needs to be carried out this is unacceptably late for many of the consultands [4]. Against this background, the advent of recombinant DNA techniques has meant a great improvement for potential carriers of hemophilia.

A number of different approaches can be taken to the diagnostic use of gene probes in hereditary diseases. In sickle cell anemia the sixth amino acid of the globin molecule has been substituted and at the DNA level this substitution leads to disappearance of a normal restriction site. The absence of this site can be easily detected by the application of the Southern blot technique [5]. Since all patients with this disease have the same mutation, only one set of reagents is required for the diagnosis. A procedure involving the use of oligonucleotide probes can also be used if large numbers of patients have the same mutation. This is the case in $\alpha$-1-antitrypsin deficiency. The diagnosis can be made by hybridizing the patient's DNA with an oligonucleotide probe complementary to the normal DNA sequence and a second probe complementary to the mutant DNA sequence [6]. In hemophilia, however, countless different mutations are responsible for the lack of clotting Factor VIII or IX. It would be impractical to establish the specific mutation in each family. So, a more universal procedure needs to be used. This procedure is restriction fragment length polymorphism (RFLP) analysis. This method is based on the occurrence of functionally neutral polymorphisms in the Factor VIII gene that can be detected by Southern blot analysis and used as markers for a mutation in the gene. Figure 1 schematically illustrates the Factor VIII molecule with its gene. Five polymorphic restriction sites have been identified, three of them intragenic (Bcl-I, Xba-I and Bgl-I [7-9]) and two of them extragenic (Taq-I and Bgl-II [10,11]). Recently, it was demonstrated that both

218

the Taq-I and the Bgl-II polymorphisms are at the telomeric side of the Factor VIII gene with the Bgl-II site being the most telomeric (Carpenter, personal communication). Recombination between the Factor VIII gene and these extragenic sites occurs with a frequency of about five percent [12]. In our studies we have used four out of these five markers [13]. The Bgl-I polymorphism does not contribute significantly to the chance of heterozygosity and we have not yet felt the need to include it in our armamentarium.

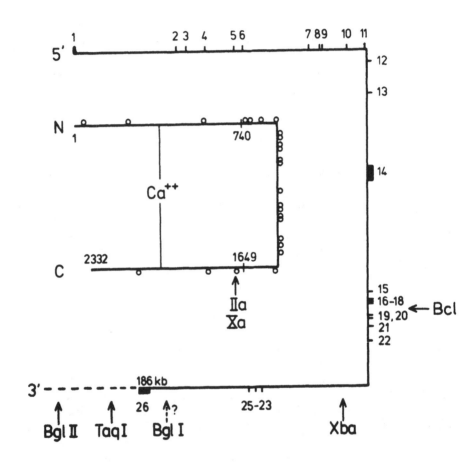

*Figure 1:* Schematic representation of Factor VIII and its gene. The inner part represents the protein with its heavily glycosylated B domain and the site of activation by thrombin (IIa) and Factor Xa. The outer part represents the gene with its 26 exons and the restriction sites for Bcl-I, Xba-I, Bgl-I, Taq-I and Bgl-II.

# Carriers

Since the introduction of DNA analysis we have examined 225 potential carriers from 68 unrelated families (Table 1). The new possibilities have led to a 100% increase in the referrals for carrier testing and prenatal diagnosis.

*Table 1.* RFLP analysis in hemophilia A.

|  | Familial | Isolated | Total |
|---|---|---|---|
| Families | 39 | 29 | 68 |
| Potential carriers | 132 | 93 | 225 |

In familial cases the use of RFLP analysis has dramatically improved our ability to distinguish carriers from non-carriers (Table 2). Eighty-six percent or 114 out of 128 possible carriers could be given near-certainty about their carrier status. In general, 60% of women is heterozygous for one of the intragenic polymorphisms and for them a diagnosis is virtually certain.

*Table 2.* Contribution of DNA analysis to results of carrier testing in familial hemophilia A. (n=128).

| Analysis | Probably carrier (p > 95%) | Probably non-carrier (p > 5%) | Doubtful (p 5-95%) |
|---|---|---|---|
| Classical | 27 | 40 | 61 |
| Classical and DNA | 45 | 69 | 14 |

Unfortunately, more than half of the consultands are related to isolated patients. If the abnormal X-chromosome and its DNA markers are not present in a female relative of the patient, carriership can be excluded. However, carriership can never be proven on the basis of DNA markers alone since each isolated patient may be the recipient of a new mutation and in that case the female relatives are probably non-carriers. A statistical diagnosis can be made if Factor VIII assays combined with DNA analysis are used in these cases. In 34 out of 90 cases carriership could be excluded while a high probability of carriership was found in nine.

In 37% of women we have to rely on one of the extragenic polymorphisms which carry a 5% risk of recombination. Our primary approach is to digest the DNA with Bcl-I, Xba-I combined with Kpn-I and with Taq-I. If the results of subsequent Southern blotting do not provide an informative situation we apply Bgl-II. In this way, the first round gives a 94% chance of heterozygosity which rises to 97% in the second round with the application of Bgl-II.

*Table 3.* Prenatal diagnosis by chorionic villous biopsy and RFLP analysis.

| Fetal sex | Diagnosis | Diagnosis based on | |
| | | intragenic RFLP | extragenic RFLP |
| --- | --- | --- | --- |
| Male | affected | 3 | 3 |
| (n=11) | unaffected | 4 | 1 |
| Female | affected | 1 | 1 |
| (n=8) | unaffected | 4 | 2 |

*Table 4.* The origin of the mutation in families with an isolated case of hemophilia A by RFLP analysis. (n=26).

| Origin of the mutation | Number of families | RFLP used for diagnoses | |
| | | intragenic | extragenic |
| --- | --- | --- | --- |
| Grandfather* | 10 | 5 | 5 |
| Grandmother | 1 | 1 | – |
| Mother | 2 | – | 2 |
| No conclusion | 13 | – | – |

* Parenthood was confirmed by HinfI/33.15 minisatellite probe analysis.

## Prenatal diagnosis

Chorionic villous biopsy allows the study of fetal cells during the ninth or the tenth week of gestation. Chromosomal analysis provides the sex of the fetus and by RFLP study it can be determined whether the unborn child carries the abnormal gene. The major advantage of this approach is that the result of the tests can be obtained well within the first trimester of the pregnancy before loving and inquisitive relatives or friends need to be informed. In addition an abortion is acceptable to many more couples during this early stage then during the 20th week which is unavoidable if the decision is based on the result of fetal blood sampling.

We have been using the same markers for prenatal diagnosis as for carrier testing [14]. The limitations of the extragenic markers are very important especially if a normal male fetus is diagnosed. In this situation, a 5% risk of a false result is unacceptable to many. If, however, an affected male is diagnosed with 95% certainty, most couples will be satisfied and decide to have the pregnancy terminated (or to accept the child in spite of the diagnosis). If the mother is informative for both of the intragenic markers Bcl-I and Xba-I we prefer the use of Bcl-I for technical reasons. Only if neither of the intragenic markers is informative we use the extragenic Taq-I marker.

A practical problem is caused by women seeking prenatal diagnosis without previous RFLP studies being carried out on themselves or their relatives. Usually, we need to have RFLP data on the consultand, her parents, an affected relative and sometimes additional relatives either affected or not. These data are required to establish carriership in the consultand and to find out whether she is heterozygous for one of the markers and to determine the linkage phase. If she is homozygous for all the markers prenatal diagnosis using RFLP's cannot be done. Moreover, it is not always easy to get all the family members together for blood sampling and usually it takes quite some effort to get the necessary results before the pregnancy is nine weeks old. During the past two years, 12 out of 19 women had not yet been tested for RFLP's when they applied to us for prenatal diagnosis.

The results of the 19 cases of prenatal diagnosis by RFLP are provided in Table 3.

## Isolated cases of hemophilia and recent mutations

Until recently, it was thought that most mothers of an isolated case of hemophilia were carrying the abnormal gene [15]. Since the introduction of RFLP analysis, however, it has been found in several instances that the abnormal X-chromosome of a patient derived from a non-affected maternal grandfather which is suggestive of a mutation in the grand-paternal sperm or in the maternal ovum. In addition, we have observed one case in which a deleted gene could be traced to the maternal X-chromosome of the mother of the patient and not to the maternal grandparents, which proves that a mutation occurred in the ovary of the maternal grandmother. The chance that a similar mutation occurs twice in the gonads of one individual is extremely small. Consequently, it is important to identify the origin of these mutations since the siblings of a recipient of such mutations are probably normal. The study of Duchenne muscular dystrophy families, however, has now disclosed the existence of germ line mosaicisms [16]. In these cases an unknown proportion of the ova or sperm cells carries the same mutation and the risk of recurrence of the disease in future children may be considerable, but has not yet been defined. Until now, such mosaicisms have not been reported for hemophilia but we consider it prudent to accept their existence and to be very careful with genetic counselling in these families. Table 4 summarizes our data on the origin of the mutations in sporadic hemophilia.

## Acknowledgements

This work was supported by a grant from the Prevention Fund, number 28-1244.

# References

1. Briët E, Bröcker-Vriends AHJT, Quadt R et al. Onderzoek naar draagsterschap van hemofilie B met behulp van restrictie-fragmentlengte-polymorfisme. Ned Tijdschr Geneeskd 1985;129:937-40.
2. Graham JB, Rizza CR, Chediak J et al. Carrier detection in hemophilia A: A cooperative international study. I. The carrier phenotype. Blood 1986;67: 1554-9.
3. Green PP, Mannucci PM, Briët E et al. Carrier detection in hemophilia A: A cooperative international study. II. The efficacy of a universal discriminant. Blood 1986;67:1560-7.
4. Mibashan RS, Rodeck CH, Thumpston JK. Prenatal diagnosis of the hemophilias. In: Bloom AL (ed). Methods in hematology: The hemophilias. Churchill Livingstone, Edinburgh 1982:176-97.
5. Orkin SH, Little PFR, Kazazian HH Jr, Boehm CD. Improved detection of the sickle mutation by DNA analysis. N Engl J Med 1982;307:32.
6. Kidd VJ, Golbus MS, Wallace RB, Kakura K, Woo SLC. Prenatal diagnosis of α1-antitrypsin deficiency by direct analysis of the mutation site in the gene. N Engl J Med 1984;310:639-42.
7. Gitschier J, Drayna D, Tuddenham EGD, White RL, Lawn RM. Genetic mapping and diagnosis of hemophilia A achieved through a Bc-II polymorphism in the factor VIII gene. Nature 1985;314:738-40.
8. Wion KL, Tuddenham EGD, Lawn RM. A new polymorphism in the Factor VIII gene for prenatal diagnosis of hemophilia A. Nucleic Acids Res 1986;11:4535-42.
9. Antonarakis SE, Waber PG, Kittur SD et al. Hemophilia A. Detection of molecular defects and of carriers by DNA analysis. N Engl J Med 1985;313: 842-8.
10. Oberlé I, Camerino G, Heilig R et al. Genetic screening for hemophilia A (classic hemophilia) with a polymorphic DNA probe. N Engl J Med 1985;312: 682-6.
11. Harper K, Pembrey ME, Davies KE, Winter RM, Hartley D, Tuddenham EGD. A clinically useful DNA probe closely linked to hemophilia A. Lancet 1984;ii:6-8.
12. Peake IR, Bloom AL. Recombination between genes and closely linked polymorphisms. Lancet 1986;i:1335-6.
13. Bröcker-Vriends AHJT, Briët E, Quadt R et al. Genotype assignment of hemophilia A by use of intragenic and extragenic restriction fragment length polymorphisms. Thromb Haemostas 1987;57:131-6.
14. Bröcker-Vriends AHJT, Briët E, Kanhai HHH et al. First trimester prenatal diagnosis of hemophilia A. Two years experience. Prenatal Diagn 1988. In press.
15. Graham JB. Genotype assignment (carrier detection) in the hemophilias. Clin in Haematol 1979;8:115-45.
16. Bakker E, van Broeckhoven Ch, Bonten EJ et al. Germline mosaicism and Duchenne muscular dystrophy mutations. Nature 1987;329:554-6.

# IN VIVO CHARACTERISTICS OF rDNA FACTOR VIII: THE IMPACT FOR THE FUTURE IN HEMOPHILIA CARE*

K.A. High**, G.C. White II**, C.W. McMillan***, B.G. Macik**, H.R. Roberts**

In the late 1940's and before, plasma was the only reliable source of blood clotting factors for replacement therapy. The physiological basis of plasma replacement therapy was initially worked out in canine models of classic hemophilia stressing the half life of Factor VIII, its distribution after infusion, and the maximal doses of Factor VIII that could be achieved in circulating blood. From this experience it became obvious that the maximal levels of Factor VIII that could be achieved with plasma were about 20% of normal or 0.2 u/ml [1]. Higher levels could not be attained because of the danger of inducing congestive heart failure. Although 20% levels of Factor VIII were sufficient to control hemarthroses, soft tissue bleeding and even major bleeding in some cases, this level was not always sufficient to control hemorrhage. Surgery, hematuria, and severe trauma to hemophilic patients frequently resulted in bleeding that required Factor VIII levels close to 100% of normal. Thus, the need for purified and concentrated Factor VIII products for classic hemophilic patients was never questioned. In fact, when plasma was the only therapeutic option, all clinical coagulationists agreed that for any clotting factor deficiencies, specific clotting factor concentrates were essential for treatment if normal hemostasis were to be achieved.

## Plasma-derived Factor VIII concentrates

This recognition led to great efforts to prepare Factor VIII concentrates. The Chapel Hill group led by Dr Brinkhous, the Oxford group led by Drs Mac-Farlane and Biggs, and the Karolinska group led by Drs B. and M. Blombäck made great strides in purifying Factor VIII from plasma [2-4]. However, the first major breakthrough occurred in 1964 when Pool and coworkers, exploiting a closed plastic bag system, succeeded in developing a simple method for separating Factor VIII rich cryoprecipitate from normal human plasma [5]. This development led to a Factor VIII product about 10 fold concentrated compared to plasma, that permitted clinicians to achieve normal circulating levels of Factor VIII in hemophilic recipients without overloading the circulation. Using cryoprecipitate as a starting product, the methods for Factor VIII purification developed in several laboratories were quickly adopted by industry

* Supported in part by grants from the National Institutes of Health: HL26309, HL01922, HL07149, CA43447.
** Dept. of Medicine and the Hemophilia Center.
*** Dept. of Pediatrics, The University of North Carolina at Chapel Hill.

*Table 1.* Advantages and disadvantages of cryoprecipitate.

| Advantages of cryoprecipitate |
| --- |
| * Relative ease of preparation (i.e. in local blood banks and hospitals)<br>* Low cost relative to concentrate in some areas of the world |

| Disadvantages of cryoprecipitate | |
| --- | --- |
| Disease transmission | Hepatitis B<br>Delta virus<br>Hepatitis NANB<br>HIV |
| Immunologic complications | Allergic<br>Alloantigens and possible<br>immunosuppression |
| Potency variation | Age of plasmas<br>Freezing/thawing technique<br>Choices of anticoagulant |
| Versatility | Necessity for freezing<br>Multiple bags must be combined<br>Difficult to heat-treat |

*Table 2.* Advantages and disadvantages of Factor VIII concentrates.

| Advantages of lyophilized commercially available concentrates |
| --- |
| High purity<br>Easy reconstitution<br>Home therapy<br>Stability<br>Easy availability<br>Accurate labelling for accurate doses |

| Disadvantages of lyophilized commercial concentrates | |
| --- | --- |
| Transmission of infectious disease | Hepatitis B, NANB<br>AIDS |
| Allogenic proteins | Immune alterations |
| Large donor pool | 2,000-20,000 donors per lot of product |
| Cost | |

so that commercial Factor VIII concentrates became widely available in the late 1960's [6]. The glycine precipitation method of Wagner was the most widely used [2]. The advantages of the commercially produced Factor VIII concentrates included increased purity, the ability to lyophilize the product, and versatility when compared to cryoprecipitate. The disadvantages included the higher incidence of all forms of hepatitis, the larger pool size of donors, and in 1978, the introduction of HIV into lots of Factor VIII prepared from large donor pools. The advantages and disadvantages of both cryoprecipitate and commercially prepared Factor VIII concentrates are shown in Tables 1 and 2.

Prior to discovery of HIV contamination of starting plasma, commercially prepared Factor VIII concentrates were already subjected to heat-treatment, usually after lyophilization. Heat was designed to free the concentrates of hepatitis viruses. After HIV was found to be the causative agent of AIDS it appeared that this type of heat-treatment attenuated HIV, but not the viruses causing either hepatitis B or non A-non B. More recent developments, including pasteurization and the use of organic solvents and detergents applied to Factor VIII concentrates, appear to render these concentrates safe in terms of transmission of viral diseases, including hepatitis B, non A-non B, and HIV. These data are summarized in Table 3. However, even the present Factor VIII preparations currently available still have large amounts of allogenic proteins; these proteins may possibly alter immune function in hemophilic recipients.

*Table 3.* Viral inactivation procedures for plasma-derived clotting factor concentrates.

| Manufacturer | Conditions | Effectiveness | |
|---|---|---|---|
| | | Hepatitis | AIDS |
| Hyland | Heat;dry;72hrs;60°C | no | yes |
| Cutter | Heat;dry;72hrs;68°C | no | yes |
| Armour | Heat;dry;30hrs;60°C | no | (?)yes |
| Alpha | Heat;dry;suspended in n-heptane;20hrs;60°C | no | yes |
| Behringwerke | Heat;solution;10hrs;60°C | (?)yes | yes |
| Immuno | Steam;10hrs;60°C;pressure;1hr;80°C | no | yes |

* Modified from Comperts, E., Reference #13.

Two recent developments have largely obviated the disadvantages of currently available Factor VIII concentrates, namely, the development of ultrapure Factor VIII preparations by monoclonal antibody purification of plasma and *in vitro* synthesis of Factor VIII by recombinant DNA techniques. The characteristics of these Factor VIII products are briefly summarized in Table 4. The proteins are pure (except for albumin added as a stabilizer) and can be treated in such a way as to render them free of live viruses. The final Factor VIII product derived by monoclonal antibody techniques still must be heat-treated or exposed to detergents and organic solvents to kill HIV and hepatitis viruses. Presumably such treatment is not necessary for Factor VIII products derived by recombinant DNA techniques. In addition, the total production of plasma-derived monoclonal purified Factor VIII concentrate is theoretically limited by the available worldwide plasma pool, whereas therapies based on recombinant DNA techniques are not.

*Table 4.* Monoclonal antibody purified plasma-derived Factor VIII and recombinant Factor VIII.

|  | Monoclonal antibody purified plasma-derived Factor VIII | Recombinant Factor VIII |
|---|---|---|
| Specific activity | 2000 u/mg protein | 5000 u/mg protein |
| Extraneous proteins | only albumin added as stabilizer | only albumin added as stabilizer |

## Isolation of the gene encoding Factor VIIIC

The basis for the production of recombinant Factor VIII was the isolation of the gene Factor VIIIC reported independently by 2 groups in late 1984 [7,8]. The cloning of the gene for Factor VIIIC proved to be a formidable task for several reasons: first, the size of the gene (186kb) made it by far the largest gene that had been characterized at the time it was reported [9]; second, the very low abundance of Factor VIII messenger RNA meant that many recombinants would need to be screened [7]; and third, the fact that the site of synthesis of the protein was not known at the time these efforts were begun meant that a circuitous cloning strategy had to be adopted.

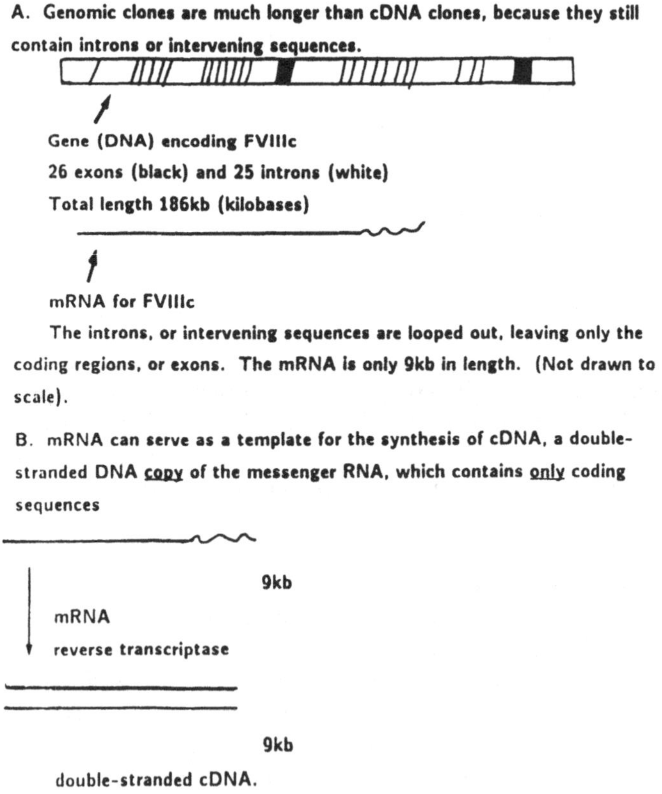

A. Genomic clones are much longer than cDNA clones, because they still contain introns or intervening sequences.

Gene (DNA) encoding FVIIIc
26 exons (black) and 25 introns (white)
Total length 186kb (kilobases)

mRNA for FVIIIc
The introns, or intervening sequences are looped out, leaving only the coding regions, or exons. The mRNA is only 9kb in length. (Not drawn to scale).

B. mRNA can serve as a template for the synthesis of cDNA, a double-stranded DNA copy of the messenger RNA, which contains only coding sequences

9kb
mRNA
reverse transcriptase

9kb
double-stranded cDNA.

*Figure 1:* Glossary of terms used to describe cloning process.

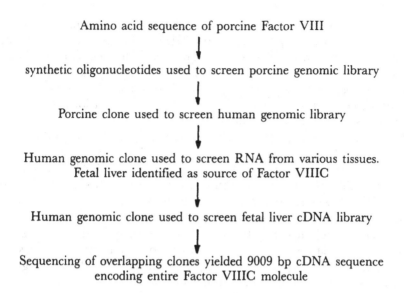

Amino acid sequence of porcine Factor VIII

↓

synthetic oligonucleotides used to screen porcine genomic library

↓

Porcine clone used to screen human genomic library

↓

Human genomic clone used to screen RNA from various tissues.
Fetal liver identified as source of Factor VIIIC

↓

Human genomic clone used to screen fetal liver cDNA library

↓

Sequencing of overlapping clones yielded 9009 bp cDNA sequence
encoding entire Factor VIIIC molecule

*Figure 2:* Molecular cloning of cDNA encoding Factor VIIIC.

The strategy used by the group at Genetics Institute [7] is depicted in Figures 1 and 2 and may be summarized as follows: since the tissue of origin of Factor VIIIC was unknown, the usual approach of constructing a cDNA library from the tissue of origin (such a library is enriched for copies of the gene in question, compared to a total genomic library) could not be utilized. Instead, genomic clones were obtained first and then used to screen RNA from a variety of tissues; Northern blots suggested liver as the best source of Factor VIIIC and the full length cDNA was obtained by screening a fetal liver cDNA library.

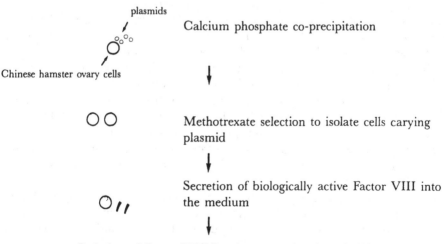

plasmids

Calcium phosphate co-precipitation

Chinese hamster ovary cells

↓

Methotrexate selection to isolate cells carying plasmid

↓

Secretion of biologically active Factor VIII into the medium

↓

Isolation of Factor VIII:C using monoclonal antibody

*Figure 3:* Schematic diagram of preparation and purification of recombinant Factor VIII in mammanlian expression system. See text for details.

Note that in order to obtain amino acid sequence information for use in constructing the probe, porcine Factor VIIIC, which could be obtained in plentiful amounts, was purified and sequenced. This sequence information was used to construct several synthetic oligonucleotides, which were then used to screen a porcine genomic library. This clone was used to obtain a human genomic clone, and the human clone used to screen various RNA sources (different tissues) as described above.

The isolation of the gene for Factor VIII permitted its use to direct the *in vitro* synthesis of recombinant Factor VIII [8]. The steps involved in *in vitro* synthesis are outlined in Figure 3. Note that Factor VIII, like other proteins requiring sophisticated post-translational modifications, cannot be expressed in the bacterial expression systems used in the production of simpler recombinant proteins, such as insulin and growth hormone. This requirement for mammalian tissue culture systems adds considerably to the expense of the product, (e.g. because of expenses of media, of monitoring cell lines, etc.). However, for very large proteins, for those requiring glycosylation, or gamma-carboxylation, bacterial systems are not adequate.*

Additional expense in the production process arises from the need to subject the recombinant protein to extremely powerful purification processes. In contrast to plasma-derived Factor VIII, a contaminant protein in a recombinant Factor VIII (rFVIII) preparation is unlikely to be of human origin, since the cell lines used are generally not human.

In the diagram shown, a recombinant plasmid carrying Factor VIII cDNA and a selectable marker (in this case the dihydrofolate reductase (DHFR) gene, which confers resistance to methotrexate on a host cell), is introduced into Chinese hamster ovary cells by calcium phosphate co-precipitation. The efficiency with which the recombinant plasmid is introduced into the recipient cells is quite low, on the order of 1 in $10^5$.

Treatment of the cells with methotrexate is thus used to select for those which have taken up the recombinant plasmid, since only those expressing the DHFR gene will survive methotrexate treatment. The transformed cells are now grown under optimal conditions of pH, $O_2$, cell density, etc. [10]. Factor VIII is secreted into the medium, from which it is purified using a monoclonal antibody. The purified rFVIII has a specific activity in the range of 7000 IU/mg protein and requires albumin for stabilization.

rFVIII produced under conditions similar to these has been analyzed extensively and found to be identical to the plasma-derived product. SDS-Page electrophoresis of recombinant and plasma derived Factor VIII, before and after thrombin cleavage, discloses no differences between plasma derived and rFVIII. rFVIII combines with von Willebrand factor and is effective in dog models [6].

The theoretical advantages of rFVIII are safety in terms of transmission of hepatitis and AIDS, and purity in terms of protein administered. There is no reason to believe that use of the product will be associated with increased incidence of inhibitors.

---

* Bacteria are capable of glycosylation, but prokaryotic and eukaryotic patterns are so different that they are not interchangeable.

rFVIII is currently undergoing testing in humans [11]. The first treatment of a human hemophilic patient occurred on March 27, 1987 in Chapel Hill, NC. Factor VIII levels of over 100% were observed and initial fall off studies were normal. Thus, the pure Factor VIII apparently combines with circulating vWF *in vivo*. Given the purity of this preparation, immunologic alterations in recipients should be minimal. The cost of rFVIII, if and when it becomes commercially available, is not yet known.

## Gene transfer therapy

Recombinant Factor VIII is produced by using the cloned gene to direct the *in vitro* synthesis of Factor VIII. Gene transfer therapy, on the other hand, refers to the actual insertion into the host's genome of a normal replacement gene. As of this writing, significant problems, including adequate levels of expression, regulation of expression, and overall safety, remain to be solved before gene transfer therapy becomes a reality.

However, hemophilia has several features which recommend it as a starting point for gene transfer trials [cf. 12]. First, unlike a number of genes already available (e.g. globin, insulin) the genes for clotting factors do not require precise regulation in order to be effective. Expression at a level as low as 5% of normal could have a therapeutic effect, and levels as high as 150% would not be harmful. Secondly, unlike many proteins which require tissue-specific expression, (not yet a realistic goal in gene transfer therapy), clotting factors could be synthesized in any tissue, so long as the tissue is capable of carrying out the necessary post-translational modifications and secreting the protein into the circulation.

## Summary

Recombinanat DNA techniques have made possible the production of a protein of high purity for replacement therapy. This product is free of viruses found in plasma-derived products and has been effective in limited clinical trials. Scaled-up production of this large and complex molecule has been complicated by the necessity for mammalian expression systems and monoclonal antibody-based purification schemes. Nevertheless, it appears likely that molecular genetic techniques will eventually result in widespread availability of a safe, effective and affordable recombinant Factor VIII.

## References

1. Roberts HR, Penick GD, Brinkhous KM. Intensive plasma therapy in the hemophilias. JAMA 1964;190:546-8.
2. Webster WP, Roberts HR, Thelin GM, Wagner RH, Brinkhous KM. Clinical use of a new glycine-precipitated antihemophilic factor fraction. Am J Med Sci 1965;250:643-61.

230

3. Macfarlane RG, Biggs R, Bidwell E. Bovine antihemophilic globulin in the treatment of hemophilia. Lancet 1954;i:1316-9.
4. Blombäck B, Blombäck M. Purification of human and bovine fibrinogen. Ark Kemi 1956;10:415-43.
5. Pool JG, Shannon AE. Production of high potency concentrates of antihemophilic globulin in a closed bag system. N Engl J Med 1965;273:1443-7.
6. Brinkhous KM, Shambrom E, Roberts HR, Webster WP, Fekete L, Wagner RH. A new high potency glycine precipitated antihemophilic factor (AHF) concentrate. JAMA 1968;205:613-5.
7. Toole JJ, Knopf JL, Wozney JM et al. Molecular cloning of a cDNA encoding human antihaemophilic factor. Nature 1984;312:342-7.
8. Wood WI, Capon DJ, Simonsen CC et al. Expression of active human Factor VIII from recombinant DNA clones. Nature 1984;312:330-7.
9. Gitschier J, Wood WI, Goralka TM et al. Characterization of the human Factor VIII gene. Nature 1984;312:326-30.
10. Martin N, Brennan A, Denome L, Shaevitz J. High productivity in mammalian cell culture. Biotechnology 1987;5:838-41.
11. rFVIII jointly manufactured and supplied by Genetics Institute and Hyland Therapeutics of Baxter Travenol. Results being prepared for separate publication.
12. Anderson WF. Prospects for human gene therapy. Science 1984;226:401-9.
13. Gomperts E. Procedures for the inactivation of viruses in clotting factor concentrates. Am J Hematol 1986;23:295-305.

# CLINICAL EXPERIENCE WITH MONOCLATE®, A MONOCLONAL ANTIBODY PURIFIED FACTOR VIII PREPARATION FROM HUMAN PLASMA

A.B. Schreiber, J.J. Petillo, K.D. Lamon

## Introduction

Monoclate® (Rorer/Armour Pharmaceuticals Division) is a highly purified Factor VIII:C preparation derived from human plasma by immunoaffinity chromatography. As described in an accompanying report in these proceedings [1], Monoclate® is a stable Factor VIII:C preparation of specific activity between 800-4500 IU/mg protein, prior to the addition of human serum albumin as a component of the parenteral formula. A key manufacturing step of the Monoclate® process is the absorption of Factor VIII:C-von Willebrand factor complexes from cryoprecipitate to monoclonal antibodies specific for von Willebrand factor, that are immobilized on a solid phase resin. In preclinical studies, the composition of Factor VIII in Monoclate® preparations appears to be indistinguishable from that in either currently commercially available impure concentrates of plasma or recombinant DNA derived material.

Acute and subacute studies in rats, rabbits and dogs have established the general and hemodynamic safety of Monoclate® infusions. Viral spiking experiments, where the manufacturing process was challenged with unusually high titers of a series of model viruses and HIV, have indicated that the affinity chromatography step provides a significant additional margin of safety. The half-life and recovery of Factor VIII bioactivity was also established as within normal ranges in hemophilic dog experiments. Prompted by this preclinical profile, we set out to assess the safety and efficacy of Monoclate® in hemophilia A patients in early 1986. The following key questions were intended to be addressed by the design of clinical studies:

1. Monoclate® represents the first Factor VIII preparation where Factor VIII:C is virtually free of von Willebrand factor. Would Factor VIII:C in Monoclate® reassociate functionally in man to reproduce normal pharmacodynamics?

2. HIV transmission by blood products, in particular plasma cryoprecipitate has caused seroconversion in a majority of hemophilia patients, with some occurrences of full-blown disease. Post-transfusion hepatitis has also been frequent among patients with hemophilia who are treated with concentrated Factor VIII prepared from pooled plasma. Would the high level of purification of Factor VIII in Monoclate® correspond to an increased safety from viral transmission in patients?

3. Small amounts of murine antibody may leak from the affinity resin used in the Monoclate® process and occasionally be found in the final product.

Product specifications for release call for less than 50 ng/100 IU Factor VIII activity. Would this amount of foreign material induce an immune response in man? If so, would this result in the occurrence of allergic reactions upon chronic treatment?

### Half-life and recovery of Monoclate®

The safety, tolerance, half-life and recovery of Monoclate® were first evaluated in seven HIV seropositive patients with severe or moderate hemophilia A. The age of the patients ranged between 16 and 39 years and their weight between 61 and 114 kg. The first infusion was well tolerated. The *in vivo* behaviour of the preparation was comparable to that observed with currently available commercial Factor VIII concentrates. The second phase half-life mean was found to be $15.2 \pm 3.2$ hours. Recovery of Factor VIII was calculated as $1.8 \pm 0.2$ IU rise/kg/dl.

The same seven patients were enrolled in a long-term study that by now has reached sixteen months of treatment on an as-needed basis. Patients each received approximately 90 infusions or 120,000 AHF units. The half-life and recovery of Factor VIII was calculated for one infusion of Monoclate® at a six month timepoint and found to be clinically and statistically indistinguishable from values at screen.

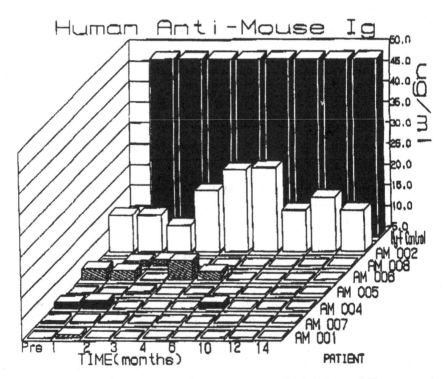

*Figure 1.* Human anti-mouse Ig antibodies in serum of adult hemophiliacs treated with Monoclate®. Black bars are data for positive control.

A battery of clinical laboratory safety assessments were performed for this ongoing study. No unexpected chemistry or hematology results were observed. ALT levels were high at screening and remained abnormally high in these patients, in which the prevalence of NANB hepatitis is maximal, though a downward trend was observed. T cell counts in individual patients were variable from month to month, with a strong trend toward stabilization. Strikingly, there was an improvement in six out of seven patients for the response to multiple skin test antigens. Three patients were anergic at screen and all demonstrated repeated, significantly positive responses after infusions with Monoclate®. In fact, the mean response for the seven patients was found to be identical to a historical age-matched cohort of normal volunteers. No drug-related adverse experiences were reported.

Results from this initial clinical study clearly demonstrate, in our opinion, that Factor VIII:C in Monoclate® rapidly reassociates with circulating von Willebrand factor *in vivo*. Further, Monoclate® appears to provide an effective procuagulant substitution therapy for adult hemophiliacs. Subjectively, Monoclate® therapy was found extremely convenient by the patients, thanks to the almost instantaneous reconstitution time, an immediate consequence of the product purity.

The viral safety of the product could not be assessed in these seven previously multiply transfused and HIV seropositive patients. As it pertains to safety concerns for murine antibody contaminants, there were no reports of hypersensitivity-related adverse experiences. A sensitive and specific radioimmunoassay was designed to follow the presence and levels of human anti-mouse Ig antibodies in the serum of these patients. The assay was validated with positive standard sera obtained from patients enrolled in clinical trials undergoing monoclonal antibody parenteral therapy for colon carcinoma [2]. In these immunotherapy trials, patients were repeatedly infused with murine antibody in amounts varying from 1 mg to 500 mg/infusion (Figure 1). They invariably developed an immune response to murine antibody and serum levels could be measured varying from 50 microgram to 150 microgram/ml. The detection level of our assay is about 4 microgram/ml of human anti-mouse Ig antibody. Six out of the seven hemophiliacs treated with Monoclate® have not presented with detectable levels of antibody over the sixteen months of observation. One patient presented detectable levels of antibody reacting with mouse Ig prior to any infusion with Monoclate®. Over the time-course study, levels remained detectable at similar levels. This patient also tested positive for rheumatoid factor. By virtue of the cross-reactivity of rheumatoid factor with the Fc portion of both human and mouse Ig, results of the assay for this patient cannot be properly assessed.

The number of patients in this study is too small to draw any firm conclusions on possible advantages of a purified preparation of Factor VIII as it relates to the immune status of hemophiliacs. The notion exists that multiply transfused patients, such as hemophiliacs, may be immunocompromised as a consequence of the enormous alloantigenic load they undergo during therapy. Several reports in the literature appear to confirm this hypothesis. For example, children with hemophilia appear to be remarkably susceptible to infection with tuberculosis when accidentally exposed to the disease [3].

There appears to be a positive correlation between disease development and the amount of replacement therapy administered. Abnormalities in T-cell subset distribution, even prior to the high prevalence of HIV infection, have been attributed to the repeated exposure to alloantigens contained in intermediate-purity plasma products [4,5]. A deficiency of the immune response at the level of antigen-dependent macrophage-T cell interaction was noted [6]. This *in vivo* observation was strengthened by laboratory work in which treatment of normal monocytes with Factor VIII concentrates was shown to lead to down regulation of Fc receptors on the monocyte membrane, which in turn leads to a reduced capacity of the cells to release oxygen radicals and bacterial killing [7]. This defect appeared to be attributable to the presence of Ig aggregates and/or immune complexes in clotting factor concentrates. The anecdotal yet remarkable resurgence of three out of seven patients from total anergy to multiple skin test antigen and the overall trend of improvement towards normalcy in all seven patients should not be dismissed lightly. This simple *in vivo* test indeed represents accurately the coordinated functionality of all immune cell subsets. This observation, which we speculate can be attributed to the purity of Factor VIII in Monoclate® prompted us to design and initiate large controlled clinical trials where the immune status of hemophiliacs is assessed. These trials are currently ongoing.

## Viral safety of Monoclate®

An open multi-center clinical study, still in progress, in eleven centers in the US and Europe, was designed to assess the effects of the chronic use of Monoclate® in pediatric hemophiliacs, previously unexposed to Factor VIII concentrates. There are currently twenty patients enrolled in the study and we here present results from an interim analysis for eleven patients that have completed six months of therapy. The age of the patients at first infusion of Monoclate® ranged from four to forty-three months. None of the eleven patients had previously been exposed to any antihemophiliac factor concentrates, but four had received cryoprecipitate from up to ten donors. Prior to entry into the study, patients were immunized against hepatitis B and all demonstrated serological findings indicative of protection without infection from the vaccination.

Monoclate® was administered by intravenous infusions, as needed for bleeding or traumatic episodes. A single lot was assigned to each patient for the six month period, a total of five lots were used. The total cumulative dose per patient ranged from 450 IU to 12,00 IU and the number of infusions from 2 to 32. The lowest total daily dosage was 110 IU and the highest was 1500 IU; the highest single dose for any infusion was 570 IU.

Clinical and laboratory safety parameters were monitored over the six-month period. These included: serum ALT levels to evaluate development of NANB hepatitis, radioimmunoassay for antibody to mouse Ig, HIV seropositivity and Factor VIII inhibitors (Table 1).

*Table 1.* Viral safety of Monoclate®.

---

11 hemophilia A patients previously unexposed to AHF
5 individual lots of Monoclate®
6 months study completed

— 2 ALT spikes over normal value, <2×normal value no evidence of NANB
  hepatitis
— no HIV seroconversion

---

Serum ALT's were obtained every two weeks. There were no remarkable patterns in the fluctuations in ALT levels (mainly within normal limits) nor were there any persistent elevations of ALT. Two patients had a single occurrence of an ALT value higher than the upper limit of normal for that particular clinical laboratory, though the abnormal value was below twice the upper limit of normalcy. These single increases in ALT were correlated with viral upper respiratory infections and/or buccal hemorrhages. It is conceivable that these may be causal for the observed elevations. All eleven patients were negative at screen and remained negative throughout the six-month study period for anti-HIV antibody. From these data, we conclude that there was no incidence of NANB hepatitis. Taking into account the five individual lots of Monoclate® used in these patients, we feel the data further strongly indicate the viral safety of the product in an absolute sense. Our results should indeed be contrasted with studies previously performed according to similar protocols where either unheated or dry heated Factor VIII concentrates were used [8,9]. In the latter studies sixteen out of eighteen patients developed persistent, extremely high levels of ALT within three months of treatment. As it pertains to HIV seroconversion, a six-month time point is too short to make conclusive statements, though data from the ongoing clinical trial extension are accumulating to confirm these findings.

None of the patients' sera had any Factor VIII inhibitors upon entry into the study. Two out of eleven patients were positive for inhibitor titer at their six-month evaluation. This relative incidence (18%) is consistent with the incidence rate associated with use of any AHF product in moderate to severe hemophilia A patients.

Two out of eleven patients had detectable human anti-mouse Ig antibody levels prior to any infusion with Monoclate® and at various time points thereafter. The clinical significance of these levels in the absence of any allergic reaction is presently unknown and may reflect a particular cross-reactivity due to 'natural' antibodies in this pediatric population [10]. All other hematological parameters were essential within normal ranges at screening at six-month determinations.

For the purpose of the trial, an adverse event was defined as any abnormal clinical sign or subjective complaint. Eight out of eleven patients reported a total of fifty-one occurrences of adverse experiences. The most frequent type was respiratory with congestion and cough. Otitis also occurred in six patients. All the occurrences of adverse experiences were judged by the caring physicians as being consistent with colds and infections known to be common in a pediatric population.

## Conclusion

Monoclate® represents a novel therapeutic modality in the treatment of hemophilia A. The highly purified Factor VIII:C in Monoclate® exhibits a pharmacodynamic behaviour similar to that from currently available impure concentrates. The administration is convenient to patients and well tolerated. The absence of occurrence of NANB hepatitis in eleven pediatric patients, previously unexposed to AHF concentrates, over a period of six months in indicative of the viral safety of the product. No clinical observations have indicated reason for safety concerns due to the potential contamination of the product with small amounts of murine antibody originating from the purification process. Preliminary results suggest a trend toward improvement of the global immune status of hemophiliacs, treated chronically with Monoclate®. These observations are currently being assessed in controlled clinical studies.

## Acknowledgement

We are indebted to Dr P. Levine (Worcester Hemophilia Center, MA) and Dr J.M. Lusher (Children's Hospital, Detroit, MI) for allowing us to refer data from their patients and gratefully acknowledge their support and help.

## References

1. Schreiber AB. Monoclonal antibodies in the production of purified proteins from human plasma. In: Smit Sibinga CTh, Das PC, Overby LR (eds). Biotechnology in bloodtransfusion. Martinus Nijhoff Publ, Dordrecht, Lancaster, Boston 1988; 117-125.
2. Shawler DL, Bartholomew RH, Smith LM, Dillman RO. Human immune response to multiple injections of murine IgG. J Immunol 1985;135:1530-5.
3. Beddall AC, Hill FGH, George RH, Williams MD, Al-Rubei K. Unusually high incidence of tuberculosis among boys with hemophilia during an outbreak of the disease in hospital. J Clin Pathol 1985;38:1163-8.
4. Lee CA, Janossy G, Ashley J, Kernoff PBA. Plasma fractionation methods and T-cell subsets in haemophilia. Lancet 1983;ii:158-60.
5. Lee CA, Kernoff PBA, Karaylannis P, Waters J, Thomas HC. Abnormal T-lymphocyte subsets in hemophilia. Relation to HLA proteins in plasma products. N Engl J Med 1984;310:1058.
6. Mannhalter JW, Zlabinger GJ, Ahmad R, Zielinski CC, Schramm W, Eibl MM. A functional defect in the early phase of the immune response observed in patients with hemophilia A. Clin Immunol Immunopathol 1986;38:390.

7. Eibl MM, Ahmad R, Wolf HM, Linnau Y, Gatz E, Mannhalter JW. A component Factor VIII preprations which can be separated from Factor VIII activity down modulates human monocyte functions. Blood 1987;69:1153-60.

8. Preston FE, Hay CRM, Dewar MS, Greaves M, Triger Dr. Non-A, non-B hepatitis and heat-treated Factor VIII concentrates. Lancet 1985;ii:213-7.

9. Manucci PM, Colombo M, Rodeghiero F. Non-A, non-B hepatitis after Factor VIII concentrate treated by heating and chloroform. Lancet 1985;ii:1013-6.

10. Ternyck T, Avrameas S. Murine natural monoclonal antibodies: A study of their polyspecificities and affinities. Immunol Rev 1986;94:99-112.

# DEPLETION OF LYMPHOCYTES FROM BONE MARROW –
# INDICATIONS, EXPECTATIONS AND CLINICAL EXPERIENCE

T.J. Hamblin

## Introduction

When S. Cosmas and S. Damian transplanted the leg of a "Blackamoor slave" to a 4th century christian, they opened a Pandora's Box of untold complexity. Bone marrow transplantation (BMT) is undoubtedly the most complicated of all transplantation procedures, a) because bone marrow is a complex mixture of tissues, and b) because both the host and the graft are immunologically competent.

The removal of lymphocytes and other cells from bone marrow grafts is an attempt to simplify the complex biological reactions taking place and in some circumstances to reduce the immunocompetence of the graft. There are, in the main, two reasons for which lymphocyte depletion is attempted:

a. T-cell depletion of bone marrow allografts to try and reduce the incidence of graft-versus-host disease (GvHD); and
b. removal of tumour cells from bone marrow autografts.

A large number of different techniques have been used for bone marrow purging and these are listed in Table 1. Most of them are effective in the circumstances in which they are used and choice between them often depends on local factors and interests. This review does not discuss the advantages and disadvantages in detail.

## T-cell depletion of bone marrow allografts

Acute GvHD is the most important complication of allogeneic BMT, occurring in approximately 40-60% of recipients of HLA-matched sibling grafts and in over 70% of grafts from matched unrelated donors (MUDs) [1]. Patients with moderate or severe GvHD have a case fatality rate of > 50%. Prevention of GvHD by post-graft treatment with methotrexate or cyclosporin or both has been less than ideal and several groups of workers have shown that the incidence of Grade II, III and IV GvHD is much less when the bone marrow is depleted of T cells by any one of a number of methods [2-4].

Unfortunately this reduction in GvHD is not matched by an improvement in survival [3]. The new life threatening complications are an increased rejection rate caused by host-versus-graft reaction and an increased relapse rate.

These data suggest that the T cells within the graft have at least two functions other than the production of GvHD; namely suppression of the host

*Table 1.* Methods of purging

| Immunological | antibody plus complement |
| | toxin |
| | radioisotope |
| | magnetic beads |
| | RBC, panning |
| Pharmacological | 4-hydroperoxycyclophosphamide |
| | mafosfamide |
| | methyl prednisolone |
| | etoposide |
| Physical | density gradients |
| | E-rosettes |
| | lectins |
| | elutriation |
| | hyperthermia |
| Preferential expansion of normal clones | double autografting |
| | circulating stem cell autografts |
| | long term bone marrow culture |
| | G-CSF |

response to the graft and a Graft-versus-Leukemia effect (GVL). It is certainly possible that yet another function is involved in the prevention of rejection of mismatched grafts. What is not known is whether these different functions can be attributed to different subsets of lymphocytes. In animals GVL is separable from GvHD [5] but this is not clearly so in humans where it may be different for different tumours. Relapse after T-depleted BMT is higher for chronic myeloid leukemia and second remission acute lymphoblastic leukemia, but the effect is less easy to demonstrate for acute myeloblastic leukemia. It has been suggested that GVL is associated with the graft NK cells, but so far attempts to use depletion regimens which leave NK cells intact have not reduced the relapse rate [6].

On the other hand rejection has been shown to occur in conjunction with GvHD, suggesting that different T-cell subsets mediate these separate effects [7]. Nadler has suggested that a host derived mature T cell bearing CD3, CD5, CD6, CD8 and HLA class II antigens but lacking CD4 and CD25 is responsible for graft rejection [8]. It is not clear what sort of cell in the graft is capable of suppressing this cell.

Current strategies in reducing rejection and relapse rates include:
a. Increasing the severity of the conditioning regimens:
750 cGy single dose TBI (Royal Free),
7 rather than 6×200 cGy fractionated TBI (Glasgow), or
1575 rather than 1200 cGy (Seattle) have all proved effective in reducing the rejection rate. The addition of total nodal irradiation or post-transplant methotrexate or cyclosporin have been unsuccessful.
b. Reducing the severity of T depletion – a T cell dose of $<10^6$/kg is all that is needed to suppress GvHD.

c. treatment of the recipient with monoclonal 'cocktails', as used in the CAMPLUS regimen for MUDs. (The marrow is lymphocyte depleted with Campath-1, while the recipient is treated with anti-CD3, CD2 and CD7, human completed fixing monoclonal antibodies.)

## Tumour cell depletion of bone marrow autografts

There is no satisfactory evidence that depleting bone marrow autografts of tumour cells prolongs survival of patients with either leukemia or lymphoma. The main obstacle to obtaining such evidence is the very high relapse rate owing to the inadequacy of the conditioning regimens, such that a randomized controlled trial with 500 patients in each area would be necessary to prove the efficacy of purging. Furthermore, only between 1 and 4% of the patients's bone marrow is returned to him, and this hugely diluted specimen may contain no tumour. Finally, small numbers of transplanted tumour cells may be unable to grow in the patient. These three objections to purging autografts may be valid but an objective study is necessary to determine whether this is so.

Since it is not known·how many tumour cells are safe to return to the patient and since in various animal models very few cells are necessary to passage the tumour, the objective of marrow purging in ABMT is to remove as many tumour cells as possible. It is extremely difficult to determine how successful a purging technique has been. Histological techniques may detect a 5% marrow infiltration, and flow cytometry perhaps 3%. Gene rearrangement studies have at best a 1% sensitivity although a new generation of gene multipliers might increase this considerably. Theoretically, immunofluorescence or immunoperoxidase is infinitely sensitive, if a slide is scanned for long enough the single contaminating cell will be found. In practice it is difficult to detect less than a 1 in 1000 contamination.

A different approach is to assay clonogenic tumour cells, bone marrow being grown in semi-solid media in conditions that encourage the growth of tumour cells rather than normal progenitors. Such tumour cell colonies may not represent the true engraftable tumour cells and thus results of these assays must be treated with circumspection.

While there is still doubt about the amount of depletion necessary to prevent the reseeding of tumour, most centres have elected to maximally deplete the marrow. For T-lymphocytes cocktails of antibodies which include anti-CD2, CD3 and CD7 and for B-lymphocyte cocktails which include anti-CD19, CD20 and possibly CD37 have been preferred. Our own experience has been with Campath-1, a rat monoclonal which fixes human complement and is cytolytic for virtually all T and B lymphocytes (Table 2). Most monoclonals do not activate human complement, and baby rabbit complement must be used. Moreover, the other marrow cells are anticomplementary, and results obtained on isolated tumour cells cannot be extrapolated to a mixture of cells in bone marrow, even when a mononuclear cell extract is obtained. A theoretical risk is that tumour cells in Go may not be killed, but having their surfaces tickled with antibodies may be enough to make them leave the safety of Go and proliferate [8].

Table 2. Killing of B-cell lymphoma cells with CAMPATH-1 and -2 rounds of human complement.

| | Total | 99% kill | 99.9% kill |
|---|---|---|---|
| Node based lymphomas* | 48 | 43 | 35 |
| Hairy cell leukemia | 4 | 1 | 1 |

\* Centroblastic/centrocytic, diffuse centroblastic, diffuse centrocytic, diffuse lymphocytic, diffuse plasmacytic and diffuse lymphoplasmacytic.

For these reasons there is probably mileage in applying antibody-toxin combinations or antibody-drug combinations to the purging of autografts. Again, the technology here is not perfect. Antibody-whole ricin molecules have about 2 logs of selectivity of targets over stem cells, and while antibody-ricin A-chain has 5 or 6 logs of selectivity, it is nothing like so efficient and killing tumour cells. What is needed is an entry molecule which will take the lethal ricin molecule from the surface to the ribosome.

Another approach to purging autografts is to look to the preferential expansion of the normal clones. Two methods have shown promise. Dexter and his group at Manchester have grown bone marrow in long-term culture [9]. Leukemic clones tend to die out under such conditions, and the end-stage cultures are then transplantable. This is a labour intensive approach making great demands on laboratory sterility. Fungal contamination is an ever present risk.

Our approach [10] has been similar to that of workers in Heidelberg, Bordeaux, Adelaide and Paris. It makes use of the fact that even heavily contaminated marrows respond to semi-ablative chemotherapy by sending a shower of marrow stem cells into the peripheral blood during the recovery phase. Such cells appear to have been biologically purged and do not contain tumour cells. They may be efficiently administered using a cell separator over 5 days.

Furthermore, they have an advantage in depopulating bone marrow [8]. Because they are also associated with a surge of more differentiated granulocyte progenitors, recovery from neutropenia is considerably hastened.

Developments in this area will include use of the recombinant growth factors FM-CSF and G-CSF, but reports on their use will have to await another meeting.

Finally looking to the future we should try to imagine ways to add a Graft-versus-Leukemia effect to bone marrow autografts. Our preliminary experiments have suggested that this may be possible with recombinant interleuking-2, either alone or with LAK cells. But this too must await another day.

# References

1. Gale RP, Champlin RE. Bone marrow transplantation in acute leukemia. Clin Haematol 1986;15:851-72.
2. Prentice HG, Blacklock HA, Janossy G et al. Depletion of T lymphocytes in donor marrow prevents significant Graft-versus-Host disease in matched allogeneic leukemic marrow transplant recipients. Lancet 1984;i;472-5.
3. Martin PJ, Hansen JA, Buckner CD et al. Effects of *in vitro* depletion of T cells in HLA identical allogeneic marrow grafts. Blood 1985;66:664-72.
4. Mitsuyasu R, Champlin R, Gale RP et al. Depletion of T lymphocytes from donor marrow for the prevention of Graft-versus-Host disease following bone marrow transplantation. Prospective randomized controlled trial. Ann Int Med 1986;105:20-6.
5. Van Bekkum DW. Graft-versus-Host disease. In: Van Bekkum DW, Löwenberg B (eds). Bone marrow transplantation, biological mechanics and clinical practice. Dekker, New York 1985:147-212.
6. Gale RP. Bone marrow purging: current status, future directions. Bone Marrow Transplant 1987;2(suppl 2):107-15.
7. Martin PJ. T cell purging with antibody – the Seattle experience. Bone Marrow Transplant 1987;2(suppl 2):53-7.
8. Nadler L. The challenge of bone marrow purging. Bone Marrow Transplant 1987;2(suppl 2):5-11.
9. Chang S, Coutinho L, Morgenstern G et al. Reconstitution of haemopoietic system with autologus marrow taken during relapse of acute myeloblastic leukemia and grown in long term culture. Lancet 1986;i:294-5.
10. Bell AJ, Figes A, Oscier DG, Hamblin TJ. Peripheral blood stem cell autografts in the treatment of lymphoid malignancies. Initial experience in three patients. Brit J Haemat 1987;66:63-8.

# HEMATOPOIETIC HORMONES IN TRANSFUSION MEDICINE

W.G. Ho

The regulation of blood cell production is a complex process of proliferation and differentiation of progenitor cells of the bone marrow in response to glycoprotein hormones termed colony stimulating factors (CSFs). The development of *in vitro* culture systems of bone marrow cells in semisolid media [1,2] led to the establishment of appropriate cell culture systems for the study of the clonal growth of hematopoietic cells. CSF research in this field has recently been intensified for reasons beyond mere scientific interest. Dysfunction of the hematopoietic system results in diseases that are major medical problems. The possibility that CSFs could function as regulators of blood cell production suggest distinct therapeutic approaches to these disorders thereby adding impetus to research.

A family of CSFs has been defined and biochemically characterized as a result of murine and human studies. There appear to be four major types of CSFs (Table 1). Two of these are relatively lineage specific; colonies grown in the presence of granulocyte-CSF (G-CSF) consist mainly of neutrophilic granulocytes [3] and their precursors while macrophage CSF (M-CSF) appears to stimulate chiefly the growth of macrophage colonies [4]. On the other hand, colonies grown in the presence of interleukin-3 (IL-3, also known as multi-CSF) contain many cell lineages [5] and colonies grown in the presence of granulocyte macrophage CSF (GM-CSF) consist of neutro-

Table 1.  Human colony-stimulating factors.

| | Other names | Molecular weight of glycoprotein | Deduced molecular weight of protein | Cell production |
|---|---|---|---|---|
| GM-CSF | CFS- | 22,000 | 14,300 | Neturophils, monocytes, esinophils |
| G-CSF | CSF- | 19,600 | 18,800 | Neutrophils |
| M-CSF | CSF-1, Urinary CSF | 70-90,000 (dimer) | 26,00 | Monotyest |
| IL-3 | Multi-CSF | 20,000 | 14,600 | Neutrophils, monocytes, eosinophils, platelets |

phils, macrophages and eosinophils [6]. However, these are not the only hematopoietic growth factors. Erythropoietin is a growth factor whose role in regulating red cell production *in vivo* has clearly been established [7]. In addition, interleuking-2 (IL-2) is a growth factor for T and B lymphocytes with important regulatory influence on lymphocyte function [8]. Other regulatory factors with as yet poorly defined functions include hematopoietin, which is believed to induce stem cells to become responsive to other CSFs [9] in a manner similar to the effects of interleukin-1 (IL-1) and interleukin-4 (IL-4) which stimulates the growth of mast cells [11] and probably interacts with other factors in the proliferation of myeloid progenitors.

## Erythropoietin and its therapeutic applications

The first hint of external influences on the regulation of erythropoiesis was suggested by Jourdanet in 1863, who observed the presence of erythrocytosis in patients living at high attitudes [12]. Over the next century following this observation, debate raged in the scientific community over the existence of the humoral substance that regulated the production of red blood cells. The issue was almost considered settled in 1950 when Reissman demonstrated in paired parabiotic rats, that when one partner was subjected to hypoxia, the other partner showed evidence of increased erythropoises [13]. However, definitive evidence of the existence of a humoral factor was not established until 1954, when Erslev demonstrated the stimulation of erythropoiesis in normal rabbits with plasma from anemic animals [7]. The existence of erythropoietin was finally accepted and subsequently became widely studied, but it was not until 1977 that erythropoietin was purified from urine [14]. The genomic and cDNA molecular clones encoding the erythropoietin were later defined [15], thereby leading to the production of recombinant human erythropoietin in quantities sufficient to allow clinical studies to be conducted.

Initial studies with erythropoietin have been carried out in end stage renal disease patients on chronic dialysis [16,17]. While hemodialysis corrects many of the metabolic disturbances of renal failure it has no influence on the anemia, hence, the rationale for use of erythropoietin in these patients. Results of these studies clearly indicate evidence of stimulation of red cell production following administration of erythropoietin. Increase in hemoglobin and hematocrit levels result in marked improvement in wellbeing, in addition to discontinuation of the need for red cell transfusions in previously transfusion-dependent patients. Erythropoietin was found to be non-toxic except for complications possibly related to the high hematocrit. These encouraging results indicate that erythropoietin may have wide application as a therapeutic agent.

Some of the potential uses of erythropoietin are indicated in Table 2. Erythropoietin has already been shown to be of definite benefit in amelior-ating the anemia of chronic renal failure. A much wider application can be envisoned with regard to surgical patients. Autologous blood storage in preparation for elective surgery has become common practice [18]. Administration of erythropoietin to individuals preparing for surgery may allow

*Table 2.* Potential uses of erythropoietin.

1. Chronic dialysis patients
2. Autologous transfusion
3. Stimulate blood production for surgery
4. Ameliorate anemia associated with chemotherapy in cancer patients
5. Increase erythropoiesis to facilitate bone marrow transplantation
6. ? Treat anemia with chronic disease
7. ? Increase hemoglobin F production in sickle cell anemia
8. ? Increase performance at high altitude of runners, etc.
9. ? Produce red cells in culture

many more units of blood to be collected for use during the surgery. In addition, use of erythropoietin during surgery and in the post operative period may markedly decrease the need for transfusions. This latter approach may have important applications in the event of emergency surgery. Erythropoietin may ameliorate the anemia associated with chemotherapy in cancer patients, as well as enhance the ionizing effects of radiation in those patients undergoing therapeutic irradiation. Erythropoietin may also stimulate erythropoiesis in patients whose bone marrow has been sub-letally irradiated as in the case of nuclear accidents, or even in the case of intentional irradiation such as bone marrow transplant recipients. Erythropoietin may also be useful in treating the anemia of chronic diseases, even though the anemia in these disorders is of multifactorial causes [19,20]. Another potential use of erythropoietin may be the prevention of crises in sickle cell anemia by the stimulation of hemoglobulin F production [21]. Other intriguing uses include the improvement in physical performance of athletes by increasing the hematocrit to supernormal levels, and the possibility of producing red blood cells by *in vitro* cultures for use in transfusion therapy.

The ability to regulate the hematocrit with erythropoietin would have far-reaching implications on blood banking It would decrease the need for transfusions in general and thereby also reduce the incidence of all complications associated with this type of replacement therapy. Instead of dealing with the collection, storage and administration of "safe" blood, the transfusion medicine specialist would be faced with maintaining the hematocrit of patients by titrating the dose of erythropoietin administered. This form of therapy would open new areas of research in determining the ideal hematocrit in man.

## Colony-stimulating factors and their applications

While erythropoietin and its effect on erythropoietin had been known for many years, the regulation of granylopoiesis and megakaryopoiesis was poorly understood. The spleen colony method of assaying for mouse pluripotent hematopoietic stem cells [22] did not allow manipulation of the milieu to properly study the factors necessary for growth of colonies. The development of semisolid culture systems for the *in vitro* growth of mouse hematopoietic stem cells [1,2] greatly facilitated research in this field. Ultimately, similar systems were developed for growing human bone marrow cells in culture thereby resulting in the identification of the four major types of CSFs and their subsequent gene sequence and cloning.

GM-CSF was the first human CSF to be cloned. The recombinant GM-CSF stimulates the production of neutrophils, monocytes and eosinophils *in vitro*. Clinical trials of the therapeutic administration of GM-CSF are currently in progress. Initial reports indicate that constant infusion of GM-CSF results in a dose-dependent increase in circulating levels of neutrophils, monocytes and eosinophils in patients with AIDS [23]. The infusions are well tolerated with only occasional reports of fever and chills. These early results indicate that GM-CSF can be used therapeutically as a regulator of granulocyte and monocyte production.

G-CSF has been purified from tumour cell lines. This G-CSF causes an increase in bone marrow and splenic production of neutrophils in mice [24]; in subhuman primates injection of G-CSF stimulates neutrophil production without apparent effect on other cell lineages [25]. Initial studies in patients undergoing chemotherapy for bladder cancer indicate that G-CSF is well tolerated and does stimulate granulopoiesis in patients with bone marrow suppression induced by chemotherapy [26].

M-CSF has so far been the only CSF demonstrated to circulate in the plasma and be excreted in the urine. It appears that M-CSF may stimulate phagocytic replication and activity [27]. Only very limited clinical trials have been conducted and no definite conclusions regarding its effects have been reached.

IL-3 stimulates the growth of multipotent stem cells including the formation of colonies of granulocytes, monocytes, eosinophils, erythroid cells and megakaryocytes. Initial studies indicate that IL-3 stimulates granulocyte and monocyte production in primates. It appears to be highly synergistic when administered together with GM-CSF.

In addition to the stimulation of production of hematopoietic cells, all the CSFs have prominent effects on the function of mature effector cells [28,29]. GM-CSF and G-CSF enhance the ability of neutrophils to phagocytose and kill organisms, while M-CSF induces similar effects on the mononuclear phagocyte. IL-3 appears to have the same effects on macrophages as well as eosinophils. Thus, CSFs play an important role in regulating the production of effector cells as well as their activity, thereby enhancing the host defense system in different ways.

The therapeutic implications of administration of CSFs (Table 3) suggest new approaches to infection control in addition to antimicrobial therapy. The numbers and function of host defense cells may be enhanced in deficient patients thereby preventing infection as well as lessening the mortality and morbidity associated with infections in these patients. Other clinical applications may be in the field of cancer therapy with amelioration of the granulocytopenia frequently produced by the myelosuppressive effects of therapy. The possibility exists of improving quality of life and prolongation of survival in AIDS patients by increasing the numbers and activity of host defense cells with CSF administration. High white counts may be useful in preventing infections in other compromised patients and may be of extreme importance

*Table 3.* Potential therapeutic applications of CSF.

1. Prevent/mitigate chemotherapy and radiation-induced leukopenia
2. Induce anti-tumor activity *in vivo* (direct cytotoxicity and ADCC)
3. Improve host defense in immunocompromized patients
4. Treat infectious and parasitic diseases
5. Treat burn patients
6. Facilitate recovery from autologous and allogeneic transplantation
7. Treat marrow failure states
8. Improve granulocyte procurement
9. Increase platelet counts in thrombocytopenia
10. Facilitate *in vitro* culture of bone marrow cells to produce mature cells for transfusion

in the management of burn patients, in the prevention of infections in surgical procedures and in the treatment of established infections including osteomyelitis, pneumonias and sepsis. While the granulocyte specific hormones will be of most benefit in pyogenic infections, those CSFs interacting with mononuclear phagocytes may be of great importance in the management of parasitic infections.

It is expected that CSFs will improve hematopoiesis in bone marrow failure states such as aplastic anemia. Also, in bone marrow transplantation, CSF may decrease the period to engraft resulting in reduced incidences of infections in these patients

The generation and direction of effector cells in cancer therapy may become more refined. Currently, trials of lymphocyte activated killer (LAK) cells show promise in this direction [30]. The action of LAK cells or other effector cells on the tumour destruction and removal may be further enhanced by priming the host defense system with CSF. IL-3 is an effective megakaryocyte CSF *in vitro* and its use in combination with the thrombopoietins may lead to stimulation of platelet production, thereby decreasing the need for platelet transfusions.

Increased availability of the various hematopoietins, as well as better understanding of their modes of action and further developments in the technology of bone marrow culture, may eventually permit the generation of blood cells *in vitro*. The blood bank of the future may actually become a blood factory whose function would be to produce all the cellular elements of blood in quantities sufficient to meet the needs of clinical application.

**References**

1. Pluznik DH, Sachs J. The cloning of normal mast cells in tissue culture. J Cell Comp Physiol 1965;66:319–24.
2. Bradley TR, Metcalf D. The growth of mouse bone marrow cells *in vitro*. Aust J Exp Biol Med Sci 1966;44:287–300.
3. Metcalf D, Nicola NA. Proliferative effects of purified granulocyte stimulating factor (G–CSF) on normal mouse hematopoietic cells. J Cell Physiol 1983;116: 198–206.

4. Stanley ER, Heard PM. Factors regulating macrophage production and growth. Purification and some properties of the colony stimulating factor from medium conditioned by mouse L-cells. J Biol Chem 1977;252:4305-12.

5. Ihle JN, Keller J, Orozlan S et al. Biologic properties of homogeneous interleukin-3. Demonstration of WEHI-3 growth factor activity, mast cell growth factor activity, P cell stimulating factor activity, colony stimulating factor activity and histamine producing cell-stimulating factor activity. J Immunol 1983;131: 282-87.

6. Metcalf D. Review: The molecular biology and functions of the granulocyte-macrophage colony stimulating factors. Blood 1986;67:257-67.

7. Erslev A. Humoral regulation of red cell production. Blood 1953;8:349-57.

8. Smith KA, Lachman LB, Oppenheim JJ, Favata MF. The functional relationship of the interleukins. J Exp Med 1980;151:1551-6.

9. Stanley ER, Bartocci A, Patinkin D, Rosendaal M, Bradley TR. Regulation of very primitive, multipotent hemopoietic cells by hemopoietin-1. Cell 1986;45: 667-74.

10. Dinarello CA. An update on human interleukin-1: from molecular biology to clinical relevance. J Clin Immunol 1985;5:287-97.

11. Yokota T, Otsaka T, Mosmann T et al. Isolation and characterization of a human interleukin cDNA clone, homologous to mouse B-cell stimulatory factor I, that expresses B-cell and T-cell stimulating activities. Proc Natl Acad Sci (USA) 1986;83:5894-8.

12. Jourdanet D. De l'anemie des altitudes et de l'anemie en general dans ses rapports avec la pression de l'atmosphere. Bailliere, Paris 1863.

13. Reissman KR. Studies of the mechanism of erythropoietic stimulation in parabiotic rats during hypoxia. Blood 1950;5:372-80.

14. Miyake T, Kung CK, Goldwasser E. Purification of human erythropoietin. J Biol Chem 1977;252:5558-64.

15. Jacobs K, Shoemaker C, Rudersdorf et al. Isolation and characterization of genomic and cDNA clones of human erythropoietin. Nature 1985;313:806-10.

16. Winearls CG, Oliver DO, Pippard MJ, Reid C, Downing MR, Cotes PM. Effect on the anemia of patients maintained by chronic hemodialysis. Lancet 1986;ii:1175-8.

17. Eschbach JW, Egrie JC, Downing MR, Browne JK, Admanson JW. Correction of the anemia of end-stage renal disease with recombinant human erythropoietin: Results of a phase I and II clinical trial. N Engl J Med 1987;316:73-8.

18. Surgenor DM. The patient's blood is the safest blood. N Engl J Med 1987;316: 542-4.

19. Erslev JA, Anema of chronic disorders. In: Williams WJ, Beutler E, Erslev AJ, Lichtman MA (eds). Hematology. 3rd ed. McGraw-Hill, New York 1985:522-8.

20. Erslev AJ, Wilson J, Caro J. Erythropoietin titers in anemic, non uremic patients. J Lab Clin Med 1987;109:429-33.

21. Al-Khatti A, Veith RW, Papyannopoulou T, Frisch EF, Goldwasser E. Stimulation of fetal hemoglobin synthesis by erythropoietin in baboons. N Engl J Med 1987;317:415-20.

22. Till JE, McCulloch EA. A direct measurement of the radiation sensitivity of normal mouse bone marrow cells. Radiat Res 1961;14:213-22.

23. Groopman JE, Mitsuyasu RT, DeLeo MJ, Oette DH, Golde DW. Effect of recombinant human granulocyte-macrophage colony stimulating factor on myelopoiesis in the acquired immunodeficiency syndrome. N Engl J Med 1987;317: 593-8.

24. Nagata S, Tsuchiya M, Asano S et al. Molecular cloning and expression of cDNA for human granulocyte colony stimulating factor. Nature 1986;319:415-7.

25. Welte K, Bonilla MA, Gillio AP et al. Recombinant human granulocyte colony-stimulating factor effects on hematopoiesis in normal and cyclophosphamide-treated primates. J Exp Med 1987;165:941-8.

26. Gabrilove JL, Jakubowski A, Grous J et al. Initial results of a study of recombinant human granulocyte colony stimulating factor (rhG-CSF) in cancer patients. Exp Hematol 1987;15:461.

27. Warren MK, Ralph P. Macrophage growth factor CSF-1 stimulates human monocyte production of interferon, tumor necrosis factor and colony stimulating activity. J Immunol 1986;7:2281-5.

28. Platzer E, Welte K, Gabrilove JL et al. Biological activities of a human pluripotent hemopoietic colony stimulating factor on normal and leukemic cells. J Exp Med 1985;162:1788-1801.

29. Lopez AF, Williamson DJ, Gamble JR et al. Recombinant human granulocyte-macrophage colony-stimulating factor stimulates in vitro mature human neutrophil and eosinophil function, surface receptor expression and survival. J Clin Invest 1986;78:1220-8.

30. Rosenberg SA, Lotze MT, Muul LM et al. Observations on the systemic administration of autologous lymphokine-activated killer cells and recombinant interleukin-2 to patients with metastatic cancer. N Engl J med 1985;313:1485-92.

# DISCUSSION

L.R. Overby, J. van der Meer

*J. Growe (Vancouver):* Dr High, you mentioned that the recombinant Factor VIII material is not identical to the native Factor VIII, it has got several of the active sites only. What I am curious about is whether there is any evidence, perhaps in the animal models studied so far, as to whether there is any kind of immunologic response inhibitor production and whether you have been following the several human patients to see if there is any change. Maybe you could also add on your comments whether the Factor VIII assays that you are doing on the patients, are assays by traditional methods, or whether there is any manipulation of these assay system for the recombinant material needed?

*K. High (Chapel Hill):* Well, let me say first that the object of the protein study was to show that actually the recombinant and the plasma derived Factor VIII are very similar in terms of *in vitro* characterization by gel electropheresis. There has been no evidence of any inhibitor formation in either animal studies or patients who have been treated so far. That was one of the greatest worries with the product, because the glycosylation patterns are not absolutely identical between the native and the recombinant Factor VIII we are using. So, one of the greatest concerns was that there might be inhibitor formation, but that has not happened. The Factor VIII activity levels that I showed you in the follow-up studies are done in our clinical coagulation laboratory using standard substrate deficient plasmas and APTT assays. There is no problem in using those same assays with the recombinant Factor VIII.

*J.D. Lutton (Valhalla):* Dr Ho, your results with the erythropoietin are very exciting and I am sure very significant to clinical medicine. I am curious to know if you have had a chance to try administration in various patients undergoing hemodialysis. Is there any difference in the response to your erythropoietin titres?

*W.G. Ho (Los Angeles):* The answer to that question is that there are now ongoing studies being conducted and no results have been reported so far. These studies are in progress in a number of institutions; for instance at UCLA and others throughout the United States.

*E. Briët (Leiden):* I would like to make a comment to Dr Schreiber. I am an ultraconservative hemophilia treater. We have been using cryoprecipitate only since the 60's and because of that only 5 out of the 80 patients have converted for the HIV virus. We do not have the impression that the seronegative patients have more infections or are more prone to common colds. To the contrary they seem to have less common colds than their unaffected siblings. I think that the arguments for the immunosuppressive effect of the proteins other than Factor VIII or IX in the concentrates are weak. The numbers are small and the data are not controlled. Jean Pierre Allain recently presented the data of a well carried out and well designed study showing that the effect was in fact the other way round, the impurer the product the better the immunology of the patient.* I feel that it is the way to go to produce pure Factor VIII concentrates. Why should we substitute more than the missing protein. I believe, however, that the immunosuppressive effect of the other proteins should not be an argument in the discussion.

*A.B. Schreiber (King of Prussia):* I am aware of the study by Dr Allain and do not fully understand why you feel that the rest of the data is pretty weak. I am further happy that you still feel that one should not infuse patients with 99.8% of irrelevant alloantigenic proteins. The immunosuppressive effects are similar to immunomodulators. When there are as many papers in the literature showing that it is immunosuppressive or immunostimulating, then there must be some people that have a different perception than you. The point I was trying to make was mainly for the population of seropositives. You in The Netherlands and some other countries have been more fortunate with your blood supply and the control thereof than we have been in the United States. There is clear data that there are many stimuli that promote the transition of HIV from a latency to active state.** The point I was trying to make is that the less attack or the less things you would infuse that could induce that activation, probably is the most logical. One does not need to be purily scientific about this, I mean if I had the choice if I were a seropositive hemophiliac or my son was, I would not hesitate to chose a product that is pure.

*E. Briët:* The study of Allain was also in HIV-positive patients, was well controlled and did not show the data that you find in an uncontrolled way. So, that does not count. But on the other hand I fully agree that we should go for pure products.

*G. Zettlmeißl:* Dr High, can you give some comments on the expression, yields of these recombinant cells, and the yields of purification by your monoclonal antibody purification method.

*K. High:* I can not answer your question on expression levels in preparation because I am not familiar with the expression levels by which the product has been produced at the company.

---

* Allain JP et al. Vox Sang 1987;53:37-43.
** Advances in host defense mechanisms. Gallin JI, Fauci AS (eds). Vol. 5. Acquired Immunodeficiency Syndrome. Raven Press, New York 1985.

*H.V. Beer (München):* Dr Schreiber, you mentioned and I found that very interesting, 20% of the normal population have antibodies to mouse protein. What is this information based on. If this is a fact, would not you expect problems with hemophiliacs with preformed mouse antibodies when they receive mouse antigen via the Factor VIII?

*A.B Schreiber:* The data on the 20% is our own data because we wanted to accumulate a large number of healthy volunteers to have a control group to validate the assay we utilized to measure the human anti-mouse antibodies. Also some data are from Ron Levy at Stanford. These antibodies are binding or recognizing epitopes with good affinity to mouse immunoglobulin epitopes. They are not part of a true immune response, so that you do not get an anamnestic response if you were to stimulate them with mouse Ig. They are the same kind of antibodies you find when you develop any diagnostic test. When you are making lots of diagnostic tests, you usually run a control group of a large number of volunteers and you determine what your background level is and then you blank that out. We do not have any positive standards and we do not know what is a normal value. We could have blanked out those 20%, as I do not think that these are true antibodies. These are cross-reactive antibodies, interference type antibodies that you have in the development of any assay for instance in analytical chemistry of new synthetic molecules that were made in the laboratory and therefore people never have been exposed to. It is the same story as when people start infusing dinitrophenyl or para-azobenzarsenate and so on.

*H.V. Beer:* Thank you. You mentioned three single point ALT elevations in three patients. Are these related to one lot or related to different lots?

*A.B. Schreiber:* That is an important point. It is why we designed to give individual lots. No they were in three different lots. These lots were also utilized in other patients. Therefore, it made us feel comfortable that the two or one other patient that had received multiple infusions of that same lot did not have any ALT elevation. The only association in the clinic that we observed and do not understand, is that those three single point elevations that did not exceed the two times the normal level, as usually defined as a parameter of NANB hepatitis, were associated with buccal hemorrhages in the patients. They had all used just a few days before that measurement tranexamic acid. Whether the hemorrhage by itself or some unknown effect of tranexamic acid gives an elevation of the ALT's is not clear, but that is the only thing that we found as an association.

*S. Moeslichan (Jakarta Selatan):* Dr Hamblin, you mentioned that monoclonal antibodies for T-cell depletion will cause increase of rejection. Is it due to disappearance of T-cells or a complex of monoclonal antibodies and T-cells. Could you advise about the use of monoclonal antibodies for T-depletion in non malignant bone marrow transplantation?

*T.J. Hamblin:* The effect of T-cell depletion is to increase the rejection rate and if you deplete an apalstic anemia or a thalassemia graft in which you use less immunosuppression in the patient, you very greatly increase the rejection rates. Therefore T-cell depletion is not appropriate in thalassemia or aplastic anemia allografts. The one piece of evidence that cyclosporin is good for prevention of Graft-versus-Host disease is in such patients. So, you do not need to do T-cell depletion. Cyclosporin is good enough suppression of GvHD in such patients.

*J. Over (Amsterdam):* Dr. High, looking at your data, do I understand correctly that you suggested that the T½ of the recombinant Factor VIII is longer than that of plasma derived Factor VIII? I think that the pair of the lines were essentially parallel and I could not see any difference in T½. I also would further suggest to extend the evaluation time from 12 hours to, for instance, 48 hours after transfusion, because the first phase of disappearance may influence the analysis of the T½ when a relatively short post-infusion period is considered.

*K. High:* There is not very much difference in the half life. It does appear to be slightly longer at least in one of the patients. But with the limited amount of patients in whom it has been examined I do not know whether that has any importance. In the second patient we did extend observation to 24 hours.

*J. Over:* Has it not been established repeatedly in the same patient?

*K. High:* No, that has only been done once in each of those patients.

*C.V. Prowse:* Dr Schreiber, you mentioned that you are useing a heat-treatment step now. Could you tell us how severe that is? You also mentioned you had set up an anti-idiotype assay. Did that yield any useful data?

*A.B. Schreiber:* The heat-treatment for the product that was currently approved is dry heat-treatment at 60°C 30 hours. We are working on other forms of heat inactivation. It is important to know that 60°C 30 hours for a purified product yields actually about two logs better viral inactivation than on impure products. Probably the virus is protected by the higher protein concentration. On the second question the purposes of the anti-idiotype assay was exactly to distinguish between natural antibodies and a true induced immune response against the idiotopes of the monoclonal used on the column. The answer is, no we have not found any positive results.

*L.R. Overby:* Dr Briët, thank you for your elegant presentation on the use of RFLP's for genetic counselling. I think we are all looking forward to having those techniques become widely available in many of the laboratories around the world. Thank you very much.

To speak for myself and the entire audience, I am sure I represent you in thanking the organisers of this conference, Dr Smit Sibinga and the staff of the Groningen Blood Centre who have taken care not only of organizing the programme, but taken care of all our personal needs. Again thank you very much and for me personally I simply must tell you what a pleasant experience this has been for me.